Sleep Medicine

Guest Editor

CHRISTIAN GUILLEMINAULT, MD

MEDICAL CLINICS
OF NORTH AMERICA

www.medical.theclinics.com

May 2010 • Volume 94 • Number 3

SAUNDERS an imprint of ELSEVIER, Inc.

W.B. SAUNDERS COMPANY
A Division of Elsevier Inc.

1600 John F. Kennedy Boulevard ● Suite 1800 ● Philadelphia, Pennsylvania 19103-2899

http://www.theclinics.com

MEDICAL CLINICS OF NORTH AMERICA Volume 94, Number 3
May 2010 ISSN 0025-7125, ISBN-13: 978-1-4377-1836-2

Editor: Rachel Glover
Developmental Editor: Theresa Collier

Medical Clinics of North America (ISSN 0025-7125) is published bimonthly by Elsevier Inc., 360 Park Avenue South, New York, NY 10010-1710. Months of issue are January, March, May, July, September, and November. Periodicals postage paid at New York, NY, and additional mailing offices. Subscription prices are USD 204 per year for US individuals, USD 361 per year for US institutions, USD 105 per year for US students, USD 259 per year for Canadian individuals, USD 469 per year for Canadian institutions, USD 165 per year for Canadian students, USD 314 per year for international individuals, USD 469 per year for international institutions and USD 165 per year for international students. To receive student/resident rate, orders must be accompanied by name of affiliated institution, date of term, and the *signature* of program/residency coordinator on institution letterhead. Orders will be billed at individual rate until proof of status is received. Foreign air speed delivery is included in all *Clinics* subscription prices. All prices are subject to change without notice. **POSTMASTER:** Send address changes to *Medical Clinics of North America*, Elsevier Health Sciences Division, Subscription Customer Service, 3251 Riverport Lane, Maryland Heights, MO 63043. **Customer Service: Telephone: 1-800-654-2452** (U.S. and Canada); **1-314-447-8871** (outside U.S. and Canada). **Fax: 1-314-447-8029. E-mail: journalscustomerservice-usa@elsevier.com** (for print support); **journalsonlinesupport-usa@ elsevier.com** (for online support).

Reprints. For copies of 100 or more of articles in this publication, please contact the Commercial Reprints Department, Elsevier Inc., 360 Park Avenue South, New York, NY 10010-1710. Tel.: 212-633-3812; Fax: 212-462-1935; E-mail: reprints@elsevier.com.

Medical Clinics of North America is also published in Spanish by McGraw-Hill Interamericana Editores S. A., P.O. Box 5-237, 06500 Mexico, D.F., Mexico.

Medical Clinics of North America is covered in *MEDLINE/PubMed (Index Medicus), Current Contents, ASCA, Excerpta Medica, Science Citation Index, and ISI/BIOMED.*

Printed in the United States of America.

GOAL STATEMENT

The goal of *Medical Clinics of North America* is to keep practicing physicians up to date with current clinical practice by providing timely articles reviewing the state of the art in patient care.

ACCREDITATION

The *Medical Clinics of North America* is planned and implemented in accordance with the Essential Areas and Policies of the Accreditation Council for Continuing Medical Education (ACCME) through the joint sponsorship of the University of Virginia School of Medicine and Elsevier. The University of Virginia School of Medicine is accredited by the ACCME to provide continuing medical education for physicians.

The University of Virginia School of Medicine designates this educational activity for a maximum of 15 *AMA PRA Category 1 Credits*™ for each issue, 90 credits per year. Physicians should only claim credit commensurate with the extent of their participation in the activity.

The American Medical Association has determined that physicians not licensed in the US who participate in this CME activity are eligible for a maximum of 15 *AMA PRA Category 1 Credits*™ for each issue, 90 credits per year.

Credit can be earned by reading the text material, taking the CME examination online at http://www.theclinics.com/home/cme, and completing the evaluation. After taking the test, you will be required to review any and all incorrect answers. Following completion of the test and evaluation, your credit will be awarded and you may print your certificate.

FACULTY DISCLOSURE/CONFLICT OF INTEREST

The University of Virginia School of Medicine, as an ACCME accredited provider, endorses and strives to comply with the Accreditation Council for Continuing Medical Education (ACCME) Standards of Commercial Support, Commonwealth of Virginia statutes, University of Virginia policies and procedures, and associated federal and private regulations and guidelines on the need for disclosure and monitoring of proprietary and financial interests that may affect the scientific integrity and balance of content delivered in continuing medical education activities under our auspices.

The University of Virginia School of Medicine requires that all CME activities accredited through this institution be developed independently and be scientifically rigorous, balanced and objective in the presentation/discussion of its content, theories and practices.

All authors/editors participating in an accredited CME activity are expected to disclose to the readers relevant financial relationships with commercial entities occurring within the past 12 months (such as grants or research support, employee, consultant, stock holder, member of speakers bureau, etc.). The University of Virginia School of Medicine will employ appropriate mechanisms to resolve potential conflicts of interest to maintain the standards of fair and balanced education to the reader. Questions about specific strategies can be directed to the Office of Continuing Medical Education, University of Virginia School of Medicine, Charlottesville, Virginia.

The faculty and staff of the University of Virginia Office of Continuing Medical Education have no financial affiliations to disclose.

The authors/editors listed below have identified no professional or financial affiliations for themselves or their spouse/partner:

Michelle Cao, DO; Jason K. M. Chau, MD, MPH, FRCS(C); Chiara De Rosa, DDS; Alex Dimitriu, MD; Ezio Fanucci, MD; Eric Frenette, MD, FRCP(C); Rachel Glover (Acquisitions Editor); Christian Guilleminault, MD, DBiol (Guest Editor); Jon-Erik C. Holty, MD, MS; Yu-Shu Huang, MD; Clair Lakkis, MD; Rachel Manber, PhD; Robert Owens, MD; Paola Pirelli, DDS; Nelson B. Powell, DDS, MD; Kannan Ramar, MD; Maurizio Saponara, MD; Bhavneesh Sharma, MD; Allison T. Siebern, PhD; Shannon S. Sullivan, MD; Ming-Horng Tsai, MD; Andrew Wolf, MD (Test Author); and Herbert J. Yue, MD.

The authors/editors listed below identified the following professional or financial affiliations for themselves or their spouse/partner:

Sean M. Caples, DO is an industry funded research/investigator for ResMed Foundation, Ventus Medical, Restore Medical, and Sleep Methods.

Atul Malhotra, MD is a consultant for Philips, Apnex, SGS, SHC, Ethicon, Pfizer, Medtronic, Itamar, and Merck; and is an industry funded research/investigator for Philips, Cephalon, and Sepracor.

Disclosure of Discussion of Non-FDA Approved Uses for Pharmaceutical Products and/or Medical Devices.
The University of Virginia School of Medicine, as an ACCME provider, requires that all faculty presenters identify and disclose any off-label uses for pharmaceutical and medical device products. The University of Virginia School of Medicine recommends that each physician fully review all the available data on new products or procedures prior to clinical use.

TO ENROLL

To enroll in the *Medical Clinics of North America* Continuing Medical Education program, call customer service at 1-800-654-2452 or visit us online at http://www.theclinics.com/home/cme. The CME program is available to subscribers for an additional fee of USD 228.

THE CLINICS ARE NOW AVAILABLE ONLINE!

Access your subscription at:
www.theclinics.com

Contributors

GUEST EDITOR

CHRISTIAN GUILLEMINAULT, MD, DBiol
Professor of Psychiatry, Behavioral Sciences and (by courtesy) Neurology, Division of Sleep Medicine, Stanford University School of Medicine; Stanford Sleep Medicine Clinic, Redwood City, California

AUTHORS

MICHELLE CAO, DO
Clinical Instructor, Division of Sleep Medicine, Stanford University School of Medicine, Stanford; Stanford Sleep Medicine Clinic, Redwood City, California

SEAN M. CAPLES, DO
Mayo Clinic, Center for Sleep Medicine, Division of Pulmonary and Critical Care Medicine, Rochester, Minnesota

JASON K.M. CHAU, MD, MPH, FRCS(C)
Assistant Professor, Department of Otolaryngology Head and Neck Surgery, University of Manitoba, Winnipeg, Manitoba, Canada

CHIARA DE ROSA, DDS
Department of Odontostomatological Sciences, University of Tor Vergata, Rome, Italy

ALEX DIMITRIU, MD
Division of Sleep Medicine, Stanford University School of Medicine, Redwood City, California

EZIO FANUCCI, MD
Department of Diagnostic Imaging Interventional Radiology, University of Tor Vergata, Rome, Italy

ERIC FRENETTE, MD, FRCP(C)
Assistant Professor of Neurology, University of Sherbrooke, Sherbrooke, Quebec, Canada

CHRISTIAN GUILLEMINAULT, MD, DBiol
Professor of Psychiatry, Behavioral Sciences and (by courtesy) Neurology, Division of Sleep Medicine, Stanford University School of Medicine; Stanford Sleep Medicine Clinic, Redwood City, California

JON-ERIK C. HOLTY, MD, MS
Staff Physician, Division of Pulmonary, Critical Care and Sleep Medicine, Department of Medicine, VA Palo Alto Health Care System, Palo Alto, California

YU-SHU HUANG, MD
Associate Professor, Division of Pediatric Psychiatry, Department of Child Psychiatry; Sleep Center; College of Medicine, Chang Gung Memorial Hospital, Taoyuan, Taiwan

CLAIR LAKKIS, MD
Fellow, Division of Sleep Medicine, Sleep Disorders Clinic, Stanford University Medical School, Redwood City, California

ATUL MALHOTRA, MD
Division of Sleep Medicine, Harvard Medical School, Brigham and Women's Hospital, Boston, Massachusetts

RACHEL MANBER, PhD
Professor, Sleep Medicine Center, Stanford University School of Medicine, Redwood City, California

ROBERT OWENS, MD
Division of Sleep Medicine, Harvard Medical School, Brigham and Women's Hospital, Boston, Massachusetts

PAOLA PIRELLI, DDS
Department of Odontostomatological Sciences, University of Tor Vergata; Via Tomacelli, Rome, Italy

NELSON B. POWELL, DDS, MD, FACS
Adjunct Clinical Professor, Department of Otolaryngology Head and Neck Surgery; Department of Psychiatry and Behavioral Science, Stanford University Sleep and Research Center, Stanford University School of Medicine, Palo Alto, Stanford, California

KANNAN RAMAR, MD
Mayo Clinic, Center for Sleep Medicine, Division of Pulmonary, Sleep and Critical Care Medicine, Mayo Clinic, Rochester, Minnesota

MAURIZIO SAPONARA, MD
Department of Neurology and Otolaryngology, University La Sapienza, Rome, Italy

BHAVNEESH SHARMA, MD
Division of Sleep Medicine, Harvard Medical School, Brigham and Women's Hospital, Boston, Massachusetts

ALLISON T. SIEBERN, PhD
Instructor, Sleep Medicine Center, Stanford University School of Medicine, Redwood City, California

SHANNON S. SULLIVAN, MD
Instructor, Stanford Sleep Medicine Center, Redwood City; Center for Sleep Sciences; Stanford University, Palo Alto, California

MING-HORNG TSAI, MD
Division of Pediatric Hematology/Oncology; Division of Pediatric Neonatology, Department of Pediatrics, Chang Gung Memorial Hospital, Yunlin; College of Medicine, Chang Gung Memorial Hospital, Taoyuan, Taiwan

HERBERT J. YUE, MD
Postdoctoral Fellow, Stanford Sleep Medicine Clinic, Stanford University School of Medicine, Redwood City, California

Contents

There has been a growing recognition of chronic pain that may be experienced by patients. There has been a movement toward treating these patients aggressively with pharmacologic and nonpharmacologic modalities. Opioids have been a significant component of the treatment of acute pain, with their increasing use in cases of chronic pain, albeit with some controversy. In addition to analgesia, opioids have many accompanying adverse effects, particularly with regard to stability of breathing during sleep. This article reviews the existing literature on the effects of opioids on sleep, particularly sleep-disordered breathing.

Breathing disorders during sleep are common in congestive heart failure (CHF). Sleep-disordered breathing (SDB) in CHF can be broadly classified as 2 types: central sleep apnea with Cheyne-Stokes breathing, and obstructive sleep apnea. Prevalence of SDB ranges from 47% to 76% in systolic CHF. Treatment of SDB in CHF may include optimization of CHF treatment, positive airway pressure therapy, and other measures such as theophylline, acetazolamide, and cardiac resynchronization therapy. Periodic limb movements are also common in CHF.

Current evidence suggests a role for obstructive sleep apnea (OSA) in the development of cardiovascular disorders. However, obesity is an active confounder in this relationship. OSA and obesity share similar pathophysiologic mechanisms potentially leading to cardiovascular disorders. Presence of OSA in obese patients may further contribute to adverse cardiovascular outcomes when compared with each condition in isolation. In this review the authors explore the complex relationship between OSA and obesity (and nonobese subjects) in the development of cardiovascular disorders.

Obstructive sleep apnea (OSA) is a prevalent condition characterized by repetitive airway obstruction during sleep with associated increased morbidity and mortality. Although CPAP is the preferred treatment, poor compliance is common. Patients intolerant of conventional OSA medical treatment may benefit from surgical therapy to alleviate pharyngeal obstruction. Case series suggest that maxillomandibular advancement has the highest surgical efficacy (86%) and cure rate (43%). Soft palate surgical techniques are less successful, with uvulopalatopharyngoplasty having an OSA surgical success rate of 50% and cure rate of 16%. Further research is needed to more thoroughly assess clinical outcomes (eg, quality of life, morbidity), better identify key preoperative patient and clinical characteristics that predict success, and confirm long-term effectiveness of surgical modalities to treat OSA.

Orthodontics and Obstructive Sleep Apnea in Children

Paola Pirelli, Maurizio Saponara, Chiara De Rosa, and Ezio Fanucci

Children who suffer from respiratory problems and obstructive sleep apnea (OSA) commonly exhibit disturbances of craniofacial morphology. A significant number have nasal obstruction associated with a narrow maxilla; maxillary constriction may increase nasal resistance and alter the tongue posture, leading to narrowing of the retroglossal airway and OSA. Sixty children with a case history of oral breathing, snoring, and night time apneas were studied. An orthognathodontic investigation was performed using radiographs that included not only the usual examinations (posteroanterior cephalographs and intraoral radiographs) but also computed tomographic scans. This article discusses the materials and methods and the results of this study.

Sleepy Driving

Nelson B. Powell and Jason K.M. Chau

Sleepiness and drowsiness are neurophysiologic states that may cause attenuation of vigilance and slowing of reaction times, and thus increase the risks of driving. This article reviews selected peer-reviewed publications from the past and present body of knowledge regarding sleepiness and drowsiness while driving and related accidents, injuries, and possible death. Comparative studies of driving drunk and driving sleepy are reviewed because both exhibit similarly dangerous driving behaviors. It is hoped that some of the information from this article could provide new interest in the necessity of education for sleepy drivers.

Advances in Narcolepsy

Michelle Cao

Narcolepsy with cataplexy is a rare but life-long and challenging disorder. Current insight into the pathophysiology of this condition seems to be autoimmune-mediated postnatal cell death of hypocretin neurons occurring by organ-specific autoimmune targeting with HLA–T-cell receptor interactions. The hypocretin system seems to have an influence on multiple organ systems beyond its wake-promoting mechanisms. The recent availability of cerebrospinal fluid hypocretin-1 analysis has led to definitive diagnostic criteria for narcolepsy with cataplexy. Pharmacologic first-line treatments for excessive daytime sleepiness and cataplexy is sodium oxybate, with modafinil for daytime sleepiness, in adults and children. Other investigative agents and treatment modalities hold promise in future directions for narcolepsy.

Kleine-Levin Syndrome is a periodic hypersomnia characterized by recurrent episodes of hypersomnia and other symptoms. This article reviews the research to date, outlines the clinical symptoms, and describes current testing and treatment. It concludes that the cause remains unknown and no treatment is effective in preventing recurrence, although modafinil may reduce duration of symptomatic episode.

Insomnia is not only the most common sleep disorder in the population, it is a frequent complaint heard overall by primary care physicians and specialists alike. Given the high prevalence of this disorder, its tendency to persist, and the frequency with which patients complain of symptoms in practice, it is imperative to have an understanding of basic sleep-wake mechanisms and the evolving field of pharmacologic approaches to enhance sleep. Currently, pharmacologic approaches are among the most widely used therapies for insomnia. This article reviews sleep-wake mechanisms, the neuroanatomic targets for sleep and wake-promoting agents, and discusses currently used agents to promote sleep and investigational hypnotics.

Emerging data underscores the public health and economic burden of insomnia evidenced by increased health risks; increased health care utilization; and work domain deficits (absenteeism and reduced productivity). Cognitive behavioral therapy for insomnia (CBTi) is a brief and effective non-pharmacologic treatment for insomnia that is grounded in the science of sleep medicine and the science of behavior change and psychological theory, and in direct comparisons with sleep medication in randomized control trials that demonstrate that CBTi has comparable efficacy with more durable long-term maintenance of gains after treatment discontinuation. The high level of empirical support for CBTi has led the National Institutes of Health Consensus and the American Academy of Sleep Medicine Practice Parameters to make the recommendation that CBTi be considered standard treatment. The aim of this report is to increase awareness and understanding of health care providers of this effective treatment option.

> REM sleep behavior disorder (RBD), formally recognized in the 1980s, is an infrequent but spectacular parasomnia characterized by dream enactment, leading to aggressive or complex behaviors. It essentially affects older men, and many years may go by before medical attention is sought. Frequent association with the α-synucleinopathies, such as Parkinson disease, has led investigators to believe that idiopathic RBD can be a harbinger of neurodegenerative diseases. Diagnosis is confirmed with a polysomnogram, which typically shows absence of normal REM sleep atonia and sometimes abnormal behavior. Treatment is achieved with clonazepam.

> Attention-deficit/hyperactivity disorder (ADHD) is a neurocognitive and behavior abnormality commonly seen in childhood and adolescence. Symptoms and consequences of ADHD and sleep problems frequently overlap, and their relationship is complex and bidirectional. To avoid inappropriate diagnosis and inadequate management, mental health professionals should assess sleep problems and disorders in children, adolescents, and adults with ADHD-related symptoms and in those with a diagnosis of ADHD. Screening for other psychiatric comorbidities and the side effects of medications, such as psychostimulants, is necessary when considering sleep complaints, because both have adverse effects on sleep.

Preface
Sleep Medicine—A
Challenging Field With
Many New Findings

Sleep disorders have finally reached a point where they are being acknowledged by the various disciplines of the medical community. The obesity epidemic, which has affected children and adults in the industrialized countries, has increased the frequency with which sleep-disordered breathing and its complications are seen. In obese individuals, in particular men, fat deposits have been found to infiltrate the abdomen, resulting in a restrictive chest bellows syndrome. In obese individuals, this restriction has a profound effect on oxygen saturation when they are awake and when they are asleep, especially in the supine position. This effect also becomes most pronounced during rapid eye movement (REM) sleep, when there is a loss of accessory muscle recruitment for breathing. Additionally, fat deposits have been noted to invade the neck, which, in combination with abdominal restriction, further increase the likelihood of upper airway collapse and obstruction during sleep.

The hyperactive adipocyte itself in these obese individuals adds its own degree of pathogenesis. The adipocyte has been found to secrete the leptin, ghrelin, adinopectin, obesin, and other peptides, which play key roles in metabolic regulation.[1] The dysregulation of these peptides in obese individuals may worsen existing health problems and may establish feedback loops, aggravating negative outcomes. Although overweight subjects with snoring and upper airway obstruction during sleep have been increasingly labeled as obstructive sleep apneic patients, it is equally important to realize that these patients present with a more complicated syndrome, in which the roles of the obese abdomen and even more of the adipocyte have yet to be fully appreciated. The cardiac and cerebrovascular associations in this syndrome have been clearly demonstrated, and nasal positive airway pressure continues to be the most viable solution for most middle-aged and older subjects. In younger subjects, maxillomandibular surgery, performed by an experienced specialist, may be the most practical option given the high rate of noncompliance with treatment in this age group.

The role of familial predisposition for the development of upper airway obstruction during sleep has also been demonstrated in many studies in the 1990s.[2–4] One of the predisposing risk factors has been the familial traits of facial anatomy and morphology. A better understanding of this risk factor has emerged in the past 10 years through the work of orthodontists and physiologists investigating the neuromuscular mechanisms of breathing. In addition to the static effects of

Med Clin N Am 94 (2010) xi–xiv
doi:10.1016/j.mcna.2010.03.009
0025-7125/10/$ – see front matter

anatomy on airway opening and collapse, the dynamic effects of dilator muscle contraction (and timing) have been found to play a key role in maintaining airway patency during breathing. In essence, upper airway constrictor muscles normally tense just before inspiration to prevent airway collapse from the negative pressures caused by inspiration. Prolonged turbulent airflow and snoring during sleep have been associated with an impairment of the sensory motor loop of the dilator response to negative intrathoracic inspiratory pressure. The possibility of such permanent neurologic sequelae[5,6] serves to underscore the importance of early diagnosis and treatment of sleep-disordered breathing in children and young adults.

A consideration in adolescents is the influence of sex hormones, often resulting in enlargement of the tongue muscles and airway soft tissues. Enlarged tonsils and adenoids are commonly identified and easily treatable causes of sleep-disordered breathing in children and young adults. A young child with snoring who is treated with adenotonsillectomy and still has some residual symptoms, however, may show a resurgence of abnormal breathing and snoring after puberty or in early adulthood due to such hormonal changes. With respect to bony or dental anatomy, well-trained orthodontists should be able to identify children with narrow bone structures early and offer treatment to enlarge the airway in eligible subjects. On the other end of the spectrum, the prevention of lifelong health problems, specifically cognitive decline and cardiovascular risk, has not yet received similar attention from the medical community.

In the fight against pain syndromes, ranging from cancer to rheumatologic diseases, as well as in the implementation of methadone programs for drug rehabilitation, the past several years have witnessed a marked increase in opioid consumption. Among many other side effects, opioids have been found to have a profound effect on breathing during sleep. For this reason, special consideration must be given to the impact of opiate use on breathing during sleep and the overall well-being of sleepy patients. Patients with heart failure or opiate use may present with similar problems during sleep: a general decrease in diaphragmatic contraction leading to hypoventilation and abnormal upper airway contraction during inspiration. Although there are tools to address these issues and noninvasively assure normal breathing, positive airway pressure may be detrimental to some heart failure patients. Specifically, in some heart failure patients, positive airway pressure may change preload and afterload in a manner that worsens the condition. There is, however, the capability of identifying these at-risk individuals and tailoring treatment appropriately.

Undoubtedly, insomnia remains one of the most common complaints for most practitioners, and prescription sleep aids place a substantial burden on health care spending. Novel hypnotic agents are continuously being developed, some of which are in entirely different drug classes from existing medications. Although the arrival of novel sleep aids is awaited, there are some closely related compounds that are already becoming available or in the final stages of investigation. Despite the promise of novel sleep agents, the past several years have shown the limited impact of these medications, especially on the complaint of poor sleep. This may be related to underlying problems that emerge during sleep but also may be related to conditioning or other factors these drugs cannot address in the long term. For this reason, behavioral treatments for insomnia have had great success and substantial results have been well documented recently.

Beyond organic illness, motor vehicle accidents continue to be a major cause of fatality in young individuals. Alcohol is a well-known cause of accidents, but increasingly, sleepiness at the wheel has emerged as an even greater contributor. Sleep deprivation, increasingly common, has been associated with an alarming frequency of "lapses of attention" and "near misses."[7] Sleep fragmentation related to shift work, regular employment, or an unrecognized organic problem may also be responsible for these accidents; the quality and quantity of sleep should always be considered. Syndromes of sleepiness, which may present with tiredness and fatigue from the time of waking, must be recognized and treated aggressively, with a constant consideration for abnormal breathing during sleep (not solely obstructive sleep apnea) as well as narcolepsy.

Since the discovery that narcolepsy was related to the destruction of a small group of cells in the lateral hypothalamus,[8] many questions have been raised. There is much ongoing research to investigate why this cell loss occurs and what results from the loss of the hypocretin/orexin peptides. The hypothesis that narcolepsy is an autoimmune disorder has recently received increasing support, with the identification of a specific T-cell receptor involved in pathogenesis.[9] In the search for treatment of daytime sleepiness and fatigue, the significant limitations of current treatments have become apparent. Commonly used amphetamine compounds, in addition to elevating blood pressure and exerting many psychiatric effects, have also been known to produce insomnia during use and rebound hypersomnia on daily end of action. Hypersomnia can also be seen periodically in Kleine-Levin syndrome (KLS), which affects adolescents and adults. Less is known about KLS than narcolepsy, but there is an understanding that the symptomatic period results from a hypoperfusion of the thalami. A prolonged period of these recurrent episodes has also been shown to result in permanent neurocognitive impairment and deficit. As with narcolepsy, there is evidence that there may be some autoimmune etiology underlying KLS, although more research is needed in this field.

Attention-deficit/hyperactivity disorder (ADHD) is a syndrome that affects children, teenagers, and adults, although there is no current objective test to confirm its diagnosis. It has also been discovered that certain sleep disorders may induce symptoms of ADHD, such as hyperactivity and inattention. The diagnostic problem is complicated by the fact that several primary psychiatric disorders may present with symptoms similar to ADHD. Before making the diagnosis of ADHD, it is of paramount importance to eliminate the possibility of sleep disorders that may present with similar behavioral elements. At this time, ADHD is probably greatly overdiagnosed and overtreated, often with potent stimulant medications. The concern is when this is done without consideration of alternative causes of hyperactivity, impulsivity, and inattention resulting from disturbed sleep.

Finally, through a better understanding of narcolepsy, with its prominent phenotype, and possibly KLS, sleep research may lead to a better understanding of autoimmune disorders in general. Research in the field of REM sleep behavior disorder (RBD) has opened a new window on neurodegenerative disorders. Significant progress has been made in understanding this condition, in which there is a loss of normal motor inhibition during REM sleep, commonly associated with dreaming. The loss of REM atonia results in dramatic presentations, in which an otherwise calm and composed individual may become a raging, aggressive, and possibly dangerous dreamer. This disappearance of physiologic muscle atonia that normally prevents acting out dreams has been associated with other neurodegenerative diseases and with delirium. Long described as an idiopathic process, RBD may actually herald the onset of several neurodegenerative disorders affecting the brainstem in a gradually ascending fashion. Schenck and colleagues[10] have demonstrated how RBD may precede the onset of Parkinson disease or dementia, specifically dementia with Lewy bodies, diseases again affecting lower brainstem structures. Can the diagnosis of RBD in middle-aged patients lead to preemptive treatment of an evolving subclinical neurodegenerative process? This will be the challenge over years to come.

Alex Dimitriu, MD
Division of Sleep Medicine
Stanford University School of Medicine
Stanford Medical Outpatient Center
450 Broadway Street, Pavillon C
Redwood City, CA 94063-5074, USA

Christian Guilleminault, MD, DBiol
Division of Sleep Medicine
Stanford University School of Medicine
Stanford Medical Outpatient Center
450 Broadway Street, Pavillon C
Redwood City, CA 94063-5074, USA

E-mail address:
cguil@leland.stanford.edu

REFERENCES

1. Meier U. Endocrine regulation of energy metabolism: review of pathobiochemical and clinical chemical aspects of leptin, ghrelin, adiponectin, and resistin. Clin Chem 2004;50(9):1511–25.
2. Mathur R, Douglas NJ. Family studies inpatients with the sleep apnea/hypopnea syndrome. Ann Intern Med 1995;222:174–8.
3. Redline S, Tishler PV, Tosteson TD, et al. The familial aggregation of obstructive sleep apnea. Am J Respir Crit Care Med 1995;151:682–7.
4. Guilleminault C, Partinen M, Hollman K, et al. Familial aggregates in obstructive sleep apnea syndrome. Chest 1995;107:1545–51.
5. Friberg D, Ansved T, Borg K, et al. Histological indications of a progressive disease in the upper airway muscles. Am J Respir Crit Care Med 1998;157:586–93.
6. Guilleminault C, Huang YS, Kirisoglu C, et al. Is obstructive sleep apnea a neurological disorder? Ann Neurol 2005;58:880–7.
7. Powell NB, Schechtman KB, Riley RW, et al. Sleepy driver near-misses may predict accident risks. Sleep 2007;30(3):331–42.
8. Thannickal TC, Moore RY, Nienhuis R, et al. Reduced number of hypocretin neurons in human narcolepsy. Neuron 2000;27:469–74.
9. Hallmayer J, Faraco J, Lin L, et al. Narcolepsy is strongly associated with the T-cell receptor alpha locus. Nat Genet 2009;41(7):859.
10. Schenck CH, Bundlie SR, Mahowald MW. Delayed emergence of a parkinsonian disorder in 38% of 29 older men initially diagnosed with idiopathic rapid eye movement sleep behaviour disorder. Neurology 1996;46:388–93.

Opioid Medication and Sleep-disordered Breathing

Herbert J. Yue, MD, Christian Guilleminault, MD, DBiol*

KEYWORDS
- Opioids • Sleep-disordered breathing
- Control of breathing • Sleep apnea

In recent years, there has been a growing recognition of chronic pain that may be experienced by patients. Historically, chronic pain has been given less importance or simply ignored by many practitioners, with deleterious effects on patients. There has been a movement toward treating these patients aggressively with pharmacologic and nonpharmacologic modalities. Opioids have been a significant component of the treatment of acute pain, with increasing use in cases of chronic pain, albeit with some controversy.[1,2] In addition to analgesia, opioids have many accompanying adverse effects, particularly with regard to stability of breathing during sleep. This article reviews the existing literature on the effects of opioids on sleep, particularly sleep-disordered breathing (SDB).

EPIDEMIOLOGY OF NARCOTIC USE

Despite the widespread use of opioids in varying aspects of medical practice, there are limited data on the specific usage or prescribing patterns of the most popular opiate medications. The Automation of Reports and Consolidated Orders System (ARCOS) is a mechanism whereby the Drug Enforcement Agency reports the amounts of opiate medications distributed on a retail basis. The data provided by ARCOS reports are limited in the sense that (1) veterinary usage is included, (2) usage of opioids for nonanalgesia indications are not specified, and (3) they do not include medications that were ultimately reordered or not distributed to patients.[3] The data subsequently represent an overestimate of the quantities of opioids used for human consumption.[3] Nevertheless, the amounts likely prescribed to patients remain substantial. In 1990, more than 2.2 million g of morphine was used medically, including 3273 g of fentanyl, 1.6 million g of oxycodone, and 118,455 g of hydromorphone.[4] When follow-up data in 1996 were evaluated, the use of fentanyl had increased by

Division of Sleep Medicine, Stanford University School of Medicine, Stanford Medical Outpatient Center, 450 Broadway Street, Pavillon C, Redwood City, CA 94063-5074, USA
* Corresponding author.
E-mail address: cguil@leland.stanford.edu

Med Clin N Am 94 (2010) 435–446
doi:10.1016/j.mcna.2010.02.007
0025-7125/10/$ – see front matter © 2010 Elsevier Inc. All rights reserved.

1168%, followed by morphine with an increase of 59%, oxycodone by 23%, and hydromorphone by 19%. The only opioid medication to drop in usage was meperidine (5.2 to 3.2 million g). This significant increase in the prescribing of opioids is important, because they are known to have deleterious effects on the control of respiration, particularly during sleep.

CONTROL OF NORMAL BREATHING WHILE AWAKE AND DURING SLEEP

Control of normal breathing is a complex interaction between central respiratory pacemakers and interactions with central and peripheral chemoreceptors and mechanoreceptors. This control is also subject to alterations by voluntary and involuntary behavioral controls. To understand the effects of opioids on SDB, it would be useful to discuss the normal control of breathing in awake and sleep states.

Central respiratory rhythm generators, as well as those responsible for other behaviors such as swallowing and suckling, are located in the pontomedullary reticular formation.[5] In neonatal animals at least, a collection of neurons called the pre-Bötzinger complex has been shown to have properties consistent with a central respiratory pacemaker. A similar structure has not yet been found in humans. The pre-Bötzinger complex is found within the rostral ventrolateral medulla oblongata and contains neurons that produce rhythmic bursts of respiratory-like activity.[5] Even when the downstream activity of these neurons is interrupted pharmacologically, the neurons continue to fire in a rhythmic pattern, supporting their potential role as central respiratory pacemakers.[5] Interruption of the pre-Bötzinger complex is associated with irregular breathing patterns, particularly during sleep.[6,7] Another area important in central respiratory pattern generation is the retrotrapezoid/parafacial respiratory nucleus, also located in the ventrolateral medulla oblongata. Neurons with pacemaker activity have also been found in this area, and it seems that both these structures (the pre-Bötzinger complex and retrotrapezoid/parafacial respiratory nucleus) are required for normal respiratory rhythm.[8,9]

Interactions between respiratory pattern generators and central and peripheral receptors are a large determinant of the control of breathing. Metabolic control of breathing involves reflex and tonic inputs from peripheral and central chemoreceptors that detect changes in carbon dioxide (CO_2)/oxygen (O_2) levels or pH. The central chemoreceptors are located in several locations, particularly the nucleus tractus solitarius, dorsal respiratory group, medullary raphe, pre-Bötzinger complex, and the retrotrapezoid/parafacial respiratory group.[5,10] These chemoreceptors are sensitive to changes in the partial pressures of carbon dioxide/pH, and increase both tidal volume and/or respiratory rate in response to hypercapnia or acidemia. Peripheral chemoreceptors consist of collections of neurons that detect changes primarily in the partial pressure of arterial oxygen, with synergistic responses to carbon dioxide/pH changes as well. These chemoreceptors are located in the carotid bodies and provide input to the nucleus tractus solitarius. Other central and peripheral receptors include central hypothalamic thermoreceptors, which provide stimulus for respiration in accordance with the energy and metabolic needs of the organism, and peripheral lung mechanoreceptors, which provide input on lung distention and volume and adjust ventilation accordingly.[5]

All these peripheral receptors have inputs on the central respiratory pattern generators, which then communicate with motor neurons that innervate the important respiratory muscles (ie, diaphragm, internal/external intercostals, and abdominal musculature). The central respiratory neurons often have a phase specificity and are active only during a particular portion of the respiratory cycle. For instance, pre-Bötzinger complex neurons are typically active only during inspiration, whereas those in the retrotrapezoid/parafacial respiratory group are active usually during exhalation.[10] There are other neurons that are active in the third phase (the postinhalation phase) and there are some whose activity spans more than 1 phase.[5]

During sleep, there are changes in the patterns and mechanics of breathing, with some well-described effects depending on the stage of sleep. Typically, during non–rapid eye movement (NREM) sleep, breathing remains regular. Although the rhythmicity remains regular, there is a small decrease in the respiratory rate with an increase in the tidal volume, which leads to an overall decrease in the total minute ventilation.[5] There is an accompanying decrease in the respiratory response to hypercapnia, although the response to hypoxemia is unchanged. This change in carbon dioxide reactivity leads to a small increase in the partial pressure of carbon dioxide levels and a small decrease in blood oxygen levels during sleep. The increase in carbon dioxide levels is also thought to serve as an additional stimulus to compensate for wakefulness-related influences.[5,11] Activity to accessory muscles of respiration and those in the upper airway is often reduced, although this is not thought to significantly alter airway resistance in normal subjects. This loss of muscle activity, however, is thought to be an important contributor to SDB in susceptible patients.

During rapid eye movement (REM) sleep, breathing is no longer regular, and there can be a large breath to breath variability in pattern and tidal volume. Typically, respiratory patterns can become irregular, with rapid increases in inspiratory muscle activity interrupted with short periods of inactivity.[5] Thresholds to hypercapnia, hypoxemia, and arousals are altered during REM sleep, with potential large increases in partial pressures of carbon dioxide and oxygen seen in susceptible individuals. All accessory muscles of respiration are essentially atonic during REM sleep, and the full maintenance of the minute ventilation (and consequently the arterial carbon dioxide and oxygen levels) is dependent on the diaphragm. It is also thought that phasic events during REM, particularly ponto-geniculo-occipital spikes, may be associated with the variability of breathing.

EFFECTS OF NARCOTICS ON BREATHING IN NORMAL INDIVIDUALS

Opioids are a group of naturally occurring and synthetic chemicals that bind to opioid receptors in the body, found primarily in the central nervous system and gastrointestinal tract. More than 1000 members of the receptor family have been reported, and they structurally act like G protein–coupled receptors.[12] Binding of an opioid ligand induces changes in the extracellular domain of the receptor, with transmission of signal through a transmembrane portion into the intracellular component of the receptor, changing it into a guanine nucleotide exchange factor. The receptor associates with a G protein and exchanges guanosine diphosphate for guanosine triphosphate, activating a downstream signaling cascade. This signaling cascade leads to changes in the cell, including opening and closing of various ion channels in the cell. The resultant flux of ions, such as those of calcium and potassium, changes the electrical balance of the cell, with resulting decreased excitability.

Four classes of opioid receptors have been described, including opioid δ receptor (DOP), opioid μ receptor (MOP), nociceptin/orphanin peptide receptor (NOP), and opioid κ receptor (KOP).[12–14] Each receptor has at least 1 associated endogenous ligand, with the overall opioid receptor system mediating physiologic processes including pain, respiration, and stress. All opioid receptor types are typically associated with analgesia, although NOP receptors have been associated with hyperalgesia when stimulated with agonists supraspinally.[15] Besides analgesia, stimulation of opioid receptors is often associated with respiratory depression, particularly with stimulation of MOP and KOP receptors. Synthetic and semisynthetic opioids bind to each receptor with varying degrees of affinity, typically with the greatest affinity for MOP receptors. Ligands may act as pure agonists, mixed agonists/antagonists, or pure antagonists. Exogenous opioids are usually metabolized hepatically, with renal clearance.

With regard to breathing, opioids cause decreases in central respiratory pattern generation with resultant decreases in respiratory rate and/or tidal volume. Much of the previous work in the literature has been performed in animals, with less information available regarding potential mechanisms in humans. In the available animal and human studies, the effects of opioids on breathing have mostly involved 2 types of studies: (1) direct instillation of opioids on chemosensitive areas such as the carotid body or brainstem or (2) systemic administration of opioids in awake and anesthetized humans and animals.[16] When opioid agonists were directly applied to medullary and pontine respiratory associated centers (including the nucleus tractus solitarius), decreases in peak activity were seen, although basal activity did not seem to change.[16,17] Opiates applied to the ventral medullary surface of animals were shown to decrease tidal volume but increase respiratory rate, whereas application to the rostral dorsal pons was shown to decrease respiratory rate.[16,18] Among the neuronal centers important for central respiratory rhythm generation, only pre-Bötzinger complex neurons are sensitive to opioids. Similar findings are also seen with opiates and peripheral chemoreceptors. When morphine was applied to the carotid bodies of anesthetized cats, decreases in chemoreceptor activity were seen that were reversed with application of an opioid antagonist (naloxone).[19]

In studies of systemic administration of opiates, there is limited applicability of animal data to human responses, because there is significant cross-species variability in responses. For instance, systemic administration of opioids in cats or goats produces respiratory stimulation, whereas in humans, opiates produce clear respiratory depression.[16] At lower doses, opiates produce a respiratory depression via reduction in tidal volume that is proportional to the dose and potency of the opiate administered.[20] At higher doses, decreases in respiratory rate and rhythm generation are seen. When morphine was given to normal human subjects, decreases in hypercapnic and hypoxic respiratory drives were also seen.[21] This effect seems to predominantly affect the respiratory response to hypoxemia; at higher doses this response is virtually ablated.[21,22] This response suggests that the action of opioids on hypoxemic respiratory drive is through effects on peripheral chemoreceptors, although a central mechanism of action has been suggested in some studies. In a study of 30 subjects randomly assigned to receive intrathecal morphine, intravenous morphine, or placebo, similar decreases in hypoxemic respiratory drive were seen.[23] Based on these studies, it seems that opiates act not only on central pattern generators but also on chemosensitive receptors that are both centrally located and in the periphery.

Although less well studied, the effects of opioids on other components involved in the control of breathing are important. For instance, there is an increase in respiratory effort in response to an increase in respiratory airway resistance or loading.[16] Administration of opiates has been shown to decrease this compensatory increase in respiratory effort.[22,24] There are also upper airway muscle reflexes that are important in maintaining airway patency. These upper airway muscles (such as the genioglossus muscles) receive tonic input during wakefulness, with phasic increases before inspiration.[25] The activity of these muscles decreases during sleep, although in normal subjects, airway patency and resistance remain essentially unchanged. However, administration of respiratory depressants (including opioids) has been associated with tendency for obstruction at the upper airway level as well as rigidity of accessory muscles of respiration (ie, intercostals and abdominal muscles). For instance, administration of a highly selective MOP agonist (fentanyl or sufentanil) has been associated not only with decreases in respiratory rate and depth of respiration but also with glottic/supraglottic obstruction.[26,27]

CLINICAL EFFECTS OF NARCOTICS ON BREATHING IN THOSE SUSCEPTIBLE TO SDB

Clinical data looking at the effects of opioids on SDB have typically consisted of case series, studies of patients on long-term oral opioids for malignant and nonmalignant reasons, or studies of patients enrolled in long-term methadone programs. Interpretation across studies is therefore difficult, because patients on long-term opioids are often concurrently prescribed antidepressants and benzodiazepines, both of which have been described to alter respiratory patterns. In a small study of 12 normal subjects, acute administration of a short-acting oral narcotic did not seem to be associated with the development of any SDB.[28] Nevertheless, a growing body of literature has described several consistent clinical findings in patients on long-term opioid therapy. Each of these findings is now examined in detail and the supporting literature is described.

Development of Central Apnea During Sleep

A significant proportion of patients taking long-term opioids develop central apnea during sleep and this seems to be a consistent finding. In one of the earliest studies, Teichtahl and colleagues[29] examined 10 patients in a methadone maintenance program and performed a clinical assessment and overnight polysomnography. They found that all 10 patients had evidence of central sleep apnea, with 6 patients having a central apnea index (CAI) greater than 5 and 4 patients with a CAI greater than 10. In a larger follow-up study of 50 patients taking long-term methadone, 30% of the patients had a CAI greater than 5, and 20% had a CAI greater than 10.[30] All the patients had been on stable doses of methadone for at least 2 months, and other potentially contributing diagnoses (such as congestive heart failure) had been excluded. Similar findings have also been described for opioids other than methadone. In 2 studies of patients enrolled in a chronic pain clinic and had been receiving a variety of opiate medications (including methadone), the investigators noted that approximately 25% of patients showed evidence of central sleep apnea, with a CAI greater than 5.[31,32]

The mechanism underlying the presence of significant central sleep apnea is not clear. Although the opioids have been presumed to be the primary culprit through their action on central respiratory pacemakers and chemoreceptors, it is not clear if excessive dosing is the only responsible mechanism. When blood toxicology tests were examined in a group of patients on long-term methadone maintenance, serum methadone levels did seem to be the most significant item correlated to the severity of central sleep apnea.[30] However, in multivariate analyses, the serum methadone level contributed to only 12% of the variance of the severity of central sleep apnea. The investigators suggested various mechanisms contributing to central sleep apnea, including prior structural damage from illicit drug use, disrupted hypoxic/hypercapnic respiratory responses, and contributions from the concurrent use of antidepressants and benzodiazepines. In a study of 50 patients receiving long-term methadone therapy, the investigators found significant decreases in the respiratory response to hypercapnia and increased ventilatory responses to hypoxia. Twenty percent of the patients had evidence of carbon dioxide retention while awake (defined as

$Pa_{CO_2}>45$), and approximately 30% had an increased alveolar-arterial oxygen gradient.[33] These ventilatory changes also seemed to be manifested through alterations in the respiratory rate and not through changes in the tidal volume.

Development of Ataxic Breathing During Sleep

Other clinical findings include the development of irregular breathing patterns in patients receiving long-term opioid therapy. In a case series of three patients receiving a variety of opiate medications, irregular breathing patterns were described, consisting of irregular respiratory pauses and gasping without periodicity, found primarily during non-REM sleep.[34] The authors felt the breathing was consistent with ataxic or Biot breathing, previously described in patients with acute neurologic disease. This pattern of breathing was first described in 1876 by Camille Biot, a French physician, in a child with tuberculous meningitis.[35] He described a respiratory pattern with pauses, distinct from Cheyne-Stokes respiration, called "rhythme meningitique." This pattern of respiration has been described for patients on opioids, who have an erratic variability in the respiratory rate and effort of breath with frequent irregular breathing. In a study of 60 patients receiving long-term opioid therapy, more than 70% of patient on opiates were observed to have ataxic or Biot breathing, compared with 5% of controls in an age- and sex-matched group.[36] This irregular breathing seemed to be related to dosing of opiates; more than 90% of subjects on a morphine dose equivalent to greater than 200 mg daily were noted to have evidence of Biot breathing.

Development of Obstructive Apneas or Hypopneas During Sleep

There does not seem to be a clear consensus in the literature regarding the development of obstructive sleep apnea syndrome in patients who receive long-term opiate treatment. As noted earlier, acute administration of an oral narcotic was not associated with increases in obstructive apneas or hypopneas in normal subjects.[28] Concurrent evaluation of upper airway function in these subjects did not find any increase in pharyngeal airway resistance while awake, although decreases in ventilatory responses to hypoxia were seen. Another case series of 3 patients noted only modest increases in the obstructive apnea and hypopnea index (AHI) in 2 patients, 1 of whom had a diagnosis of obstructive sleep apnea before being prescribed previous opiate therapy.[37] In a study of 50 subjects on long-term methadone therapy, no statistically significant increases in the occurrence of obstructive sleep apnea compared with a control group were seen.[30] In contrast, Farney and colleagues[34] described 3 patients on long-term sustained-release opioid medications with markedly prolonged obstructive hypopneas during sleep, each lasting greater than 5 minutes on average. These obstructive hypopneas were associated with severe oxyhemoglobin desaturations and seen exclusively during NREM sleep. Another 2 case series of 6 and 10 subjects, respectively, noted that obstructive respiratory events accounted for between 16% and 80% of the increase in the AHI.[29,38] A recent study of 71 patients on long-term methadone maintenance therapy with subjective sleep complaints noted that 35% of the study population had evidence of obstructive sleep apnea on an overnight home polysomnogram. The investigators did not observe significant central sleep apnea in their cohort, with approximately 15% of subjects having a CAI greater than 5. When methadone levels and concurrent drug use were tested, neither seemed to be correlated with the degree of central sleep apnea. In 2 separate studies from the same pain clinic, 35% and 57% of the subjects had evidence of either pure or mixed obstructive sleep apnea.[31,32] The degree of SDB correlated most with the dose of methadone in statistical analyses, although the investigators did not specifically look at obstructive versus central events during sleep.

Development of Hypoxemia

Hypoxemia in patients taking long-term opioids has been variably described in the literature, with many groups reporting an increased incidence of significant oxyhemoglobin desaturation during sleep among patients receiving long-term opioid therapy compared with control groups.[29,31,36] The increase in nocturnal hypoxemia, however, is not entirely explained by a concurrent increase in SDB. In a study of 98 patients on long-term opioid medications, 72% had evidence of nocturnal oxyhemoglobin desaturation, defined as an arterial oxyhemoglobin saturation during sleep of (1) less than 90% for 5 minutes with a nadir of 85% or less or (2) greater than 30% of the total sleep time.[31] Ten percent of the subjects with significant nocturnal desaturations did not have evidence of sleep apnea on overnight polysomnography. When the investigators examined for the incidence of significant desaturations during sleep among subjects with varying degrees of SDB, they found only a moderate increase in the incidence of sleep-associated desaturations with increased SDB severity (60% in subjects with an AHI in the mild range vs 80% of subjects with an AHI in the moderate to severe range). There was a statistically significant correlation, albeit a weak one, between the morphine equivalent dose and the time spent in sleep with an oxyhemoglobin saturation less than 90% ($R = .237, P = .023$). Ten percent of the subjects also had evidence of hypoxemia during wakefulness that worsened during sleep. Similar findings were seen in a study of 60 patients on long-term opioid use, with a statistically significant difference in average arterial oxygen saturation in awake subjects compared with a control group.[36]

EFFECTS OF NARCOTICS ON SLEEP ARCHITECTURE

Not much is known about the effects of opioids on sleep architecture. Early studies in animals have demonstrated disruption in sleep associated with opioid administration, including decreases in total sleep time and REM sleep.[39] More recent studies in human subjects have primarily demonstrated decreases in slow wave and REM sleep, with concurrent increases in stage 2 sleep.[40] Similar findings were also noted in a study of 42 subjects who were administered a one-time dose of either extended-release morphine or methadone.[41] Another study in patients who underwent abdominal surgery and subsequently received narcotics for pain relief reported an absence of REM sleep for the first few nights, with a large rebound in REM sleep later in their convalescence.[42] Others have found a suggestion of increased nocturnal arousals in patients on long-term opioids, albeit measured via limb electromyogram.[43] It seems that the changes in REM and slow wave sleep are the most consistent, although a significant amount of variability in the findings remains. In addition, most of the studies available in the literature consist of case series, without accompanying control groups. Many of the previous studies have also relied on abnormal subjects for the studies, specifically previous narcotic addicts, as the study population. Such a focus limits the interpretation of these studies as well as issues such as variability in scoring of sleep studies, doses of opioids used, and types of narcotics used (ie, short- vs long-acting). More work is necessary to further delineate the changes in sleep architecture with opioid medications.

TREATMENT

Currently, there is no clear consensus on the treatment of opioid-associated SDB. As noted earlier, patients may have several disturbances in their respiratory patterns during sleep, including characteristics of central sleep apnea, obstructive sleep apnea, ataxic breathing, or a combination of all 3 types. Several nocturnal ventilatory strategies have been tried with varying degrees of success, including continuous positive airway pressure (CPAP) support, bilevel therapy (usually with a backup rate), and adaptoservo ventilation (ASV). In the case series of 3 patients on long-term opioid medication with evidence of sleep-disordered breathing discussed earlier, the investigators attempted titration with CPAP therapy with limited success.[34] Although the number of respiratory events decreased, the patients were reported to have continued severe hypoxemia that necessitated supplemental oxygen. Despite relative tolerance of increasing CPAP pressures, the patients continued to have a large number of central respiratory events, and there was some suggestion that the CPAP may have worsened the central sleep apnea. Similar findings were reported in another case series of 6 patients on long-term methadone maintenance.[38] Five of the 6 subjects agreed to proceed with a CPAP titration, and in 4 of these subjects, significant central apneas persisted despite titration up to a CPAP pressure of 20 cm H_2O. In 1 subject, it seemed that the CPAP was effective at a pressure of 20 cm H_2O, although the patient was unable to tolerate therapy. Two case series of 5 and 22 patients on long-term opioids with SDB noted increases in the CAI with CPAP treatment, with an average increase of 10 to 20 central events per hour.[34,44] Although CPAP may be beneficial in relieving the airway obstruction potentially associated with opioid use, it does not seem to be able to successfully treat any concurrent central sleep apnea and may be associated with increased frequency of central apneas during sleep.

Bilevel therapy with a backup rate has also been suggested as a treatment for patients with mixed central and obstructive sleep apnea, although there have not been many studies published on the subject. In the case series reported by Alatarr and colleagues,[38] patients who failed CPAP therapy because of efficacy or tolerance issues were then offered a bilevel titration, with timed backup rates of 12 to 16. Four patients agreed to proceed and were successfully titrated, with subsequent improvement in reports of daytime sleepiness. Three of these 4 patients required supplemental oxygen despite a successful titration. Bilevel therapy has been examined in patients with mixed obstructive and central sleep apnea as well as obesity hypoventilation syndromes with some success, although there are no comparisons available on the use of bilevel therapy and other modalities (such as CPAP or ASV) in patients with opioid-associated SDB.[45–49] However, the authors have completed work on an unpublished study on more than 40 patients with a combination of obstructive sleep apnea and long-term opioid intake. Bilevel therapy with a backup rate was successful in controlling all patients with a 6 months follow-up compared with CPAP (Christian Guilleminault, unpublished data, 2010).

There has been growing interest in the use of ASV pressure support as a new modality in the treatment of SDB in patients receiving long-term opioid treatment. ASV machines work by varying the amount of ventilatory support, with the goal of avoiding hyperventilation and keeping the patient's partial pressure of carbon dioxide above the apneic threshold. These machines typically operate using an algorithm that measures the patient's minute ventilation on a running and spontaneous basis. Pressure support is adjusted dynamically to decrease in times of increased patient respiratory effort and increase during times of decreased patient respiratory effort. There has been a growing literature examining their use in Cheyne-Stokes respiration, central sleep apnea, and mixed obstructive/central sleep apnea syndromes with positive results.[50–54] Two case series have examined the use of ASV in patients on long-term opioid therapy with conflicting results. Javaheri and colleagues[44] examined 5 consecutive patients referred for an evaluation for obstructive sleep apnea who were also concurrently taking long-term opioid medication. All patients underwent an overnight diagnostic polysomnogram followed by a CPAP titration. CPAP was found to be an ineffective therapy in all patients, and they underwent a third night study with titration with ASV. The average AHI decreased from 70 to 20 with ASV; the remainder consisted entirely of hypopneas. The CAI, which had increased with CPAP therapy (from 26 to 37), was 0 at the end of the ASV titration. In contrast, Farney and colleagues[55] performed a retrospective analysis of 22 patients on long-term opioid use who were referred for SDB and had been tested with ASV. The average AHI decreased from 66.6 at baseline to 54.2 with ASV but was not statistically significant. Although the obstructive apnea index decreased significantly, the hypopnea index was observed to increase. There was no statistically significant change in the CAI, and the investigators noted that ataxic breathing continued. Unlike in the study by Javaheri and colleagues,[44] the end expiratory pressure was not titrated in the subjects in the study by Farney and colleagues,[55] suggesting a possible rationale for the relatively ineffective control of obstructive events in their study. Further research is necessary to determine the role of ASV in the treatment of opioid-associated SDB.

SUMMARY

The use of opioid medication is increasing with the potential for adverse effects on respiration, especially during sleep. Opioids seem to affect the control of breathing on many levels, including alterations in the central respiratory pacemaker function as well as effects on central and peripheral chemoreceptors. The use of opioids has been associated with abnormal breathing patterns in susceptible patients, including development of central sleep apnea, obstructive sleep apnea, ataxic breathing, and hypoxemia. The optimal treatment for these patients with opioid-associated SDB is not well-known, although equipment using positive-airway-pressure during sleep clearly provides benefit to these subjects. Further work is necessary to elucidate the mechanisms of SDB in patients on long-term opioid medication as well as how best to treat them.

REFERENCES

1. Ballantyne JC, Mao J. Opioid therapy for chronic pain. N Engl J Med 2003;349: 1943.
2. Portenoy RK. Opioid therapy for chronic nonmalignant pain: a review of the critical issues. J Pain Symptom Manage 1996;11:203.
3. Gilson AM, Ryan KM, Joranson DE, et al. A reassessment of trends in the medical use and abuse of opioid analgesics and implications for diversion control: 1997–2002. J Pain Symptom Manage 2004;28(2):176–88.
4. Joranson DE, Ryan KM, Gilson AM, et al. Trends in medical use and abuse of opioid analgesics. JAMA 2000;283(13):1710–4.
5. Kubin L. Respiratory physiology: CNS ventilatory control. In: Opp MR, Kilduff TS, Armitage R, et al, editors. SRS basic of sleep guide, 1st edition. Westchester (IL): Sleep Research Society; 2005. p. 81–8.
6. McKay LC, Feldman JL. Unilateral ablation of pre-Bötzinger complex disrupts breathing during sleep but not wakefulness. Am J Respir Crit Care Med 2008; 178:89–95.
7. McKay LC, Janczewski WA, Feldman JL. Sleep-disordered breathing after targeted ablation of pre Bötzinger complex neurons. Nat Neurosci 2005;8:1142–4.

8. Janczewski WA, Feldman JL. Distinct rhythm generators for inspiration and expiration in the juvenile rat. J Physiol 2006;570(Pt 2):407–20.

9. Onimaru H, Homma I. A novel functional group for respiratory rhythm generation in the ventral medulla. J Neurosci 2003;23:1426–78.

10. Walker JM, Farney RJ. Are opioids associated with sleep apnea? A review of the evidence. Curr Pain Headache Rep 2009;13(2):120–6.

11. Feldman JL, Mitchell GS, Nattie EE. Breathing: rhythmicity, plasticity, chemosensitivity. Annu Rev Neurosci 2003;26:239–66.

12. Martin TJ, Eisenach JC. Pharmacology of opioid and nonopioid analgesics in chronic pain states. J Pharmacol Exp Ther 2001;299(3):811–7.

13. Inturrisi CE. Clinical pharmacology of opioids for pain. Clin J Pain 2002;18:S2–13.

14. Pattinson KT. Opioids and the control of respiration. Br J Anaesth 2008;100:747–58.

15. Lambert DG. The nociceptin/orphanin FQ receptor: a target with broad therapeutic potential. Nat Rev Drug Discov 2008;7(8):694–710.

16. Santiago TV, Edelman NH. Opioids and breathing. J Appl Physiol 1985;59(6): 1675–85.

17. Denavit-Saubié M, Champagnat J, Zieglgänsberger W. Effects of opiates and methionine-enkephalin on pontine and bulbar respiratory neurones of the cat. Brain Res 1978;155(1):55–67.

18. Pokorski M, Grieb P, Wideman J. Opiate system influences central respiratory chemosensors. Brain Res 1981;211(1):221–6.

19. McQueen DS, Ribeiro JA. Inhibitory actions of methionine-enkephalin and morphine on the cat carotid chemoreceptors. Br J Pharmacol 1980;71(1): 297–305.

20. Eckenhofff JE, Oech R. The effects of narcotics and antagonists upon respiration and circulation in man. Clin Pharmacol Ther 1960;1:483–524.

21. Weil JV, McCullough RE, Kline JS, et al. Diminished ventilatory response to hypoxia and hypercapnia after morphine in normal man. N Engl J Med 1975; 292:1103–6.

22. Kryger MH, Yacoub O, Dosman J, et al. Effect of meperidine on occlusion pressure responses to hypercapnia and hypoxia with and without external inspiratory resistance. Am Rev Respir Dis 1976;114:333–40.

23. Bailey PL, Lu JK, Pace NL, et al. Effects of intrathecal morphine on the ventilatory response to hypoxia. N Engl J Med 2000;343(17):1228–34.

24. Santiago TV, Goldblatt K, Winters A, et al. Respiratory consequences of methadone: the response to added resistance to breathing. Am Rev Respir Dis 1980; 122:623–8.

25. Remmers JE, DeGroot WJ, Sauerland EK, et al. Pathogenesis of upper airway occlusion during sleep. J Appl Physiol 1978;44:931–8.

26. Drummond GB. Comparison of decreases in ventilation caused by enflurane and fentanyl during anaesthesia. Br J Anaesth 1984;55:825–35.

27. Bennett JA, Abrams JT, Van Riper DF, et al. Difficult or impossible ventilation after sufenidil-induced anaesthesia is caused primarily by vocal cord closure. Anesthesiology 1997;87:1070–4.

28. Robinson RW, Zwillich CW, Bixler EO, et al. Effects of oral narcotics on sleep-disordered breathing in healthy adults. Chest 1987;91:197–203.

29. Teichtahl H, Prodromidis A, Miller B, et al. Sleep-disordered breathing in stable methadone programme patients: a pilot study. Addiction 2001;96(3): 395–403.

30. Wang D, Teichtahl H, Drummer O, et al. Central sleep apnea in stable methadone maintenance treatment patients. Chest 2005;128(3):1348–56.

31. Mogri M, Desai H, Webster L, et al. Hypoxemia in patients on chronic opiate therapy with and without sleep apnea. Sleep Breath 2009;13(1): 49–57.

32. Webster LR, Choi Y, Desai H, et al. Sleep-disordered breathing and chronic opioid therapy. Pain Med 2008;9(4):425–32.

33. Teichtahl H, Wang D, Cunnington D, et al. Ventilatory responses to hypoxia and hypercapnia in stable methadone maintenance treatment patients. Chest 2005; 128(3):1339–47.

34. Farney RJ, Walker JM, Cloward TV, et al. Sleep-disordered breathing associated with long-term opioid therapy. Chest 2003;123(2):632–9.

35. Biot MC. Contribution a l'etude du phenomene respiratoire de Cheyne-Stokes. Lyon Med 1876;23:517–28 561–7 [in French].

36. Walker JM, Farney RJ, Rhondeau SM, et al. Chronic opioid use is a risk factor for the development of central sleep apnea and ataxic breathing. J Clin Sleep Med 2007;3(5):455–61.

37. Mogri M, Khan MI, Grant BJ, et al. Central sleep apnea induced by acute ingestion of opioids. Chest 2008;133:1484–8.

38. Alattar MA, Scharf SM. Opioid-associated central sleep apnea: a case series. Sleep Breath 2009;13(2):201–6.

39. Nash P, Colasanti B, Khazan N. Long-term effects of morphine on the electroencephalogram and behavior of the rat. Psychopharmacologia 1973;29(3): 271–6.

40. Shaw IR, Lavigne G, Mayer P, et al. Acute intravenous administration of morphine perturbs sleep architecture in healthy pain-free young adults: a preliminary study. Sleep 2005;28(6):677–82.

41. Dimsdale JE, Norman D, DeJardin D, et al. The effect of opioids on sleep architecture. J Clin Sleep Med 2007;3(1):33–6.

42. Knill RL, Moote CA, Skinner MI, et al. Anesthesia with abdominal surgery leads to intense REM sleep during the first postoperative week. Anesthesiology 1990; 73(1):52–61.

43. Staedt J, Wassmuth F, Stoppe G, et al. Effects of chronic treatment with methadone and naltrexone on sleep in addicts. Eur Arch Psychiatry Clin Neurosci 1996;246(6):305–9.

44. Javaheri S, Malik A, Smith J, et al. Adaptive pressure support servoventilation: a novel treatment for sleep apnea associated with use of opioids. J Clin Sleep Med 2008;4(4):305–10.

45. Kushida CA, Chediak A, Berry RB, et al. Positive Airway Pressure Titration Task Force, American Academy of Sleep Medicine. Clinical guidelines for the manual titration of positive airway pressure in patients with obstructive sleep apnea. J Clin Sleep Med 2008;4(2):157–71.

46. Kuźniar TJ, Morgenthaler TI. Treatment of complex sleep apnea syndrome. Curr Treat Options Neurol 2008;10(5):336–41.

47. Ogawa A, Iwase T, Yamamoto T, et al. Improvement of Cheyne-Stokes respiration, central sleep apnea and congestive heart failure by noninvasive bilevel positive pressure and medical treatment. Circ J 2004;68(9):878–82.

48. Arzt M, Wensel R, Montalvan S, et al. Effects of dynamic bilevel positive airway pressure support on central sleep apnea in men with heart failure. Chest 2008; 134(1):61–6.

49. Fietze I, Blau A, Glos M, et al. Bi-level positive pressure ventilation and adaptive servo ventilation in patients with heart failure and Cheyne-Stokes respiration. Sleep Med 2008;9(6):652–9.

50. Teschler H, Döhring J, Wang YM, et al. Adaptive pressure support servo-ventilation: a novel treatment for Cheyne-Stokes respiration in heart failure. Am J Respir Crit Care Med 2001;164(4):614–9.

51. Randerath WJ, Galetke W, Kenter M, et al. Combined adaptive servo-ventilation and automatic positive airway pressure (anticyclic modulated ventilation) in coexisting obstructive and central sleep apnea syndrome and periodic breathing. Sleep Med 2009;10(8):898–903.

52. Randerath WJ, Galetke W, Stieglitz S, et al. Adaptive servo-ventilation in patients with coexisting obstructive sleep apnoea/hypopnoea and Cheyne-Stokes respiration. Sleep Med 2008;9(8):823–30.

53. Banno K, Okamura K, Kryger MH. Adaptive servo-ventilation in patients with idiopathic Cheyne-Stokes breathing. J Clin Sleep Med 2006;2(2):181–6.

54. Szollosi I, O'Driscoll DM, Dayer MJ, et al. Adaptive servo-ventilation and deadspace: effects on central sleep apnoea. J Sleep Res 2006;15(2):199–205.

55. Farney RJ, Walker JM, Boyle KM, et al. Adaptive servoventilation (ASV) in patients with sleep disordered breathing associated with chronic opioid medications for non-malignant pain. J Clin Sleep Med 2008;4(4):311–9.

Sleep in Congestive Heart Failure

Bhavneesh Sharma, MD*, Robert Owens, MD, Atul Malhotra, MD

KEYWORDS

- Congestive heart failure • Sleep apnea
- Positive airway pressure therapy • Cheyne-Stokes respiration

Congestive heart failure (CHF) is the leading cause of hospitalization in those older than 65 years in the United States. More than 5 million Americans have CHF, with an annual incidence approaching 10 per 1000 among the United States population older than 65. The disease is costly and deadly. More than 5% of the national health care budget dollars are spent on CHF.[1] The 5-year mortality associated with CHF still remains high at 50%, despite recent advances in treatment.[2] CHF results in approximately 300,000 deaths each year.

Breathing disorders during sleep are common in CHF.[3–5] Sleep-disordered breathing (SDB) in CHF can be broadly classified as 2 types: central sleep apnea with Cheyne-Stokes breathing (CSA-CSB), and obstructive sleep apnea (OSA). The 2 can occur together. CSB is characterized by crescendo-decrescendo changes in tidal volume that result in central apneas (lack of airflow without respiratory effort) as shown in **Fig. 1**. OSA is characterized by repeated pharyngeal airway collapse during sleep, resulting in repetitive episodes of oxygen desaturation episodes despite ongoing respiratory effort, and arousals (**Fig. 2**). Three to four percent of women and 6% to 9% of men in the general population have OSA, when defined as an apnea-hypopnea index (AHI; number of apneas and hypopneas per hour of sleep) greater than 5 events per hour accompanied by daytime sleepiness or cardiovascular morbidity such as hypertension.[6] CHF may contribute to SDB by various mechanisms, including increased pharyngeal wall edema and unstable ventilatory control (discussed in a later section). OSA may also impair cardiac function acutely by increasing afterload, caused by increased ventricular transmural pressure during ongoing respiratory efforts; and chronically by OSA's association with increased sympathetic

A.M. has received consulting and/or research funding from Philips, Pfizer, NMT, Apnex, Cephalon, Itamar, Sepracor, Restore/Medtronic, Ethicon, SGS, Novartis. He has an established investigator award from the American Heart Association, and is Principal Investigator on NIH HL73146 R01 HL085188-01A2 R01 HL090897-01A2 K24 HL 093218 – 01 A1.

Division of Sleep Medicine, Harvard Medical School, Brigham and Women's Hospital, 75 Francis Street # Asb1, Boston, MA 02115-6106, USA

* Corresponding author.

E-mail address: bhavneesh@hotmail.com

Med Clin N Am 94 (2010) 447–464

doi:10.1016/j.mcna.2010.02.009

0025-7125/10/$ – see front matter

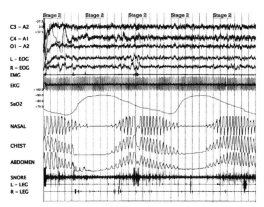

Fig. 1. Polysomnogram showing Cheyne-Stokes breathing. There are crescendo-decrescendo changes in tidal volume that result in central apneas (as shown in the chest and abdominal respiratory movements in the polysomnogram).

activity.[7] OSA further complicates CHF by contributing to hypertension, myocardial infarction, stroke, and nocturnal arrhythmias.

In this article, the authors discuss the epidemiology of SDB in CHF, the pathophysiology of CSA and OSA in CHF, and the clinical consequences and management of SDB in CHF, including positive airway pressure (PAP).

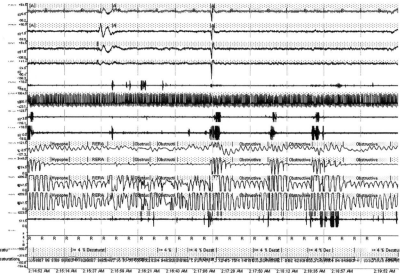

Fig. 2. Polysomnogram showing obstructive sleep apnea. There are repetitive episodes of oxygen desaturation episodes despite ongoing respiratory effort (as shown by thoracic and abdominal respiratory movements), and arousals. Apnea exists when airflow is less than 20% of baseline for at least 10 seconds in adults. Hypopnea exists when airflow decreases at least 30% from baseline, there is diminished airflow lasting at least 10 seconds, at least 90% of the duration of diminished airflow is spent with airflow that is at least 30% less than baseline, and decreased airflow is accompanied by at least 4% oxyhemoglobin desaturation. Respiratory effort related arousals (RERAs) exist when there is a sequence of breaths that lasts at least 10 seconds, is characterized by increasing respiratory effort or flattening of the nasal pressure waveform, and leads to an arousal from sleep, but does not meet the criteria of an apnea or hypopnea.

EPIDEMIOLOGY OF SLEEP-DISORDERED BREATHING IN CONGESTIVE HEART FAILURE

Prevalence of SDB in CHF is difficult to estimate, as there are various criteria used to define sleep apnea, including the threshold of AHI, definition of hypopnea, and the criteria used to differentiate CSA from OSA. Most studies to date have focused on systolic (low ejection fraction) CHF. In the first study using polysomnography in systolic CHF patients by Javaheri and colleagues,[3] the prevalence of SDB (defined by AHI ≥ 20 events/h) was 51% (40% CSA and 11% OSA). A large retrospective study in 450 subjects with systolic CHF reported a 61% prevalence of SDB using criteria of 15 events/h or greater. The prevalence of OSA was higher in this study (32%) than that of CSA (29%), likely due to the criteria used to define hypopnea or selection bias due to the retrospective nature of the study.[5] Another study demonstrated a 55% prevalence of CSB in CHF patients with left ventricular ejection fraction (LVEF) less than 40%.[8] Most of these studies were done before the current heart failure treatment guidelines were formulated and implemented, and did not necessarily not reflect current prevalence in the setting of widespread use of, for example, β-blockers in the treatment of CHF.

Recent studies have continued to show a high prevalence of SDB in patients with CHF treated with current guideline-based therapy. In the largest study done in systolic CHF patients treated with current guidelines, SDB was present in 76% of patients (40% had CSA and 36% had OSA)[9]—a prevalence and distribution generally confirmed by other studies.[10–12] Between 1997 and 2004, the prevalences of OSA and CSA did not change significantly despite increased use of β-blockers and spironolactone, and an increase in LVEF. This relatively high prevalence of SDB in CHF does not reflect referral bias to sleep clinics: the prevalence was still 61% in 108 consecutive stable CHF patients on maximal therapy assessed in a heart failure clinic population, that is, with no referral bias to a sleep clinic (31% had CSA-CSB and 30% had OSA).[13] Thus, SDB prevalence in CHF has remained high despite medical advances in the treatment of CHF. The sustained high prevalence of SDB appears to be independent of the effect of improved survival, and thus increasing age (a risk factor for the development of SDB), in this population.

To the authors' knowledge, only one study has carefully investigated the prevalence of SDB in patients with stable diastolic (preserved ejection fraction) heart failure. In this study 55% of patients had SDB, predominantly OSA.[14] The causal pathways mediating this association are unclear but given the strong link between OSA and hypertension, diastolic dysfunction may well be related to left ventricular hypertrophy resulting from hypertension. Unlike systolic heart failure, SDB may be a cause, rather than an effect, of diastolic heart failure.

Table 1 provides a summary of prevalence data in the literature. Prevalence of SDB ranges from 47% to 76% in systolic CHF. CSA is usually more common than OSA, particularly in studies in which men outnumber women. The factors associated with SDB in CHF in these epidemiologic studies are summarized in **Table 2**.

PATHOPHYSIOLOGY OF SLEEP-DISORDERED BREATHING IN CONGESTIVE HEART FAILURE
Mechanisms of CSA-CSB in Heart Failure

Prolonged circulation time secondary to low cardiac output in systolic CHF was traditionally thought to be the main cause of CSB. It was hypothesized that delayed transmission of changes in arterial blood gases to central and peripheral chemoreceptors would cause ventilatory undershoot and overshoot. However, it has been shown that there is no difference in cardiac output, LVEF, or blood circulation time from the lungs

Table 1
Clinical studies showing prevalence of sleep-disordered breathing (SDB) in congestive heart failure (CHF)

First Author	Year	Number of CHF Patients	Characteristics of CHF Patients	Definition of SDB	Results
Javaheri[3]	1998	81	LVEF <45%	AHI >20/h	51% Prevalence of SDB (CSA = 40%, OSA = 11%)
Sin[5]	1999	450	Known CHF, NYHA class II–IV	AHI ≥15/h	61% Prevalence of SDB (CSA = 29%, OSA = 32%)
Lanfranchi[8]	1999	62	LVEF ≤35% NYHA class II–III	Studied only CSA	55% Prevalence of CSB
Oldenburg[9]	2007	700	LVEF ≤40%, NYHA class ≥II	AHI ≥5/h	76% Prevalence of SDB (CSA = 40%, OSA = 36%)
Yumino[10]	2009	218	LVEF ≤45%	AHI ≥15/h	47% Prevalence of SDB (CSA = 21%, OSA = 26%)
Schulz[11]	2007	203	LVEF <40%, NYHA class II–III	AHI ≥10/h	71% Prevalence of SDB (CSA = 28%, OSA = 43%)
MacDonald[13]	2008	108	LVEF <40%, NYHA class II–IV	AHI ≥15/h	61% Prevalence of SDB (CSA = 31%, OSA = 30%)
Chan[14]	1997	20	Diastolic CHF, NYHA class II–III	AHI ≥10/h	55% Prevalence of SDB (OSA = 35%, CSA = 20%)
Padeletti[12]	2009	29	Decompensated CHF (mean LVEF = 20%)	AHI ≥15/h	76% Prevalence of SDB, predominantly CSA-CSB

Abbreviations: AHI, apnea-hypopnea index; CSA, central sleep apnea; CSB, Cheyne-Stokes breathing; LVEF, left ventricular ejection fraction; NYHA, New York Heart Association; OSA, obstructive sleep apnea.

Table 2	
Factors associated with SDB in CHF	
Central Sleep Apnea	**Obstructive Sleep Apnea**
Severity of NYHA functional class	Obesity
Atrial fibrillation	Habitual snoring
Awake hypocapnia ($PaCO_2$ <36 mm Hg)	
Nocturnal ventricular arrhythmias	
LVEF <20%	

to chemoreceptors in carefully matched CHF patients with and without CSA-CSB,[15] challenging the hypothesis that prolonged circulatory time plays a key role in CSA-CSB in patients with CHF.

CSA in CHF is predominantly caused by instability of ventilatory control systems. Patients with CSA-CSB have increased peripheral and central chemoresponsiveness that promotes hyperventilation and hypocapnia.[16–19] Patients with CSA-CSB in CHF typically have a chronic respiratory alkalosis due to hyperventilation during both wakefulness and sleep. An important factor contributing to chronic hyperventilation is pulmonary vagal irritant receptor stimulation by pulmonary venous congestion.[20–23] Hyperventilation often drives the P_{CO_2} below the apneic threshold, leading to decreased central respiratory drive. Patients with CSA-CSB in CHF also have abnormal cerebrovascular reactivity to CO_2 leading to a greater tendency to develop ventilatory undershoot in response to a greater degree of alkalosis than normal, causing central apnea.[24]

Mechanisms of OSA in Heart Failure

Patients with CSA-CSB in CHF have also been found to have obstructive apnea episodes at the end of central apneas in almost one-third of patients.[25] Direct fiberoptic observation has shown episodes of upper airway narrowing and closure during central apneas.[26] This narrowing could be the effect of reduced neural output to the upper airway muscles during the nadir of ventilation, in addition to an anatomically narrow upper airway.[26]

OSA alone can also occur in CHF. Like other patients with OSA, obesity and age are significant risk factors. Obesity may be a marker for narrowing of the upper airway because of deposition of pharyngeal fat or reduced end-expiratory lung volume. However, the prevalence of obesity in CHF patients is not very high, most patients being clinically overweight (mean body mass index [BMI; body weight divided by height squared] 28 kg/m^2)[3] and mildly obese.[5] CHF patients may have increased risk for OSA due to extracellular fluid overload. Pharyngeal edema and narrowing may develop during supine sleep with redistribution of fluid from the legs. This observation was supported by the observed improvement in OSA after diuretic therapy in a group of patients with diastolic CHF and OSA.[27] The mechanisms of SDB in CHF are summarized in **Table 3**.

DIAGNOSIS OF SLEEP-DISORDERED BREATHING IN CONGESTIVE HEART FAILURE

An in-laboratory overnight polysomnogram with an attendant technician is the gold standard for diagnosing SDB. CHF patients commonly have both central and obstructive apneas occurring together, although 1 of the 2 SDB patterns may predominate.[3,5] Patients with CHF who report snoring, excessive daytime

Table 3
Principal mechanisms contributing to SDB in CHF

Central Sleep Apnea	Obstructive Sleep Apnea
Pulmonary vagal afferent receptor stimulation[19]	Obesity
Increased central chemoresponsiveness[17]	Reduced neural output to upper airway muscles[26]
Abnormal cerebrovascular reactivity to P_{CO_2}[23]	Pharyngeal edema[27]
	Upper airway anatomic abnormalities

somnolence or fatigue, and poor sleep quality should have their sleep assessed by polysomnography in a sleep laboratory. Paroxysmal nocturnal dyspnea may actually reflect CSA-CSB, with an arousal during a period of hyperpnea. Polysomnography could also be considered in patients with heart failure who have nocturnal angina, recurrent arrhythmias, refractory heart failure symptoms, or in whom an abnormal respiratory pattern has been witnessed. Questionnaires like the Epworth Sleepiness Scale (ESS),[28] the Berlin Questionnaire,[29] and the Maislin Questionnaire[30] can be used to screen patients for SDB; however, CHF patients typically do not report excessive daytime sleepiness. CHF patients have less subjective daytime sleepiness as measured by ESS despite having less total sleep time compared with subjects without CHF.

A variety of portable home polysomnograph devices are also available to diagnose SDB, but none is currently recommended.[31,32] Home nocturnal oximetry has 85% sensitivity and 93% specificity to diagnose SDB in CHF, but may not distinguish between CSA and OSA accurately.[33] Home respiratory telemonitoring might constitute a potential low-cost alternative to traditional polysomnography in the evaluation and management of SDB in CHF patients.[34] Heart rate variation in response to apnea events has been used to diagnose SDB in patients with CHF.[35] Thoracic impedance monitoring has been used to measure cardiac output variation in response to apnea events in CHF patients with SDB.[36] These new techniques are not being used widely to diagnose SDB in CHF patients, and the authors await further data before giving any definitive recommendations.

PATHOPHYSIOLOGICAL CONSEQUENCES OF SLEEP-DISORDERED BREATHING IN CONGESTIVE HEART FAILURE

CSB results in recurrent hypoxemia, hypercapnia, and hypocapnia, and increased negative intrathoracic pressure. These changes cause release of inflammatory mediators, increases in transmural pressure in cardiac chambers, and diminished oxygen delivery to tissues. The mean overnight urinary norepinephrine excretion (UNE) level is significantly elevated in CHF patients with either OSA or CSA-CSB compared with those with CHF and no SDB, indicating increased overnight sympathetic activity.[7] CSA-CSB is associated with nocturnal ventricular arrhythmias—premature ventricular contractions (PVCs), couplets, and ventricular tachycardia—which decrease significantly when CSA is suppressed using continuous positive airway pressure (CPAP).[37] PVCs may be seen more in the hypercapnic phase of CSA than the apneic phase.[38] In addition, atrial fibrillation is also common in CHF patients with CSA,[3,39] although the causal relationship is unclear.

Whether these nocturnal arrhythmias or CSA-CSB affect outcome is unknown. Although patients with CSA-CSB and CHF have worse quality of life than those without CSA-CSB,[40] CSA is not clearly associated with increased mortality in CHF patients.[15,41] Thus, the data remain controversial as to whether CSA has independent prognostic utility in CHF.

OSA and potential relationships to cardiovascular function have been better studied. Ongoing respiratory efforts against an occluded upper airway cause intrathoracic pressure swings that increase systolic transmural pressure, increase left ventricular afterload, and thus reduce cardiac output.[42] OSA has been shown to cause left ventricular systolic[43,44] and diastolic[45] dysfunction even in patients without a history of CHF, which improved after nocturnal CPAP treatment for 6 months. Increased sympathetic activity during OSA results in increased heart rate, vasoconstriction, and increased peripheral resistance.[46] OSA is also a well-recognized independent risk factor for hypertension[47] and coronary artery disease,[48] which may worsen CHF. OSA may yield acceleration of atherosclerosis by causing inflammation and endothelial dysfunction. This finding is supported by the observation that OSA patients have high plasma C-reactive protein concentrations (in some but not all studies)[49] and increased reactive oxygen species production in neutrophils.[50] Thus OSA may exacerbate CHF through a variety of mechanisms.

TREATMENT OF SLEEP-DISORDERED BREATHING IN CONGESTIVE HEART FAILURE

The first step in the management plan for a patient with SDB and CHF should be optimization of CHF treatment. As discussed earlier, use of diuretics[27] reduced OSA in CHF patients, and lowering of the pulmonary capillary wedge pressure can improve CSA. Captopril[51] and carvedilol[52,53] may also reduce CSA in CHF patients.

General measures such as avoiding supine sleep, attempting to reduce weight if obese, and avoidance of the use of benzodiazepines and alcoholic beverages before bedtime may decrease the likelihood of upper airway occlusion during sleep, thus reducing OSA in CHF patients. Treatment of OSA with a mandibular advancement device in mild to moderate stable CHF reduced AHI and plasma brain natriuretic peptide level, but there was no improvement in LVEF or health-related quality of life.[54] Despite these alternative therapies, many patients will require PAP to eliminate apneas.

Positive Airway Pressure

Positive airway pressure devices have been successfully used to treat OSA in stable CHF patients. Nocturnal CPAP use in patients with CHF and OSA can result in reductions in left ventricular transmural pressure, which may increase LVEF.[55] CPAP use has been shown to improve LVEF in some[56–59] (but not all[60]) studies, improve quality of life, and to lower overnight UNE,[57] daytime systolic blood pressure, and left ventricular end-systolic diameter[58] in patients with stable systolic CHF and OSA. Negative results in one study may be explained by the low CPAP use (mean CPAP usage was 3.5 h/night). In a meta-analysis of randomized controlled trials comparing the effect of nocturnal CPAP therapy on LVEF in patients with stable systolic CHF and OSA, the pooled odds ratio for improvement in LVEF after CPAP therapy was 7.3.[61] The effect is probably rapid: significant improvement in LVEF was also seen after 3 days of PAP therapy in patients with decompensated CHF and OSA.[62–64] The results of the randomized controlled trials evaluating PAP therapy in CHF and OSA are summarized in **Table 4**.

In various studies with a follow-up period of 1 to 3 months, CPAP was an effective treatment for CHF with CSA-CSB, improving SDB,[65–67] LVEF,[65,66,68] and

Table 4
Randomized controlled trials studying effect of positive airway pressure therapy in patients with CHF and obstructive sleep apnea

First Author	Year	Number of CHF Patients	Intervention	Duration of Intervention	Control	Results
Egea[56]	2008	60	CPAP	3 mo	Sham CPAP	Improvement in LVEF
Mansfield[57]	2004	55	CPAP	3 mo	Medical therapy for CHF	Significant improvement in LVEF and QOL, reduction in overnight UNE
Kaneko[58]	2003	24	CPAP	1 mo	Medical therapy for CHF	Improvement in LVEF, reduction in LVESD
Smith[60]	2007	26	Autotitrating CPAP	6 wk	Sham CPAP	Improvement in daytime sleepiness, but not in LVEF or exercise capacity
Khayat[62]	2009	46	Autotitrating CPAP	3 d	Medical therapy for decompensated CHF	Significant improvement in LVEF

Abbreviations: CPAP, continuous positive airway pressure; LVEF, left ventricular ejection fraction; LVESD, left ventricular end-systolic diameter; QOL, quality of life; UNE, urinary norepinephrine excretion.

inspiratory muscle strength,[66] and decreasing urinary norepinephrine levels.[67] CPAP treatment was associated with a 60% relative risk reduction in mortality-cardiac transplantation rate in patients on CPAP therapy for a mean of 2.2 years.[65] In another study with longer follow-up, LVEF and sleep quality were significantly improved after 3 months of CPAP use in CHF patients, and the improvement persisted after 12 months.[69]

The Canadian Continuous Positive Airway Pressure Trial for Congestive Heart Failure Patients with Central Sleep Apnea (CANPAP) studied 258 CHF patients with CSA with nocturnal CPAP for 2 years (n = 128) against a control group without CPAP (n = 130).[68] The CPAP group had the expected decrease in AHI, but improvements were also seen in UNE levels, mean nocturnal oxygen saturation, LVEF, and 6-minute walk distance compared with the control group after 3 months. However, these changes did not lead to differences between the 2 groups in terms of number of hospitalizations, quality of life, or transplant-free survival (primary outcome). There was actually an early increase in mortality in the CPAP-treated group, although later survival was better then the control group. A major finding of this trial is that CSA suppression by CPAP was not adequate (CPAP reduced the mean AHI to 19 events per hour of sleep, which remained above the trial inclusion threshold of 15 events/h). In a post hoc analysis, the patients whose CSA was suppressed below 15 events/h with CPAP treatment experienced a greater increase in LVEF and did have better transplant-free survival at 3 months compared with control subjects.[70] These results suggested that in CHF patients, CPAP might improve both LVEF and heart transplant–free survival if CSA is suppressed soon after its initiation. However, the improvement in apnea may simply be a marker of less severe underlying disease, emphasizing the need for further randomized trials.

Other technologies exist for treatment of apneas in CHF, although outcome data such as with CPAP are not yet available. For example, bilevel ventilation has been found to be equally as effective as CPAP in improving sleep quality, New York Heart Association functional class, and circulation time in patients with CSA and CHF.[71] Flow-targeted dynamic bilevel positive airway pressure (BPAP) was found to reduce AHI to a significantly lower level than untreated, CPAP, or fixed BPAP groups, and also reduced AHI below threshold level of 15 events/h in all CHF patients who had residual CSA after treatment with CPAP and fixed BPAP.[72] Adaptive servoventilation (ASV) is a new technology that adjusts the delivered pressure support according to the measured air flow of the patient. Use of ASV in systolic CHF patients with CSA caused a significant reduction in the AHI[73,74] and UNE level,[74] and improved LVEF,[73] quality of life, and cardiopulmonary exercise testing parameters.[75] ASV suppressed CSA-CSB better than CPAP and nocturnal O_2 in CHF patients.[76] Several ongoing clinical trials are further investigating the effect of ASV on various parameters including survival, LVEF, exercise capacity, and quality of life in patients with CHF and CSA or CPAP-refractory sleep apnea.[77–79] The CANPAP II study has recently been funded to test the hypothesis that these newer devices may be useful in treating SDB in CHF. However, at the present time hard outcome data are generally lacking for these newer devices. A summary of controlled studies evaluating use of PAP in CHF patients with CSA is shown in **Table 5**.

These studies show the importance of keeping a high index of suspicion for SDB in patients with CHF. PAP devices thus may be used in CHF patients with SDB who have symptoms of excessive daytime sleepiness or other comorbidities like hypertension; however, their use to improve CHF outcome (including survival and LVEF) is not recommended at present. It is clear that further research is needed in this area.

Table 5
Controlled trials studying effect of positive airway pressure therapy in patients with CHF and central sleep apnea/Cheyne-Stokes breathing

First Author	Year	Number of CHF Patients	Intervention	Duration of Intervention	Control	Results
Sin[65]	2000	66	CPAP	3 mo	Medical therapy for CHF	Improvement in LVEF, reduction in combined mortality-cardiac transplantation rate
Granton[66]	1996	17	CPAP	3 mo	Medical therapy for CHF	Improvement in LVEF and inspiratory muscle strength (MIP)
Naughton[67]	1995	35	CPAP	1 mo	Medical therapy for CHF	Reduction in UNE and PNE level
Bradley[68]	2005	258	CPAP	3 mo	Medical therapy for CHF	Improvement in exercise capacity, LVEF and mean oxygen saturation; no difference in survival after 2 years follow-up. Better heart transplant–free survival in CSB-suppressed group in post hoc analysis[80]
Köhnlein[71]	2002	35	Bilevel ventilation, CPAP	2 wk	Crossover design	Significant and equivalent improvement in sleep quality, circulation time, and NYHA class with both bilevel ventilation and CPAP
Arzt[70]	2008	14	BPAP, CPAP, dynamic BPAP	Consecutive night use of all 3 PAP devices	BPAP, CPAP	Dynamic BPAP suppressed CA-CSB better than CPAP or BPAP
Pepperell[74]	2003	30	ASV	1 mo	Subtherapeutic level of ASV	Improvement in LVEF; reduction in serum BNP and urinary catecholamine excretion
Hastings[75]	2008	19	ASV	6 mo	Medical therapy for CHF	Improvement in LVEF and QOL
Teschler[76]	2001	14	ASV, BPAP, CPAP, nocturnal O_2	1 night	Crossover design	ASV suppressed CSA-CSB better than CPAP and nocturnal O_2, but not BPAP; LVEF not measured

Abbreviations: ASV, adaptive servoventilation; BNP, brain natriuretic peptide; BPAP, bilevel positive airway pressure; CPAP, continuous positive airway pressure; CSB, Cheyne-Stokes breathing; LVEF, left ventricular ejection fraction; MIP, maximal inspiratory pressure; NYHA, New York Heart Association; PNE, peripheral norepinephrine excretion; QOL, quality of life; UNE, urinary norepinephrine excretion.

Nocturnal Oxygen Therapy

Nocturnal oxygen therapy has been shown to reduce central sleep apnea in CHF. Treatment with oxygen was found to improve exercise capacity,[80–83] decrease overnight urinary norepinephrine secretion,[80] and decrease muscle sympathetic activity[84] in CHF patients with CSA. In addition, nocturnal oxygen also improved LVEF and quality of life in CHF patients.[82,83]

Supplemental CO_2 Therapy

Adding dead space (as a form of supplemental CO_2) using a facemask attached to a cylinder of adjustable volume improved CSA and sleep quality in CHF patients.[85] Several researchers have investigated either inspiring CO_2 or adding dead space, but these approaches are rarely used clinically. Inspired CO_2 can lead to considerable insomnia, and was classically used by psychiatrists to induce panic attacks in diagnostic testing. Thus, these treatment approaches remain theoretical at the present time.

Theophylline

Oral theophylline therapy for 5 days in stable CHF patients (LVEF <45%) improved SDB in a study,[86] although the mechanism by which theophylline improves CSA in CHF is unclear. At therapeutic serum concentrations, theophylline competes with adenosine at some of its receptor sites. In the central nervous system, adenosine is a respiratory depressant, and theophylline stimulates respiration by antagonizing adenosine. It is therefore conceivable that an increase in ventilation as a result of treatment with theophylline results in a decreased number of episodes of central apnea during sleep.[87] In addition, theophylline is likely a potent inotrope in the short term, when the agent is given to methylxanthine-naïve hearts. Because there are no controlled long-term studies, theophylline is not commonly used to treat CSA, perhaps in part due to its arrhythmogenic potential.

Acetazolamide

Use of acetazolamide orally before bedtime daily for 6 nights resulted in significant reduction in AHI and improved sleep quality.[16] Acetazolamide is a mild diuretic and thus may decrease pulmonary venous congestion in CHF, which contributes to CSA. In addition, acetazolamide induces nonanion gap metabolic acidosis, which stimulates breathing; this results in reduction in the apneic threshold to P_{CO_2}, which decreases the likelihood of developing central sleep apnea.[88]

Atrial Overdrive Pacing

Atrial overdrive pacing (AOP) in patients with central or obstructive sleep apnea who had received permanent atrial-synchronous ventricular pacemakers for symptomatic sinus bradycardia decreased apneas and hypopneas significantly in a single study.[89] However, another study failed to show any beneficial effect.[90] Atrial overdrive pacing exerted a mild effect on apnea-hypopnea events in CHF patients with OSA, but the results were less effective than for CPAP therapy.[91]

Left Ventricular Assist Device

Correction of CSA and significant improvement in exercise capacity and symptoms after implantation of a left ventricular assist device in CHF patients was reported in one study.[92]

Cardiac Resynchronization Therapy

Cardiac resynchronization therapy (CRT), which improves cardiac output by coordinating right and left ventricular contraction, leads to a reduction of CSA and to increased sleep quality in patients with CHF and SDB.[93] CRT also improved cardiac function and reduced the AHI in patients with both OSA and CHF.[94] CRT combined with AOP resulted in a significant but minor additional improvement of CSA compared with CRT alone.[95] Both AOP and CRT may reduce SDB by increasing cardiac output, thus decreasing pulmonary venous congestion. Decrease in pharyngeal wall edema may also decrease OSA in these patients. The ongoing Impact of Resynchronization Therapy on Sleep Disordered Breathing in Advanced Congestive Heart Failure (IMPACT) trial is further investigating the effect of CRT with or without AOP on SDB and sleep quality in patients with CHF and SDB.[96]

Cardiac Transplantation

Thirteen CHF patients with CSA were studied before and after successful cardiac transplantation, there was improvement in SDB after 6 months of follow-up, but CSA persisted in 3 patients and 4 patients acquired OSA after 13 months.[97] A similar study confirmed that 36% of CHF patients who had successful cardiac transplantation developed OSA, likely due to weight gain and fat deposition secondary to the use of steroids for immunosuppression. A suggested algorithm for managing SDB in CHF is shown in **Fig. 3**.

PERIODIC LIMB MOVEMENTS AND CONGESTIVE HEART FAILURE

The prevalence of periodic limb movements (PLMs; defined as a PLM index >5 events/h) in adult systolic CHF patients was 19% in one study.[98] The proportion of stable CHF patients with moderately severe PLM (>25/h) was significantly higher (52%) than control subjects (11%) in another study by Hanly and colleagues.[99] Proposed hypotheses for the high prevalence of PLMs in CHF patients are (a) electrolyte and acid-base abnormalities associated with CHF, and (b) stimulation of a spinal reflex in conjunction with cortical inhibition during sleep secondary to reduced peripheral blood flow due to CHF.[100] The clinical relevance or prognostic value of these findings is unknown.

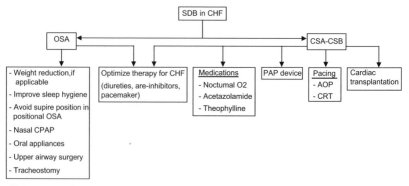

Fig. 3. A suggested algorithm for management of sleep-disordered breathing in congestive heart failure.

SUMMARY

CHF and SDB are common diseases, and they frequently exist together. CHF may contribute to SDB, and SDB in turn further worsens CHF. CHF patients with SDB have a worse prognosis and may have increased mortality. Optimum treatment of CHF as per guidelines is the first step in the management of SDB in CHF. PAP may improve AHI as well as LVEF in CHF patients with OSA. Positive pressure ventilation may also improve LVEF and survival in the subgroup of CHF patients in whom CSA is adequately suppressed. Newer devices may be more successful than conventional positive pressure ventilation in suppressing CSA in CHF; however, long-term clinical trials are required to show efficacy of these novel treatments in improving survival in CHF patients with SDB.

REFERENCES

1. Hunt SA, Baker DW, Chin MH, et al. ACC/AHA Guidelines for the evaluation and management of chronic heart failure in the adult: executive summary: a report of the American College of Cardiology/American Heart Association Task Force on Practice Guidelines. Circulation 2001;104(24):2996–3007.
2. Levy D, Kenechaiah S, Larson MG, et al. Long-term trends in the incidence of and survival with heart failure. N Engl J Med 2002;347(18):1397–402.
3. Javaheri S, Parker TJ, Liming JD, et al. Sleep apnea in 81 ambulatory male patients with stable heart failure. Types and their prevalences, consequences, and presentations. Circulation 1998;97(21):2154–9.
4. Tremel F, Pépin JL, Veale D, et al. High prevalence and persistence of sleep apnoea in patients referred for acute left ventricular failure and medically treated over 2 months. Eur Heart J 1999;20(16):1201–9.
5. Sin DD, Fitzgerald F, Parker JD, et al. Risk factors for central and obstructive sleep apnea in 450 men and women with congestive heart failure. Am J Respir Crit Care Med 1999;160(4):1101–6.
6. Punjabi NM. The epidemiology of adult obstructive sleep apnea. Proc Am Thorac Soc 2008;5(2):136–43.
7. Solin P, Kaye DM, Little PJ, et al. Impact of sleep apnea on sympathetic nervous system activity in heart failure. Chest 2003;123(4):1119–26.
8. Lanfranchi PA, Braghiroli A, Bosimini E, et al. Prognostic value of nocturnal Cheyne-Stokes respiration in chronic heart failure. Circulation 1999;99(11): 1435–40.
9. Oldenburg O, Lamp B, Faber L, et al. Sleep-disordered breathing in patients with symptomatic heart failure: a contemporary study of prevalence in and characteristics of 700 patients. Eur J Heart Fail 2007;9(3):251–7.
10. Yumino D, Wang H, Floras JS, et al. Prevalence and physiological predictors of sleep apnea in patients with heart failure and systolic dysfunction. J Card Fail 2009;15(4):279–85.
11. Schulz R, Blau A, Börgel J, et al. Sleep apnoea in heart failure. Eur Respir J 2007;29(6):1201–5.
12. Padeletti M, Green P, Mooney AM, et al. Sleep disordered breathing in patients with acutely decompensated heart failure. Sleep Med 2009;10(3):353–60.
13. MacDonald M, Fang J, Pittman SD, et al. The current prevalence of sleep disordered breathing in congestive heart failure patients treated with beta-blockers. J Clin Sleep Med 2008;4(1):38–42.
14. Chan J, Sanderson J, Chan W, et al. Prevalence of sleep-disordered breathing in diastolic heart failure. Chest 1997;111(6):1488–93.

15. Findley LJ, Zwillich CW, Ancoli-Israel S, et al. Cheyne-Stokes breathing during sleep in patients with left ventricular heart failure. South Med J 1985;78(1):11–5.

16. Bradley TD. Crossing the threshold: implications central sleep apnea. Am J Respir Crit Care Med 2002;165(9):1203–4.

17. Javaheri S. Acetazolamide improves central sleep apnea in congestive heart failure: a double-blind, prospective study. Am J Respir Crit Care Med 2006; 173(2):234–7.

18. Solin P, Roebuck T, Johns DP, et al. Peripheral and central ventilatory responses in central sleep apnea with and without congestive heart failure. Am J Respir Crit Care Med 2000;162(6):2194–200.

19. Javaheri S. A mechanism of central sleep apnea in patients with heart failure. N Engl J Med 1999;341(13):949–54.

20. Solin P, Bergin P, Richardson M, et al. Influence of pulmonary capillary wedge pressure on central sleep apnea in heart failure. Circulation 1999;99(12): 1574–9.

21. Lorenzi-Filho G, Azevedo ER, Parker JD, et al. Relationship of carbon dioxide tension in arterial blood to pulmonary wedge pressure in heart failure. Eur Respir J 2002;19(1):37–40.

22. Paintal AS. Vagal sensory receptors and their reflex effects. Physiol Rev 1973; 53(1):159–227.

23. Oldenburg O, Bitter T, Wiemer M, et al. Pulmonary capillary wedge pressure and pulmonary arterial pressure in heart failure patients with sleep-disordered breathing. Sleep Med 2009;10(7):726–30.

24. Xie A, Skatrud JB, Khayat R, et al. Cerebrovascular response to carbon dioxide in patients with congestive heart failure. Am J Respir Crit Care Med 2002;165(3):371–8.

25. Dowdell WT, Javaheri S, McGinnis W. Cheyne-Stokes respiration presenting a sleep apnea syndrome: clinical and polysomnographic features. Am Rev Respir Dis 1990;141(4 Pt 1):871–9.

26. Badr S, Toiber F, Skatrud J, et al. Pharyngeal narrowing/occlusion during central sleep apnea. J Appl Physiol 1995;78(5):1806–15.

27. Bucca CB, Brussino L, Battisti A, et al. Diuretics in obstructive sleep apnea with diastolic heart failure. Chest 2007;132(2):440–6.

28. Johns MW. A new method for measuring daytime sleepiness: the Epsworth sleepiness scale. Sleep 1991;14(6):540–5.

29. Netzer NC, Stoohs RA, Netzer CM, et al. Using the Berlin questionnaire to identify patients at risk for the sleep apnea syndrome. Ann Intern Med 1999;131(7): 485–91.

30. Maislin G, Pack AI, Kribbs NB, et al. A survey screen for prediction of apnea. Sleep 1995;18(3):158–66.

31. Chesson AL Jr, Berry RB, Pack A. Practice parameters for the use of portable monitoring devices in the investigation of suspected obstructive sleep apnea in adults. Sleep 2003;26(7):907–13.

32. American Thoracic Society/American College of Chest Physicians/American Academy of Sleep medicine Taskforce Steering Committee. Executive summary on the systematic review and practice parameters for portable monitoring in the investigation of suspected sleep apnea in adults. Am J Respir Crit Care Med 2004;169(10):1160–3.

33. Sériès F, Kimoff RJ, Morrison D, et al. Prospective evaluation of nocturnal oximetry for detection of sleep-related breathing disturbances in patients with chronic heart failure. Chest 2005;127(5):1507–14.

34. Mortara A, Pinna GD, Johnson P, et al. Home telemonitoring in heart failure patients: the HHH study (Home or Hospital in Heart Failure). Eur J Heart Fail 2009;11(3):312–8.

35. Tateishi O, Shouda T, Sakai T, et al. Apnea-related heart rate variability in congestive heart failure patients. Clin Exp Hypertens 2003;25(3):183–9.

36. Yasuda Y, Umezu A, Horihata S, et al. Modified thoracic impedance plethysmography to monitor sleep apnea syndromes. Sleep Med 2005;6(3):215–24.

37. Javaheri S. Effects of continuous positive airway pressure on sleep apnea and ventricular irritability in patients with heart failure. Circulation 2000;101(4):392–7.

38. Leung RS, Diep TM, Bowman ME, et al. Provocation of ventricular ectopy by Cheyne-Stokes respiration in patients with heart failure. Sleep 2004;27(7):1337–43.

39. Javaheri S. Sleep disorders in systolic heart failure: a prospective study of 100 male patients. The final report. Int J Cardiol 2006;106(1):21–8.

40. Carmona-Bernal C, Ruiz-García A, Villa-Gil M, et al. Quality of life in patients with congestive heart failure and central sleep apnea. Sleep Med 2008;9(6):646–51.

41. Javaheri S, Shukla R, Zeigler H, et al. Central sleep apnea, right ventricular dysfunction, and low diastolic blood pressure are predictors of mortality in systolic heart failure. J Am Coll Cardiol 2007;49(20):2028–34.

42. Luo Q, Zhang HL, Tao XC, et al. Impact of untreated sleep apnea on prognosis of patients with congestive heart failure. Int J Cardiol 2009. [Epub ahead of print].

43. Bradley TD, Hall MJ, Ando S, et al. Hemodynamic effects of simulated obstructive apneas in humans with and without heart failure. Chest 2001;119(6):1827–35.

44. Shahar E, Whitney CW, Redline S, et al. Sleep disordered breathing and cardiovascular disease: cross-sectional results of The Sleep Heart Health Study. Am J Respir Crit Care Med 2001;163(1):19–25.

45. Arias MA, García-Río F, Alonso-Fernández A, et al. Obstructive sleep apnea syndrome affects left ventricular diastolic function: effects of nasal continuous positive airway pressure in men. Circulation 2005;112(3):375–83.

46. Somers VK, Dyken ME, Clary MP, et al. Sympathetic neural mechanisms in obstructive sleep apnea. J Clin Invest 1995;96(4):1897–904.

47. Nieto FJ, Young TB, Lind BK, et al. Association of sleep-disordered breathing, sleep apnea, and hypertension in a large community-based study. JAMA 2000;283(14):1829–36.

48. Butt M, Dwivedi G, Khair O, et al. Obstructive sleep apnea and cardiovascular disease. Int J Cardiol 2010;139(1):7–16.

49. Shamsuzzaman AS, Winnicki M, Lanfranchi P, et al. Elevated C-reactive protein in patients with obstructive sleep apnea. Circulation 2002;105(21):2462–4.

50. Schulz R, Mahmoudi S, Hattar K, et al. Enhanced release of superoxide from polymorphonuclear neutrophils in obstructive sleep apnea. Impact of continuous positive airway pressure therapy. Am J Respir Crit Care Med 2000;162(2 Pt 1):566–70.

51. Walsh JT, Andrews R, Starling R, et al. Effects of captopril and oxygen on sleep apnoea in patients with mild to moderate congestive cardiac failure. Br Heart J 1995;73(3):237–41.

52. Tamura A, Kawano Y, Kadota J, et al. Carvedilol reduces the severity of central sleep apnea in chronic heart failure. Circ J 2009;73(2):295–8.

53. Tamura A, Kawano Y, Naono S, et al. Relationship between beta-blocker treatment and the severity of central sleep apnea in chronic heart failure. Chest 2007;131(1):130–5.

54. Eskafi M, Cline C, Nilner M, et al. Treatment of sleep apnea in congestive heart failure with a dental device: the effect on brain natriuretic peptide and quality of life. Sleep Breath 2006;10(2):90–7.

55. Johnson CB, Beanlands RS, Yoshinaga K, et al. Acute and chronic effects of continuous positive airway pressure therapy on left ventricular systolic and diastolic function in patients with obstructive sleep apnea and congestive heart failure. Can J Cardiol 2008;24(9):697–704.

56. Egea CJ, Aizpuru F, Pinto JA, et al. Cardiac function after CPAP therapy in patients with chronic heart failure and sleep apnea: a multicenter study. Sleep Med 2008;9(6):660–6.

57. Mansfield DR, Gollogly NC, Kaye DM, et al. Controlled trial of continuous positive airway pressure in obstructive sleep apnea and heart failure. Am J Respir Crit Care Med 2004;169(3):361–6.

58. Kaneko Y, Floras JS, Usui K, et al. Cardiovascular effects of continuous positive airway pressure in patients with heart failure and obstructive sleep apnea. N Engl J Med 2003;348(13):1233–41.

59. Tkacova R, Rankin F, Fitzgerald FS, et al. Effects of continuous positive airway pressure on obstructive sleep apnea and left ventricular afterload in patients with heart failure. Circulation 1998;98(21):2269–75.

60. Smith LA, Vennelle M, Gardner RS, et al. Auto-titrating continuous positive airway pressure therapy in patients with chronic heart failure and obstructive sleep apnoea: a randomized placebo-controlled trial. Eur Heart J 2007; 28(10):1221–7.

61. Sharma B, Karbowitz S, Feinsilver S. A meta-analysis of randomized controlled trials evaluating the effect of nocturnal continuous airway pressure (CPAP) therapy on ejection fraction in patients with systolic congestive heart failure and obstructive sleep apnea. Sleep 2009;32:A175.

62. Khayat RN, Abraham WT, Patt B, et al. In-hospital treatment of obstructive sleep apnea during decompensation of heart failure. Chest 2009;134(4):991–7.

63. Krachman SL, D'Alonzo GE, Berger TJ, et al. Comparison of oxygen therapy with nasal continuous positive airway pressure on Cheyne-Stokes respiration during sleep in congestive heart failure. Chest 1999;116(6):1550–7.

64. Yasuma F. [Effects of continuous positive airway pressure on Cheyne-Stokes breathing in congestive heart failure]. Nihon Kokyuki Gakkai Zasshi 2002; 40(10):801–5 [in Japanese].

65. Sin DD, Logan AG, Fitzgerald FS, et al. Effects of continuous positive airway pressure on cardiovascular outcomes in heart failure patients with and without Cheyne-Stokes respiration. Circulation 2000;102(1):61–6.

66. Granton JT, Naughton MT, Benard DC, et al. CPAP improves inspiratory muscle strength in patients with heart failure and central sleep apnea. Am J Respir Crit Care Med 1996;153(1):277–82.

67. Naughton MT, Benard DC, Liu PP, et al. Effects of nasal CPAP on sympathetic activity in patients with heart failure and central sleep apnea. Am J Respir Crit Care Med 1995;152(2):473–9.

68. Bradley TD, Logan AG, Kimoff RJ, et al. Continuous positive airway pressure for central sleep apnea and heart failure. N Engl J Med 2005;353(19):2025–33.

69. Yasuma F. Cheyne-Stokes respiration in congestive heart failure: continuous positive airway pressure of 5-8 cm H_2O for 1 year in five cases. Respiration 2005;72(2):198–201.

70. Arzt M, Floras JS, Logan AG, et al. Suppression of central sleep apnea by continuous positive airway pressure and transplant-free survival in heart

failure: a post hoc analysis of the Canadian Continuous Positive Airway Pressure for Patients with Central Sleep Apnea and Heart Failure Trial (CANPAP). Circulation 2007;115(25):3173–80.

71. Köhnlein T, Welte T, Tan LB, et al. Assisted ventilation for heart failure patients with Cheyne-Stokes respiration. Eur Respir J 2002;20(4):934–41.

72. Arzt M, Wensel R, Montalvan S, et al. Effects of dynamic bilevel positive airway pressure support on central sleep apnea in men with heart failure. Chest 2008; 134(1):61–6.

73. Oldenburg O, Schmidt A, Lamp B, et al. Adaptive servoventilation improves cardiac function in patients with chronic heart failure and Cheyne-Stokes respiration. Eur J Heart Fail 2008;10(6):581–6.

74. Pepperell JC, Maskell NA, Jones DR, et al. A randomized controlled trial of adaptive ventilation for Cheyne-Stokes breathing in heart failure. Am J Respir Crit Care Med 2003;168(9):1109–14.

75. Hastings PC, Vazir A, Meadows GE, et al. Adaptive servo-ventilation in heart failure patients with sleep apnea: a real world study. Int J Cardiol 2010;139(1): 17–24.

76. Teschler H, Döhring J, Wang YM, et al. Adaptive pressure support servo-ventilation: a novel treatment for Cheyne-Stokes respiration in heart failure. Am J Respir Crit Care Med 2001;164(4):614–9.

77. Zhang XL. Treatment of Cheyne Stokes respiration with adaptive servo ventilation and bilevel ventilators in patients with chronic heart failure. Available at: http://www.ClinicalTrials.gov. Identifier: NCT00725595. Accessed December 12, 2009.

78. Hetland A. Chronic heart failure—Cheyne Stokes respiration—CS2 (3C-Study). Available at: http://www.ClinicalTrials.gov. Identifier: NCT00563693. Accessed December 12, 2009.

79. Teschler H, Cowie M. Treatment of predominant central sleep apnoea by adaptive servo ventilation in patients with heart failure (Serve-HF). Available at: http://www.ClinicalTrials.gov. Identifier: NCT00733343. Accessed December 12, 2009.

80. Staniforth AD, Kinnear WJ, Starling R, et al. Effect of oxygen on sleep quality, cognitive function and sympathetic activity in patients with chronic heart failure and Cheyne-Stokes respiration. Eur Heart J 1998;19(6):922–8.

81. Sasayama S, Izumi T, Seino Y, et al. Effects of nocturnal oxygen therapy on outcome measures in patients with chronic heart failure and Cheyne-Stokes respiration. Circ J 2006;70(1):1–7.

82. Sasayama S, Izumi T, Matsuzaki M, et al. Improvement of quality of life with nocturnal oxygen therapy in heart failure patients with central sleep apnea. Circ J 2009;73(7):1255–62.

83. Toyama T, Seki R, Kasama S, et al. Effectiveness of nocturnal home oxygen therapy to improve exercise capacity, cardiac function and cardiac sympathetic nerve activity in patients with chronic heart failure and central sleep apnea. Circ J 2009;73(2):299–304.

84. Andreas S, Bingeli C, Mohacsi P, et al. Nasal oxygen and muscle sympathetic nerve activity in heart failure. Chest 2003;123(2):366–71.

85. Khayat RN, Xie A, Patel AK, et al. Cardiorespiratory effects of added dead space in patients with heart failure and central sleep apnea. Chest 2003; 123(5):1551–60.

86. Javaheri S, Parker TJ, Wexler L, et al. Effect of theophylline on sleep-disordered breathing in heart failure. N Engl J Med 1996;335(8):562–7.

87. Cherniack NS. Sleep apnea and its causes. J Clin Invest 1984;73(6):1501–6.

88. Nakayama H, Smith CA, Rodman JR, et al. Effect of ventilatory drive on carbon dioxide sensitivity below eupnea during sleep. Am J Respir Crit Care Med 2002; 165(9):1251–60.

89. Garrigue S, Bordier P, Jaïs P, et al. Benefit of atrial pacing in sleep apnea syndrome. N Engl J Med 2002;346(6):404–12.

90. Lüthje L, Unterberg-Buchwald C, Dajani D, et al. Atrial overdrive pacing in patients with sleep apnea with implanted pacemaker. Am J Respir Crit Care Med 2005;172(1):118–22.

91. Sharafkhaneh A, Sharafkhaneh H, Bredikus A, et al. Effect of atrial overdrive pacing on obstructive sleep apnea in patients with systolic heart failure. Sleep Med 2007;8(1):31–6.

92. Vazir A, Hastings PC, Morrell MJ, et al. Resolution of central sleep apnoea following implantation of a left ventricular assist device. Int J Cardiol 2010; 138(3):317–9.

93. Sinha AM, Skobel EC, Breithardt OA, et al. Cardiac resynchronization therapy improves central sleep apnea and Cheyne-Stokes respiration in patients with chronic heart failure. J Am Coll Cardiol 2004;44(1):68–71.

94. Skobel EC, Sinha AM, Norra C, et al. Effect of cardiac resynchronization therapy on sleep quality, quality of life, and symptomatic depression in patients with chronic heart failure and Cheyne-Stokes respiration. Sleep Breath 2005;9(4): 159–66.

95. Stanchina ML, Ellison K, Malhotra A, et al. The impact of cardiac resynchronization therapy on obstructive sleep apnea in heart failure patients: a pilot study. Chest 2007;132(2):433–9.

96. Shalaby A. Impact of resynchronization therapy on sleep disordered breathing in advanced congestive heart failure (IMPACT). Available at: http://www.ClinicalTrials.gov. Identifier: NCT00521534. Accessed December 12, 2009.

97. Mansfield DR, Solin P, Roebuck T, et al. The effect of successful heart transplant treatment of heart failure on central sleep apnea. Chest 2003;124(5):1675–81.

98. Javaheri S, Abraham WT, Brown C, et al. Prevalence of obstructive sleep apnoea and periodic limb movement in 45 subjects with heart transplantation. Eur Heart J 2004;25(3):260–6.

99. Hanly PJ, Zuberi-Khokhar N. Periodic limb movements during sleep in patients with congestive heart failure. Chest 1996;109(6):1497–502.

100. Skomro R, Silva R, Alves R, et al. The prevalence and significance of periodic leg movements during sleep in patients with congestive heart failure. Sleep Breath 2009;13(1):43–7.

Cardiovascular Consequences of Obese and Nonobese Obstructive Sleep Apnea

Kannan Ramar, MD*, Sean M. Caples, DO

KEYWORDS

- Obstructive sleep apnea • Obesity
- Cardiovascular consequences

Obstructive sleep apnea (OSA) continues to garner widespread attention, mostly because of its health-related consequences such as cardiovascular disorders and associated comorbid symptoms such as daytime sleepiness and snoring. OSA is characterized by repeated episodes of partial or complete upper airway closure during sleep, resulting in frequent arousals and sleep fragmentation, apneas and hypopneas, and intermittent hypoxemia. These perturbations can lead to chronic cardiovascular disorders such as hypertension. Among the many risk factors in the pathogenesis of OSA, obesity is one of the most important.[1] Obesity, per se, may also predispose to cardiovascular disorders. In this review, the authors explore the complex interactions between obesity, cardiovascular diseases, and OSA.

OBESITY AND CARDIOVASCULAR DISEASE
Mechanisms

There are various mechanisms by which obesity can lead to cardiovascular disorders. Obesity appears to be a chronic inflammatory state, as evidenced by elevated levels of serum markers of systemic inflammation such as C-reactive protein (CRP) and interleukin 6 (IL-6), which can predispose to cardiovascular disorders. Leptin is a novel adipocyte-derived hormone that induces weight loss by decreasing appetite and increasing energy expenditure. Obesity appears to predispose to leptin resistance resulting in elevated plasma leptin levels. Elevated leptin levels are independent risk factors for cardiovascular disorders by promoting platelet aggregation, insulin

Disclosure: Dr Caples supported by research grants from ResMed Foundation, Ventus Medical, Restore Medical and NHLBI HL99534Z-01.
Division of Pulmonary, Sleep and Critical Care Medicine, Center for Sleep Medicine, Mayo Clinic, 200 First Street South West, Rochester, MN 55901, USA
* Corresponding author.
E-mail address: ramar.kannan@mayo.edu

resistance, and increased sympathetic neural activity.[2] Insulin resistance is commonly seen in obesity and is also a predictor for cardiovascular diseases. Insulin stimulates leptin production and the presence of insulin resistance increases the risk for development of diabetes, as well as alterations in lipids, coagulation, fibrinolysis, and inflammation, subsequently predisposing to endothelial dysfunction and atherosclerosis.[3] Increased insulin resistance in the peripheral tissues in obesity predisposes to increased sympathetic neural activity.[4] Obesity is one of the key variables that constitutes metabolic syndrome.[5] Metabolic syndrome confers an increased risk for atherosclerosis and cardiovascular disorders.[6] The shift in diet from fiber rich foods to a more Western diet, along with inactivity, has predisposed the general population to obesity. Obesity is also associated with high circulating levels of triglycerides, low high-density lipoprotein (HDL) cholesterol, and plasma concentrations of apolipoprotein B-containing lipoproteins, all being risk factors for increased cardiovascular disorders.[7–9]

Obesity also has adverse effects on cardiovascular hemodynamics.[10] Obesity increases total blood volume and cardiac output, resulting in increased cardiac workload.[11] Increased sympathetic neural activity in obesity may conceivably induce an overall increase in heart rate. Combined with the increased cardiac workload, this can lead to hemodynamic consequences. There is an increase in ventricular filling pressures and volumes leading to left ventricular chamber dilation and hypertrophy.[11,12] In addition to left ventricular chamber enlargement, obesity leads to left atrial enlargement due to increased blood volume and abnormal diastolic filling.[11,13] All these perturbations may result in increased cardiovascular morbidity such as hypertension, congestive heart failure, atrial fibrillation, and arrhythmias.

Cardiovascular Consequences of Obesity

The link between obesity and cardiovascular disease has been well established. The epidemiologic link between obesity and incident hypertension was established by the Framingham study, in which 2027 men and 2267 women were followed up for 8 years.[14] In another Framingham study of 5881 participants who were followed up over a 14-year period, every 1 kg/m^2 increment in body mass index (BMI; weight in kilograms divided by height in meters squared) led to a 5% to 7% increased risk of congestive heart failure.[15] More than 30% of obese patients had heart failure, and the probability increased significantly with increasing duration of obesity.[16] Obesity is a major component of the metabolic syndrome, and is an independent risk factor for atherosclerosis and the development of coronary artery disease (CAD).[17,18] Due to the hemodynamic effects of obesity as explained here, obesity may also contribute to the higher prevalence of atrial fibrillation (AF). In the prospective Framingham cohort study of 5282 participants who were followed for a mean of 13.7 years, obesity was associated with a 50% increased risk for AF.[19] In a recent meta-analysis, obese patients had a 49% increased risk of developing AF that increased in parallel with increasing BMI.[20] Obesity increases the risk of sudden cardiac death,[21] with substantial evidence supporting the occurrence of frequent complex ventricular arrhythmias even in the absence of heart failure or left ventricular dysfunction.[11] The annual rate of sudden cardiac death is nearly 40 times higher than that in the matched nonobese population.[22]

Because OSA is strongly associated with both obesity and cardiovascular disease, it may plausibly represent an important mediator between obesity and cardiovascular disease themselves. Unfortunately, the presence of OSA is often not assessed in studies examining the relationship between obesity and cardiovascular disorders. In a recent meta-analysis of 40 cohort studies, although obesity led to increased cardiovascular mortality, the presence of OSA was not evaluated in any of these studies.[23]

OSA AND CARDIOVASCULAR DISEASE

There has recently been increasing evidence from longitudinal cohort studies and a limited number of randomized controlled studies that OSA may play a causal role in the pathophysiology of certain cardiovascular diseases such as systemic hypertension, with increasing evidence shown in others such as heart failure, stroke, and cardiac arrhythmias. However, a few caveats should be noted. First, the OSA literature on cardiovascular diseases has historically been dominated by case series and case-control studies, both of which are vulnerable to hidden biases and have poor discriminating power to determine the cardiovascular risk imparted purely by OSA independent of confounders such as obesity. Second, aside from several small continuous positive airway pressure (CPAP) trials in the setting of systemic hypertension, there remains a paucity of controlled interventional trials assessing the impact of OSA treatment on hard cardiovascular end points and outcomes. Third, the current metric to characterize OSA, the apnea-hypopnea index (AHI; number of apneas and hypopneas per hour of sleep), has its shortcomings. While probably the best composite measurement of OSA severity, the AHI does not quantify other processes operative in the pathophysiology of cardiovascular disease, such as the degree and duration of oxyhemoglobin desaturation or sleep disruption that may occur independently of frank apneas and hypopneas, for example, during snore arousals or periodic limb movements.

Pathophysiology

OSA results in repetitive partial or complete closure of the upper airway during sleep, despite ongoing respiratory efforts. Each such event is associated with oxyhemoglobin desaturation followed by central nervous system arousal to reestablish upper airway patency, followed by reoxygenation. Acute repetitive stressors associated with these cascade of events include nocturnal hypoxemia, increased sympathetic neural activity,[24] production of reactive oxygen radicals following reoxygenation,[25] and swings in intrathoracic pressure due to respiratory efforts against a collapsed upper airway.[26]

The swings in intrathoracic pressure during each of these apneic/hypopneic events can be extreme (up to -80 cm of water), resulting in an increase in cardiac afterload (by increasing the left ventricular transmural pressure, and thereby the left ventricular wall stress/tension) and impaired left ventricle relaxation, thereby contributing to decreased stroke volume and cardiac output.[26–28]

Presence of hypoxemia during these obstructive apneic events results in repetitive bursts of sympathetic neural activity, with increased activity noted even during the day, along with elevated catecholamine levels.[24,29] Arousals from OSA also lead to increases in heart rate and blood pressure.[30,31] All these factors result in an increase in oxygen demand. Following arousals from apnea and resumption of breathing, there is reoxygenation. This repetitive hypoxemia-reoxygenation has been thought to result in release of free radicals that activates nuclear factor κB, which has been implicated in upregulation of proinflammatory genes and adhesion molecules resulting in endothelial dysfunction, platelet activation, and possibly atherosclerosis.[32] This inflammatory pathway could increase blood pressure independently of activation of the sympathetic neural activity.[33] Platelet activation and aggregation as well as morning levels of fibrinogen concentration are increased in OSA patients and tend to decrease after one night of CPAP use.[34,35] Vibration produced from snoring, which is commonly seen in patients with OSA, may lead to carotid vessel wall damage, perhaps resulting in the formation of atherosclerotic plaques.[36] The effects of all these perturbations can potentially result in chronic cardiovascular homeostatic dysregulation resulting in systemic hypertension, congestive heart failure, arrhythmias such as AF, strokes, sudden cardiac death, and pulmonary hypertension. In the next sections, the authors assess the causal role of OSA in the pathophysiology of hypertension, heart failure, and cardiac arrhythmias.

Systemic hypertension

There is strong evidence from both animal models[37] and human epidemiologic studies that OSA is one of the causative factors in systemic hypertension. Large prospective longitudinal studies help us understand the link between OSA and hypertension (HTN). The Wisconsin Sleep Cohort Study is a population-based longitudinal study that was initiated in the 1980s, and looked at the natural history of sleep-disordered breathing in adults. Cross-sectional analysis of baseline polysomnograms (PSG) and blood pressure data were collected in 1060 adults in the 30- to 60-year age range. The study showed a linear increase in blood pressure with increasing AHI, and an odds ratio of 1.8 for HTN at an AHI of 15 or more.[38] Compelling evidence for the link between OSA and HTN came from their prospective 4-year follow-up data, which showed an increasing odds of developing HTN independent of known confounding factors.[39] The Sleep Heart Health Study (SHHS) also demonstrated a dose-response relationship between HTN and indices of OSA severity even after adjustment for confounding factors.[40] These associations were evident in both sexes, all age groups, all ethnic groups, and in obese and nonobese subjects. Subsequent analysis showed that AHI was significantly associated with systolic and diastolic HTN for subjects younger than 60 years (odds ratio for AHI between 15 and 29.9/h was 2.38 and odds ratio for AHI more than 30/h was 2.24) but not for those older than 60 years.[41]

CPAP has been shown to acutely attenuate sympathetic drive and nocturnal blood pressure in patients with OSA.[24,42,43] However, the data regarding effects on daytime blood pressure have been more difficult to interpret. Several observational studies, often uncontrolled and from highly select populations, have suggested improvements in daytime blood pressure control with the use of CPAP. Because of these shortcomings, and an apparent true placebo effect realized in the measurement of blood pressure, several randomized, placebo-controlled trials (RCTs) have been performed, yielding variable and sometimes inconsistent results. The generalization of the studies is somewhat limited, because they comprise small sample sizes and the majority of subjects are normotensive at baseline. However, some findings are worth mentioning. With the largest study to date, Pepperell and colleagues[44] found a small but significant reduction in blood pressure in a largely normotensive cohort over only 4 weeks of therapy. Becker and colleagues,[45] in a controlled trial comparing therapeutic with subtherapeutic CPAP, found fairly dramatic reductions in mean blood pressure (9.9 ± 11.4 mm Hg) in a small cohort with severe OSA (mean AHI >60/h) treated for more than 60 days, the longest trial to date. Potential limitations to the study include a high dropout rate and the fact that about two-thirds were treated with various antihypertensive medications. A point that does stand out, suggesting the importance of treatment-dose effect, is that subtherapeutic CPAP reduced the AHI by 50% but did not result in any reduction in blood pressure.

Whereas excessive daytime sleepiness is a common and potentially dangerous consequence of OSA, it is not a universal symptom. There is evidence to suggest that sleepiness may be an important mediator of some of the systemic effects of OSA. That is, in the absence of sleepiness even severe OSA, as quantified by the AHI, does not always translate to reductions in blood pressure after CPAP treatment, regardless of whether normotension or hypertension exists at baseline. In a randomized controlled trial, Barbe and colleagues[46] showed that in normotensives with severe sleep apnea by AHI criteria but no daytime sleepiness, CPAP treatment imparted no reductions in blood pressure. Similar findings were recently reported by the Oxford group but in a cohort of hypertensive sleep apneics.[47] Even mild subjective sleepiness confers some blood pressure benefit with the use of CPAP.[48]

Finally, the results of a randomized trial comparing ambulatory blood pressure in moderately severe sleep apneics following treatment with therapeutic CPAP, sham CPAP, or supplemental oxygen are notable.[49] Whereas therapeutic CPAP resulted in blood pressure reductions, supplemental oxygen, despite normalizing oxygen saturation, did not. This finding suggests that hypoxia-mediated mechanisms may not fully explain the acute and chronic effects of sleep apnea on the vasculature. It may well be that central nervous system arousals, which are attenuated, if not abolished with CPAP therapy, are equally important, perhaps through effects on sympathetic output or hemodynamics.

A recent meta-analysis of 12 RCTs of blood pressure reduction with CPAP treatment in OSA,[50] confirmed by a subsequent article,[51] while confirming heterogeneity of study design and population, showed the pooled effect of CPAP treatment in patients with OSA (both normotensive and hypertensive) had a net significant reduction in mean blood pressure of 1.5 to 2 mm Hg. The results also suggest a greater antihypertensive effect in those with hypertension and daytime sleepiness at baseline. However, there were differences in the severity of OSA in these treatment trials and differences in inclusion/exclusion criteria.

Because chronic conditions such as OSA-associated hypertension could reasonably lead to vascular remodeling and other structural cardiovascular changes, it is entirely feasible that short-term controlled studies may fail to disclose the true effects of faithful CPAP therapy on hypertension and its consequences. Furthermore, given the prevalence of hypertension and its effects on the development of other cardiovascular diseases, including heart failure and stroke, the results of small changes in blood pressure and decreases in nocturnal blood pressure may be far reaching.

Heart failure

Observational data support the potential importance of OSA in cardiovascular outcomes. Case-control studies suggest that OSA may lead to cardiac structural changes, plausibly explained as an adaptive response to the consequent physiologic stressors.[52,53] Incident AF, an important risk factor for heart failure, is associated with the degree of oxyhemoglobin desaturation in OSA.[54] A study of mortality in a pure heart failure population with OSA suggested higher death rates in those who were noncompliant with CPAP compared with those who had mild or no OSA.[55] Similar inferences might be drawn from a 10-year cohort study by Marin and colleagues,[56] who showed an increase in fatal and nonfatal cardiovascular events in patients with severe, untreated OSA.

Given the high rate of coexistence of OSA and heart failure, one cannot exclude the possibility that cardiac function may modulate upper airway function, hence predisposing to OSA. Cardinal features of heart failure include circulatory overload and dependent edema resulting from organ hypoperfusion and associated neurohormonal imbalances. There is evidence to suggest that tissue edema, especially position-dependent redistribution, may influence upper airway dimensions and mechanics. Using computed tomography images, Shepard and colleagues[57] found that, in men with known OSA, experimental changes in central venous pressure were associated with alterations in upper airway cross-sectional area. The most significant changes were observed with reductions in central venous pressure (by blood pressure cuff inflation of the legs), where increases in airway cross-sectional area were seen at end-inspiratory tidal volume.

Two controlled, short-term interventional trials of CPAP for OSA in the setting of heart failure have been performed, both yielding various positive results.[58,59] Using a randomized, parallel comparative design, the control groups were composed of subjects optimally medically managed, though not subjected to placebo. The intervention was applied after a full, second-night in-laboratory polysomnographic titration of CPAP. Kaneko and colleagues[58] reported an approximately 9% increase in left ventricular ejection fraction (LVEF) and significant reductions in blood pressure after just 1 month of CPAP therapy. Mansfield and colleagues,[59] studying a group of subjects with somewhat less severe degrees of both heart failure and OSA than the subjects of Kaneko and colleagues,[58] applied CPAP therapy for 3 months and showed significant improvements in LVEF and reductions in urinary catecholamines, but no changes in blood pressure.

In contrast, a third controlled CPAP interventional trial showed no such changes in any cardiovascular end points, including ejection fraction, blood pressure, and exercise capacity.[60] Notwithstanding potential methodological shortcomings that may limit the applicability of the results, including a cross-over design and use of an auto-titrating CPAP machine without confirmatory follow-up PSG, the trial showed significant improvements in daytime symptoms in this group with fairly severe OSA. Unfortunately, with average CPAP use of just over 3 hours per night, it also underscores the well-identified challenges of maintaining adherence to CPAP treatment. It is clear that larger, long-term interventional trials of CPAP treatment, as well as its alternatives, are needed.

Cardiac arrhythmias

Several observational studies have shown an association between OSA and various nocturnal arrhythmias. Recent data from the SHHS, after adjusting for many confounders, showed that, compared with subjects with a respiratory disturbance index (RDI; number of respiratory events per hour) less than 5, those with severe OSA (RDI $\geq$ 30) had a higher rate of AF, nonsustained ventricular tachycardia, and ectopic ventricular beats.[61] Bradyarrhythmias are commonly encountered in OSA, may correlate with the severity of disordered breathing, can occur with a structurally normal heart, and may be attenuated by effective CPAP therapy.[62,63] The aforementioned SHHS data, however, show similar rates of bradycardias and conduction delays between subjects with severe OSA and those without significant OSA.

Mounting data strengthen the association between OSA and AF, 2 disorders that often coexist.[64] Continuous cardiac monitoring with an atrial defibrillator showed that the onset of nearly 75% of episodes of persistent atrial fibrillation in OSA patients occurred in the overnight hours (8 PM to 8 AM).[65] Retrospective analysis shows that, within 12 months of successful therapeutic electrical cardioversion for atrial fibrillation, untreated sleep apneics were found to have an arrhythmia recurrence rate double that of patients treated with CPAP.[66] Recent review of 17 years of PSG data from a population-based cohort suggests that nocturnal hypoxemia associated with OSA influences the incidence of atrial fibrillation.[54] Because none of these observational data can convincingly implicate OSA as an independent cause of new-onset atrial fibrillation, further longitudinal cohort studies and outcome-based interventional trials are needed to characterize the relationship between OSA and atrial arrhythmias.

INTERACTION BETWEEN OBESITY AND OSA ON CARDIOVASCULAR CONSEQUENCES

Coexistence of Obesity and OSA

Obesity and OSA often coexist, with more than 40% of obese patients having significant OSA and 70% of OSA patients being obese.[67-69] As obesity and OSA tend to commonly coexist, and as each of them have been shown to have similar cardiovascular consequences as previously mentioned, it is important to consider their relative roles and their relative importance of shared common pathways that lead to cardiovascular consequences. Obesity and OSA, independent of each other, can affect similar biologic pathways that predispose to cardiovascular diseases such as predisposing to insulin resistance and oxidative stress.[70-73] It is therefore possible that any cardiovascular end point might be explained by obesity without needing to consider OSA, but unfortunately most studies in obese patients assessing the relationship with cardiovascular outcomes did not assess for OSA and exclude it as a possible confounder.

Obesity as a Risk Factor for OSA

Obesity is one of the main risk factors in the pathogenesis of OSA,[1] and the prevalence of OSA is increasing with increasing prevalence of obesity, particularly central (visceral) obesity.[74,75] A 10% increase in weight gain is associated with a 6-fold increase in the odds of developing OSA.[76] Similarly, another study showed a 4-fold increase in OSA risk with every 6 kg/m² increment in BMI.[77] The causal relationship between obesity and OSA is further supported by some observational studies that show that weight loss leads to a decrease in OSA severity[76,78,79] **(Fig. 1)**. The severity of OSA, as estimated by the AHI, increases with obesity.[76,80] The severity of OSA is an important predictor of cardiovascular morbidity.[39]

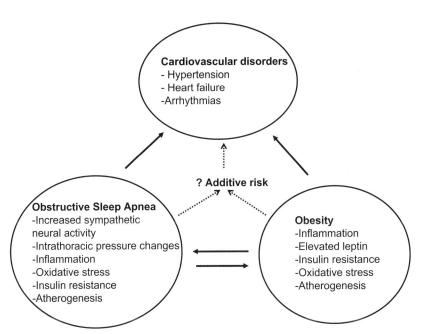

Fig. 1. The interaction between obesity and OSA, and its cardiovascular consequences. Note some of the similar pathogenetic mechanisms between OSA and obesity for cardiovascular consequences. Combination of OSA and obesity probably increases the risk for cardiovascular disorders.

OSA as a Risk Factor for Obesity

Patients with OSA may be predisposed to weight gain. In fact there are data to suggest that newly diagnosed OSA patients have difficulty losing weight and may actually be predisposed to excessive weight gain, compared with similarly matched obese subjects without OSA.[81,82] The reasons are likely multifactorial. Patients with OSA tend to be hypersomnolent and fatigued, leading to decreased physical activity. Also, obese patients with OSA have leptin resistance so that the weight-reducing effects of leptin are blunted, resulting in a cycle of weight gain and worsening OSA. CPAP use in OSA has been associated with loss of visceral fat.[83] Based on the available evidence thus far, it appears that there may be a relation between obesity and OSA that could mutually enhance the progression and severity (see **Fig. 1**).

Role of Visceral Fat

Visceral fat distribution, irrespective of the overall BMI, appears to be a stronger predictor for cardiovascular disorders.[70] Most of the studies assessing the link between OSA and cardiovascular disorders try to control for overall obesity, but not for visceral obesity. Also, visceral fat is a risk factor for OSA and is increased in OSA patients compared with BMI-matched controls.[75,84] CPAP therapy has shown to decrease visceral fat accumulation in OSA patients even without an overall decrease in BMI.[83] Therefore, visceral fat could be a confounding variable that is not routinely measured in studies assessing OSA and cardiovascular disorders.

Does the Presence of OSA in Obese Patients Place Them at a Higher Risk for Cardiovascular Events than Obese Patients Without OSA?

Some of the basic molecular mechanisms may suggest that OSA in obese patients may place them at higher risk for cardiovascular outcomes (see **Fig. 1**) than obese patients without OSA, though such assertions await firm clinical evidence. Plasma levels of leptin in OSA patients are even higher than in similarly matched obese but non-OSA subjects,[85,86] indicating that the presence of OSA in obese subjects potentiates further leptin resistance and, potentially, cardiovascular disease. Obesity and OSA also predispose to alterations in renal hemodynamics, resulting in sodium retention and volume expansion.[87,88] The renin-angiotensin system is activated in obesity and there is a positive correlation between BMI and plasma aldosterone, angiotensinogen, plasma rennin activity, and plasma angiotensin-converting enzyme activity[89,90] OSA is also associated with significantly higher levels of angiotensin II and aldosterone compared with healthy controls.[90] Therefore it is possible that the activation of the renin-angiotensin-aldosterone system may be augmented by the presence of OSA in obese patients; further studies are needed to confirm this hypothesis. Similarly, oxidative stress has been documented in both OSA and obese patients independent of each other (see **Fig. 1**). Oxidative stress results in vasoconstriction by blocking nitric oxide synthase enzyme, inactivating nitric oxide, activation of angiotensin II, and a resulting increase of endothelin-1.[91,92] Whether OSA exerts a cumulative effect on oxidative stress in obese patients remains to be established, and whether treatment of OSA interrupts these processes to result in tangible improvements in outcomes is unknown.

Does the Presence of OSA in Obese Patients Place Them at a Higher Risk for Cardiovascular Events than OSA Patients Without Obesity?

Although obesity might increase the risk for cardiovascular events in OSA patients compared with OSA without underlying obesity, the authors are unaware of literature to date that specifically compares these 2 groups. The authors propose that experimental models exist that may help answer the question. For example, one might assess cardiovascular outcomes in Asians, who have a lower BMI but have craniofacial features that place them at risk for the development of OSA, with and without obesity for the same degree of OSA severity.

The degree of oxyhemoglobin desaturations and the cumulative burden of nocturnal hypoxia, important predictors of cardiovascular morbidity,[93] are not well reflected in the classic AHI metric but may be important variables that may distinguish risk of obesity from OSA. In a recent, novel model of intermittent hypoxia in humans, healthy adults developed significant increases in mean awake blood pressure when exposed to intermittent hypoxia during sleep over a 2-week period.[94] As hypoxia appears to be a significant predictor of cardiovascular consequences secondary to OSA, could the presence of obesity augment hypoxia compared with nonobese subjects with similar severity of OSA? In fact, in a recent study obesity was found to be an important predictor on the severity of oxyhemoglobin desaturation during the obstructive apneic and hypopneic events, independent of other confounding variables such as age, gender, event duration, sleep position, and baseline oxyhemoglobin saturation.[95] Therefore, obese OSA patients can potentially be at higher risk for cardiovascular morbidity and mortality compared with nonobese OSA patients for the same severity of OSA derived from the AHI. Of course, this will need to be addressed in future prospective studies.

SUMMARY

The current evidence suggests a role for OSA in the development of cardiovascular disorders, though obesity is almost certainly an active confounder in this relationship. OSA and obesity share pathophysiologic mechanisms potentially leading to cardiovascular disorders (see **Fig. 1**). It may therefore be hypothesized that the presence of OSA in obese patients may further contribute to adverse cardiovascular outcomes when compared with each condition in isolation. These concepts do raise some important questions. Does OSA, in the absence of obesity, lead to adverse cardiovascular outcomes? Are there independent or additive benefits of CPAP therapy and weight loss with regard to cardiovascular outcomes? Similarly, does treatment of OSA in the obese subjects confer the same advantages on cardiovascular function as in nonobese subjects with OSA, or does the presence of obesity attenuate the impact of CPAP on cardiovascular outcomes? Future studies are clearly needed to answer such questions.

REFERENCES

1. Young T, Palta M, Dempsey J, et al. The occurrence of sleep-disordered breathing among middle-aged adults. N Engl J Med 1993;328:1230.
2. Wallace AM, McMahon AD, Packard CJ, et al. Plasma leptin and the risk of cardiovascular disease in the West of Scotland Coronary Prevention Study (WOSCOPS). Circulation 2001;104:3052.
3. McFarlane SI, Banerji M, Sowers JR. Insulin resistance and cardiovascular disease. J Clin Endocrinol Metab 2001;86:713.
4. Abate N. Obesity and cardiovascular disease. Pathogenetic role of the metabolic syndrome and therapeutic implications. J Diabetes Complications 2000;14:154.
5. Expert panel on detection, evaluation, and treatment of high blood cholesterol in adults. Executive summary of the third report of the National Cholesterol Education Program (NCEP) expert panel on detection, evaluation, and treatment of high blood cholesterol in adults (adult treatment panel III). JAMA 2001;285:2486.

6. Eckel RH, Grundy SM, Zimmet PZ. The metabolic syndrome. Lancet 2005;365: 1415.

7. Gaziano JM, Hennekens CH, O'Donnell CJ, et al. Fasting triglycerides, high-density lipoprotein, and risk of myocardial infarction. Circulation 1997;96:2520.

8. Genest JJ Jr, Martin-Munley SS, McNamara JR, et al. Familial lipoprotein disorders in patients with premature coronary artery disease. Circulation 1992;85: 2025.

9. Jeppesen J, Hein HO, Suadicani P, et al. Triglyceride concentration and ischemic heart disease: an eight-year follow-up in the Copenhagen Male Study. Circulation 1998;97:1029.

10. Alpert MA. Obesity cardiomyopathy: pathophysiology and evolution of the clinical syndrome. Am J Med Sci 2001;321:225.

11. Messerli FH, Nunez BD, Ventura HO, et al. Overweight and sudden death. Increased ventricular ectopy in cardiopathy of obesity. Arch Intern Med 1987; 147:1725.

12. Lavie CJ, Milani RV, Ventura HO, et al. Disparate effects of left ventricular geometry and obesity on mortality in patients with preserved left ventricular ejection fraction. Am J Cardiol 2007;100:1460.

13. Lavie CJ, Amodeo C, Ventura HO, et al. Left atrial abnormalities indicating diastolic ventricular dysfunction in cardiopathy of obesity. Chest 1987;92: 1042.

14. Garrison RJ, Kannel WB, Stokes J 3rd, et al. Incidence and precursors of hypertension in young adults: the Framingham Offspring Study. Prev Med 1987;16:235.

15. Kenchaiah S, Evans JC, Levy D, et al. Obesity and the risk of heart failure. N Engl J Med 2002;347:305.

16. Alpert MA, Terry BE, Mulekar M, et al. Cardiac morphology and left ventricular function in normotensive morbidly obese patients with and without congestive heart failure, and effect of weight loss. Am J Cardiol 1997;80:736.

17. Hubert HB, Feinleib M, McNamara PM, et al. Obesity as an independent risk factor for cardiovascular disease: a 26-year follow-up of participants in the Framingham Heart Study. Circulation 1983;67:968.

18. Lavie CJ, Milani RV. Obesity and cardiovascular disease: the Hippocrates paradox? J Am Coll Cardiol 2003;42:677.

19. Wang TJ, Parise H, Levy D, et al. Obesity and the risk of new-onset atrial fibrillation. JAMA 2004;292:2471.

20. Wanahita N, Messerli FH, Bangalore S, et al. Atrial fibrillation and obesity—results of a meta-analysis. Am Heart J 2008;155:310.

21. Poirier P, Giles TD, Bray GA, et al. Obesity and cardiovascular disease: pathophysiology, evaluation, and effect of weight loss: an update of the 1997 American Heart Association scientific statement on obesity and heart disease from the obesity committee of the council on nutrition, physical activity, and metabolism. Circulation 2006;113:898.

22. Kannel WB, Plehn JF, Cupples LA. Cardiac failure and sudden death in the Framingham Study. Am Heart J 1988;115:869.

23. Romero-Corral A, Montori VM, Somers VK, et al. Association of bodyweight with total mortality and with cardiovascular events in coronary artery disease: a systematic review of cohort studies. Lancet 2006;368:666.

24. Somers VK, Dyken ME, Clary MP, et al. Sympathetic neural mechanisms in obstructive sleep apnea. J Clin Invest 1995;96:1897.

25. Li C, Jackson RM. Reactive species mechanisms of cellular hypoxia-reoxygenation injury. Am J Physiol Cell Physiol 2002;282:C227.

26. Shiomi T, Guilleminault C, Stoohs R, et al. Leftward shift of the interventricular septum and pulsus paradoxus in obstructive sleep apnea syndrome. Chest 1991;100:894.

27. Stoohs R, Guilleminault C. Cardiovascular changes associated with obstructive sleep apnea syndrome. J Appl Physiol 1992;72:583.

28. Virolainen J, Ventila M, Turto H, et al. Effect of negative intrathoracic pressure on left ventricular pressure dynamics and relaxation. J Appl Physiol 1995;79:455.

29. Narkiewicz K, Kato M, Phillips BG, et al. Nocturnal continuous positive airway pressure decreases daytime sympathetic traffic in obstructive sleep apnea. Circulation 1999;100:2332.

30. O'Donnell CP, Allan L, Atkinson P, et al. The effect of upper airway obstruction and arousal on peripheral arterial tonometry in obstructive sleep apnea. Am J Respir Crit Care Med 2002;166:965.

31. Schneider H, Schaub CD, Chen CA, et al. Effects of arousal and sleep state on systemic and pulmonary hemodynamics in obstructive apnea. J Appl Physiol 2000;88:1084.

32. Ryan S, Taylor CT, McNicholas WT. Selective activation of inflammatory pathways by intermittent hypoxia in obstructive sleep apnea syndrome. Circulation 2005; 112:2660.

33. Vongpatanasin W, Thomas GD, Schwartz R, et al. C-reactive protein causes downregulation of vascular angiotensin subtype 2 receptors and systolic hypertension in mice. Circulation 2007;115:1020.

34. Bokinsky G, Miller M, Ault K, et al. Spontaneous platelet activation and aggregation during obstructive sleep apnea and its response to therapy with nasal continuous positive airway pressure. A preliminary investigation. Chest 1995; 108:625.

35. Steiner S, Jax T, Evers S, et al. Altered blood rheology in obstructive sleep apnea as a mediator of cardiovascular risk. Cardiology 2005;104:92.

36. Lee SA, Amis TC, Byth K, et al. Heavy snoring as a cause of carotid artery atherosclerosis. Sleep 2008;31:1207.

37. Brooks D, Horner RL, Kozar LF, et al. Obstructive sleep apnea as a cause of systemic hypertension. Evidence from a canine model. J Clin Invest 1997;99:106.

38. Young T, Peppard P, Palta M, et al. Population-based study of sleep-disordered breathing as a risk factor for hypertension. Arch Intern Med 1997;157:1746.

39. Peppard PE, Young T, Palta M, et al. Prospective study of the association between sleep-disordered breathing and hypertension. N Engl J Med 2000; 342:1378.

40. Nieto FJ, Young TB, Lind BK, et al. Association of sleep-disordered breathing, sleep apnea, and hypertension in a large community-based study. Sleep Heart Health Study. JAMA 1829;283:2000.

41. Haas DC, Foster GL, Nieto FJ, et al. Age-dependent associations between sleep-disordered breathing and hypertension: importance of discriminating between systolic/diastolic hypertension and isolated systolic hypertension in the Sleep Heart Health Study. Circulation 2005;111:614.

42. Ali NJ, Davies RJ, Fleetham JA, et al. The acute effects of continuous positive airway pressure and oxygen administration on blood pressure during obstructive sleep apnea. Chest 1992;101:1526.

43. Dimsdale JE, Loredo JS, Profant J. Effect of continuous positive airway pressure on blood pressure: a placebo trial. Hypertension 2000;35:144.

44. Pepperell JC, Ramdassingh-Dow S, Crosthwaite N, et al. Ambulatory blood pressure after therapeutic and subtherapeutic nasal continuous positive airway

pressure for obstructive sleep apnoea: a randomised parallel trial. Lancet 2002; 359:204.

45. Becker HF, Jerrentrup A, Ploch T, et al. Effect of nasal continuous positive airway pressure treatment on blood pressure in patients with obstructive sleep apnea. Circulation 2003;107:68.

46. Barbe F, Mayoralas LR, Duran J, et al. Treatment with continuous positive airway pressure is not effective in patients with sleep apnea but no daytime sleepiness. A randomized, controlled trial. Ann Intern Med 2001;134:1015.

47. Robinson GV, Smith DM, Langford BA, et al. Continuous positive airway pressure does not reduce blood pressure in nonsleepy hypertensive OSA patients. Eur Respir J 2006;27:1229.

48. Hui DS, To KW, Ko FW, et al. Nasal CPAP reduces systemic blood pressure in patients with obstructive sleep apnoea and mild sleepiness. Thorax 2006;61: 1083.

49. Norman D, Loredo JS, Nelesen RA, et al. Effects of continuous positive airway pressure versus supplemental oxygen on 24-hour ambulatory blood pressure. Hypertension 2006;47:840.

50. Haentjens P, Van Meerhaeghe A, Moscariello A, et al. The impact of continuous positive airway pressure on blood pressure in patients with obstructive sleep apnea syndrome: evidence from a meta-analysis of placebo-controlled randomized trials. Arch Intern Med 2007;167:757.

51. Bazzano LA, Khan Z, Reynolds K, et al. Effect of nocturnal nasal continuous positive airway pressure on blood pressure in obstructive sleep apnea. Hypertension 2007;50:417.

52. Otto ME, Belohlavek M, Romero-Corral A, et al. Comparison of cardiac structural and functional changes in obese otherwise healthy adults with versus without obstructive sleep apnea. Am J Cardiol 2007;99:1298.

53. Usui K, Parker JD, Newton GE, et al. Left ventricular structural adaptations to obstructive sleep apnea in dilated cardiomyopathy. Am J Respir Crit Care Med 2006;173:1170.

54. Gami AS, Hodge DO, Herges RM, et al. Obstructive sleep apnea, obesity, and the risk of incident atrial fibrillation. J Am Coll Cardiol 2007;49:565.

55. Wang H, Parker JD, Newton GE, et al. Influence of obstructive sleep apnea on mortality in patients with heart failure. J Am Coll Cardiol 2007;49:1625.

56. Marin JM, Carrizo SJ, Vicente E, et al. Long-term cardiovascular outcomes in men with obstructive sleep apnoea-hypopnoea with or without treatment with continuous positive airway pressure: an observational study. Lancet 2005; 365:1046.

57. Shepard JW Jr, Pevernagie DA, Stanson AW, et al. Effects of changes in central venous pressure on upper airway size in patients with obstructive sleep apnea. Am J Respir Crit Care Med 1996;153:250.

58. Kaneko Y, Floras JS, Usui K, et al. Cardiovascular effects of continuous positive airway pressure in patients with heart failure and obstructive sleep apnea. N Engl J Med 2003;348:1233.

59. Mansfield DR, Gollogly NC, Kaye DM, et al. Controlled trial of continuous positive airway pressure in obstructive sleep apnea and heart failure. Am J Respir Crit Care Med 2004;169:361.

60. Smith LA, Vennelle M, Gardner RS, et al. Auto-titrating continuous positive airway pressure therapy in patients with chronic heart failure and obstructive sleep apnoea: a randomized placebo-controlled trial. Eur Heart J 2007;28: 1221.

61. Mehra R, Benjamin EJ, Shahar E, et al. Association of nocturnal arrhythmias with sleep-disordered breathing: the Sleep Heart Health Study. Am J Respir Crit Care Med 2006;173:910.

62. Grimm W, Koehler U, Fus E, et al. Outcome of patients with sleep apnea-associated severe bradyarrhythmias after continuous positive airway pressure therapy. Am J Cardiol 2000;86:688.

63. Guilleminault C, Connolly SJ, Winkle RA. Cardiac arrhythmia and conduction disturbances during sleep in 400 patients with sleep apnea syndrome. Am J Cardiol 1983;52:490.

64. Gami AS, Pressman G, Caples SM, et al. Association of atrial fibrillation and obstructive sleep apnea. Circulation 2004;110:364.

65. Mitchell AR, Spurrell PA, Sulke N. Circadian variation of arrhythmia onset patterns in patients with persistent atrial fibrillation. Am Heart J 2003;146:902.

66. Kanagala R, Murali NS, Friedman PA, et al. Obstructive sleep apnea and the recurrence of atrial fibrillation. Circulation 2003;107:2589.

67. van Boxem TJ, de Groot GH. Prevalence and severity of sleep disordered breathing in a group of morbidly obese patients. Neth J Med 1999;54:202.

68. Vgontzas AN, Tan TL, Bixler EO, et al. Sleep apnea and sleep disruption in obese patients. Arch Intern Med 1994;154:1705.

69. Young T, Peppard PE, Gottlieb DJ. Epidemiology of obstructive sleep apnea: a population health perspective. Am J Respir Crit Care Med 2002;165:1217.

70. Fox CS, Massaro JM, Hoffmann U, et al. Abdominal visceral and subcutaneous adipose tissue compartments: association with metabolic risk factors in the Framingham Heart Study. Circulation 2007;116:39.

71. Ip MS, Lam B, Ng MM, et al. Obstructive sleep apnea is independently associated with insulin resistance. Am J Respir Crit Care Med 2002;165:670.

72. Punjabi NM, Shahar E, Redline S, et al. Sleep-disordered breathing, glucose intolerance, and insulin resistance: the Sleep Heart Health Study. Am J Epidemiol 2004;160:521.

73. Rader DJ. Effect of insulin resistance, dyslipidemia, and intra-abdominal adiposity on the development of cardiovascular disease and diabetes mellitus. Am J Med 2007;120:S12.

74. Grunstein R, Wilcox I, Yang TS, et al. Snoring and sleep apnoea in men: association with central obesity and hypertension. Int J Obes Relat Metab Disord 1993;17:533.

75. Shinohara E, Kihara S, Yamashita S, et al. Visceral fat accumulation as an important risk factor for obstructive sleep apnoea syndrome in obese subjects. J Intern Med 1997;241:11.

76. Peppard PE, Young T, Palta M, et al. Longitudinal study of moderate weight change and sleep-disordered breathing. JAMA 2000;284:3015.

77. Young T, Shahar E, Nieto FJ, et al. Predictors of sleep-disordered breathing in community-dwelling adults: the Sleep Heart Health Study. Arch Intern Med 2002;162:893.

78. Schwartz AR, Gold AR, Schubert N, et al. Effect of weight loss on upper airway collapsibility in obstructive sleep apnea. Am Rev Respir Dis 1991;144:494.

79. Smith PL, Gold AR, Meyers DA, et al. Weight loss in mildly to moderately obese patients with obstructive sleep apnea. Ann Intern Med 1985;103:850.

80. Newman AB, Foster G, Givelber R, et al. Progression and regression of sleep-disordered breathing with changes in weight: the Sleep Heart Health Study. Arch Intern Med 2005;165:2408.

81. Phillips BG, Hisel TM, Kato M, et al. Recent weight gain in patients with newly diagnosed obstructive sleep apnea. J Hypertens 1999;17:1297.
82. Phillips BG, Kato M, Narkiewicz K, et al. Increases in leptin levels, sympathetic drive, and weight gain in obstructive sleep apnea. Am J Physiol Heart Circ Physiol 2000;279:H234.
83. Chin K, Shimizu K, Nakamura T, et al. Changes in intra-abdominal visceral fat and serum leptin levels in patients with obstructive sleep apnea syndrome following nasal continuous positive airway pressure therapy. Circulation 1999;100:706.
84. Vgontzas AN, Papanicolaou DA, Bixler EO, et al. Sleep apnea and daytime sleepiness and fatigue: relation to visceral obesity, insulin resistance, and hypercytokinemia. J Clin Endocrinol Metab 2000;85:1151.
85. Ip MS, Lam KS, Ho C, et al. Serum leptin and vascular risk factors in obstructive sleep apnea. Chest 2000;118:580.
86. Shimizu K, Chin K, Nakamura T, et al. Plasma leptin levels and cardiac sympathetic function in patients with obstructive sleep apnoea-hypopnoea syndrome. Thorax 2002;57:429.
87. Hall JE. Mechanisms of abnormal renal sodium handling in obesity hypertension. Am J Hypertens 1997;10:49S.
88. Hall JE, Brands MW, Henegar JR. Mechanisms of hypertension and kidney disease in obesity. Ann N Y Acad Sci 1999;892:91.
89. Engeli S, Sharma AM. The renin-angiotensin system and natriuretic peptides in obesity-associated hypertension. J Mol Med 2001;79:21.
90. Moller DS, Lind P, Strunge B, et al. Abnormal vasoactive hormones and 24-hour blood pressure in obstructive sleep apnea. Am J Hypertens 2003;16:274.
91. Somers MJ, Harrison DG. Reactive oxygen species and the control of vasomotor tone. Curr Hypertens Rep 1999;1:102.
92. Wilcox CS. Reactive oxygen species: roles in blood pressure and kidney function. Curr Hypertens Rep 2002;4:160.
93. Punjabi NM, Newman AB, Young TB, et al. Sleep-disordered breathing and cardiovascular disease: an outcome-based definition of hypopneas. Am J Respir Crit Care Med 2008;177:1150.
94. Tamisier R, Gilmartin GS, Launois SH, et al. A new model of chronic intermittent hypoxia in humans: effect on ventilation, sleep, and blood pressure. J Appl Physiol 2009;107:17.
95. Peppard PE, Ward NR, Morrell MJ. The impact of obesity on oxygen desaturation during sleep-disordered breathing. Am J Respir Crit Care Med 2009;180:788.

Surgical Options for the Treatment of Obstructive Sleep Apnea

Jon-Erik C. Holty, MD, MS[a],*, Christian Guilleminault, MD, DBiol[b]

KEYWORDS

• Obstructive sleep apnea • Sleep apnea syndromes • Surgery

Obstructive sleep apnea (OSA) is a highly prevalent condition characterized by increased nocturnal airflow resistance resulting in repetitive episodes of pharyngeal collapse during sleep.[1] Approximately 20% of adults in the United States have OSA (defined as an apnea-hypopnea index (AHI) ≥ 5/h) with up to 10% having moderate to severe disease (AHI ≥ 15/h).[2,3] In addition, between 3% and 10% of children have OSA (AHI ≥ 1/h).[4–7] Obesity, male gender, advancing age, and mandibular-maxillary insufficiency are well-characterized risk factors.[8] OSA predisposes to increased cardiovascular and cerebrovascular morbidity and mortality, and is associated with excessive daytime sleepiness and neurocognitive underperformance.[8] Untreated, the 15-year mortality for adults with severe disease is approximately 30% with adjusted mortality hazards ratios of 1.4, 1.7, and 3.8 for mild, moderate, and severe disease, respectively (P-trend = 0.004).[2]

Conventional nonsurgical OSA therapy necessitates indefinite positive airway pressure (eg, continuous positive airway pressure [CPAP] or bilevel therapy) that works by pneumatically stenting open the upper airway, thus preventing apneas and hypopneas during sleep.[9–11] CPAP is an effective treatment modality for OSA, improving symptoms (eg, excessive daytime sleepiness, quality of life) and reducing cardiovascular mortality.[12,13] Unfortunately, more than 50% of patients with OSA are intolerant of and ultimately reject CPAP therapy.[14,15] Common complaints include mask discomfort and leak, rhinorrhea, conjunctivitis, dry mouth, nasal congestion, aerophagia, claustrophobia, and chest wall discomfort.[6] Individuals intolerant of CPAP therapy have a 10% absolute increased mortality risk (compared with adherent subjects) at 5 years.[16,17]

Contract/Grant Support: None.
Conflict of interest: None.
[a] Division of Pulmonary, Critical Care and Sleep Medicine, Department of Medicine, VA Palo Alto Health Care System, 3801 Miranda Avenue, Palo Alto, CA 94304, USA
[b] Division of Sleep Medicine, Stanford University School of Medicine, Stanford Medical Outpatient Center, 450 Broadway Street, Pavillon C, Redwood City, CA 94063-5074, USA
* Corresponding author.
E-mail address: jholty@stanford.edu

Med Clin N Am 94 (2010) 479–515
doi:10.1016/j.mcna.2010.02.001
0025-7125/10/$ – see front matter. Published by Elsevier Inc.

Effective surgical therapies for OSA predate the first reported use of CPAP by Sullivan and colleagues[9] in 1981 and Rapoport and colleagues[18] in 1982. Tracheostomy was employed as early as 1969[19] and Kuo and colleagues[20] in 1979 (and later Bear and Priest[21] in 1980) reported the results of mandibular advancement for the treatment of OSA. In 1952, Ikematsu[22] began removing excessive oropharyngeal tissue to alleviate snoring and reported the results of his palatopharynoplasty with partial uvulectomy in 152 habitual snorers in 1962. In the late 1970s, Fujita and colleagues[23] adapted Ikematsu's procedure and introduced the uvulopalatopharyngoplasty as a new surgical approach to treat OSA.[24] Because the anatomic cause of OSA is heterogeneous with most OSA patients having multiple concurrent pharyngeal abnormalities,[25–27] surgical procedures have evolved to address specific anatomic airflow limitations and to augment the effectiveness of existing procedures. This review describes the pathophysiology of OSA, the rationale for surgery, and the various surgical techniques used to treat OSA.

PATHOPHYSIOLOGY OF OSA

Patients with OSA have nocturnal airflow restriction resulting from upper-airway collapse between the naso- and hypopharynx.[28] During normal breathing, contraction of the diaphragm results in an increased thoracic volume that generates negative intrapleural pressure drawing air down to the alveoli. During a normal negative pressure inspiration, upper-airway reflexes phasically activate pharyngeal muscles (eg, genioglossus, tensor palatini, geniohyoid, stylohyoid) to dilate and stiffen the upper airway to maintain patency.[29–32] Pharyngeal dilator muscle activity is reduced in normal and OSA individuals during sleep.[30,33] However, patients with OSA have anatomically smaller upper airways and diminished pharyngeal dilator tone resulting in clinically significant airflow limitation (eg, apneas and hypopneas) during nocturnal negative pressure inspiration.[28,34,35] Most individuals with OSA have multiple pharyngeal abnormalities[25] with anatomic airway narrowing primarily in the lateral dimension.[36,37]

In addition, patients with OSA are often obligatory mouth breathers during sleep.[38] Nasal breathing (compared with mouth breathing) is more efficient because the nasal cavity has a more constant resistance (compared with the oral cavity) and because stimulation of nasal receptors is involved in activating the pharyngeal dilators.[39] In normal individuals, a transition from nasal to oral breathing results in a greater risk of pharyngeal collapse because of greater negative inspiratory pressures needed to overcome increased airway resistance.[39] Experimental nasal obstruction[40–42] or inhibiting the nasopharyngeal reflex (by applying topical anesthesia)[43] causes nocturnal apneas, hypopneas, and oxygen desaturation in normal individuals.

OSA is in part a neurologic disorder of the upper airway.[30,33,44,45] Pharyngeal collapse is often caused by abnormal activation of pharyngeal dilator muscles from dysfunctional pharyngeal reflexes.[46] In patients with nocturnal upper-airway resistance, repetitive vibratory trauma (eg, snoring) and tremendous swings in pharyngeal pressures (caused by apneas and hypopneas) during sleep results in pathologic injury to the pharyngeal dilator muscles and nerves.[33,47,48] This irreversible damage predisposes the upper airway to inspiratory collapse during sleep.[45,49–51]

RATIONAL FOR OSA SURGERY

The aim of OSA surgery is to eliminate airway collapse and reduce airway resistance during sleep without causing impairment to the normal functions of the upper airway and associated structures. Indications for surgery depend on: (1) the severity of OSA and comorbid medical conditions; (2) the severity of symptoms (eg, excessive daytime sleepiness); and (3) the anatomic location(s) causing obstruction. General indications for surgery include moderate-severe OSA, severe excessive daytime sleepiness (even when the AHI is ≤20/h), OSA with comorbid conditions (eg, arrhythmias, hypertension), OSA with anatomic airway abnormalities, and failure of medical OSA management.[52] Upper-airway abnormalities amenable to surgery include those within the nasal cavity (eg, deviated septum, polyps, hypertrophic turbinates, collapsible nasal valves), nasopharynx (eg, stenosis, adenoids), oropharynx (eg, palatine tonsils, elongated uvula, redundant mucosal folds, low hanging palate, webbing), and hypopharynx (eg, lingual tonsils, large tongue base, redundant aryepiglottic folds) **(Table 1)**. Relative contraindications to surgery include morbid obesity (except for bariatric surgery and tracheostomy), severe or unstable cardiopulmonary disease, active alcohol/illicit drug abuse, older age, unstable psychological problems, or unrealistic expectations from surgical therapy.

All adult OSA patients should be offered a nonsurgical treatment option (eg, CPAP) before proceeding to surgery. Even in patients electing to proceed directly to surgery, a trial of CPAP therapy may be helpful as this is a noninvasive means to determine the expected extent of symptom abatement after surgery. Preoperative CPAP is indicated in patients with severe OSA (AHI >40/h with severe nocturnal oxygen desaturation <80%) and should be continued postoperatively until 2 weeks before the postoperative polysomnogram.[53]

In children, early recognition of OSA and prompt correction of anatomic upper-airway abnormalities is paramount. By the age of 4 years, 60% of the adult craniofacial skeleton is attained, with 90% by age 12 years.[54–56] Children with pharyngeal obstruction (eg, tonsillar hypertrophy, turbinate enlargement) protect the patency of the airway by sleeping in the prone or side position with an extended, flexed head, and an anteriorally displaced tongue.[57] Anterior displacement of the tongue is associated with narrower upper and shorter lower dental arches,[57–61] posterior displacement of the mandible,[60,62] with resultant development of mandibular retrusion, increased overjet, and facial height[63–68] (all known risk factors for OSA).[58,69] Thus, early recognition

Table 1		
Anatomic location of pharyngeal obstruction in relationship to surgical procedure		
Anatomic Treatment Effect	**Anatomic Obstruction**	**Surgical Procedure**
1. Bypass upper airway	Collapsed airway	Tracheostomy
2. Soft tissue removal	Nasal cavity	Polypectomy, radiofrequency ablation of the turbinates
	Nasopharynx	Adenoidectomy
	Oropharynx	Tonsillectomy
		Uvulopalatopharyngoplasty
		Laser-assisted uvulopalatoplasty
	Hypopharynx	Midline glossectomy
		Tongue base reduction
3. Skeletal/soft tissue modification	Nasal cavity	Septoplasty
	Oropharynx	Rapid maxillary expansion
	Hypopharynx	Mandibular advancement
		Genioglossal advancement
		Hyoid myotomy suspension
	Oro- and hypopharynx	Maxillomandibular advancement

and surgical correction of significant airway obstruction in children is necessary to prevent abnormal craniofacial development and the irreversible damage to the pharyngeal dilator reflexes that potentially can lead to the lifelong consequences of OSA.

In adults and children, preoperative upper airway assessment is necessary to determine the level of obstruction (anywhere between the nose and epiglottis) and plan the optimal surgical approach. Preoperative fiberoptic endoscopy (performed with a Müller maneuver) and cephalometric analysis are helpful to classify the type of airway obstruction and identify obstructions of the hypopharynx.[26,70] Computed tomography may have added benefit.[71] The anatomy of the upper airway is classified into 3 general obstructive types (Fujita classification): (1) type 1: narrow oropharynx (eg, large tonsils, enlarged uvula, pillar webbing) with normal palatal arch position; (2) type 2: low arched palate with relatively large tongue; further subdivide into 2a (predominantly oropharyngeal abnormality) and 2b (abnormality involves oro- and hypopharynx); (3) type 3: hypopharyngeal obstruction (eg, retrognathia, floppy epiglottis, enlarged linguinal tonsils) with normal oropharynx.[72,73] The type of obstruction is often modified whether nasal obstruction concurrently exits. Surgical procedures address specific upper-airway abnormalities (eg, uvulopalatopharyngoplasty for type 1, genioglossus advancement for type 3, maxillomandibular advancement for combined type 1, 2 and 3). Preoperative pharyngeal anatomy, OSA severity, and patient preference (eg, recovery time, prolonged facial paresthesias, and malocclusion) are all contributing factors influencing the surgical decision.

SURGICAL SUCCESS

Various surgical procedures are now available to increase the posterior airspace and treat OSA in CPAP intolerant patients. However, no surgical treatment is 100% effective. Similar to previous reviews of OSA surgery,[74,75] we defined surgical success as an AHI less than 20 and a reduction in AHI of 50% or more after surgery.[76] Where possible, we provide surgical cure rates (defined as an AHI <5/h in adults and <1/h in children).[77]

PHARYNGEAL SURGICAL PROCEDURES

Individual surgical procedures are described in the following sections for the treatment of OSA organized by the treatment effect on the anatomic airway obstruction (eg, bypassing the upper airway obstruction, removal of soft tissue structures, or skeletal (or soft tissue) modification) (see **Table 1**).

Procedures that Bypass the Upper Airway Obstruction

Tracheostomy

In 1965, Valero and Alroy[78] reported improvement in nocturnal oxygenation in a patient with progressive respiratory failure secondary to traumatic micrognathia. Kuhlo and colleagues in 1969[19] followed by Lugaresi and colleagues in 1970[79,80] were the first to effectively treat OSA (or Pickwickian syndrome) by means of a tracheostomy. By bypassing the upper airway, tracheostomy is purported to be curative for OSA.[81] Although many studies purport resolution of airway obstruction after tracheostomy,[82–85] relatively few studies report pre- and posttracheostomy polysomnography parameters (eg, AHI) (**Table 2**).[81,86–91]

The largest case series (n = 50) reported complete resolution of obstructive apneas after tracheostomy.[81] Of 9 studies evaluating 61 patients, tracheostomy was highly effective at eliminating obstructive apneas (apnea index went from

Table 2
Efficacy of tracheostomy for OSA[a]

Study	Demographics			Apnea Index[b]			AHI (REM)[c]			Apnea-Hypopnea Index (NREM)[c]		
	N	Age (y)	Follow-up (mo)	Pre-Trach	Post-Trach	P-value[d]	Pre-Trach	Post-Trach	P-value[d]	Pre-Trach	Post-Trach	P-value[d]
Haapaniemi et al, 2001[86]	7	53.4 ± 9.8	60.9 ± 30.7	–	–		–	–		–	–	
Kim et al, 1998[87]	23	47.0 ± 12.4	–	–	–		58.5 ± 34.1	26.0 ± 31.2		92.5 ± 39.1	19.8 ± 26.3	
Fletcher, 1989[95]	1	–	51.0	114.0	0.0		–	–		–	–	
Fletcher et al, 1987[88]	8	55.4 ± 6.8	9.0 ± 3.2	84.6 ± 38.7	0.0 ± 0.0		–	–		–	–	
Guilleminault et al, 1981[81]	4	–	30.0 ± 6.9	94.5 ± 19.8	0.4 ± 0.5		–	–		–	–	
Sugita et al, 1980[90]	1	40.0	3.0	77.0	0.0		–	–		–	–	
Weitzman et al, 1980[96]	10	47.5 ± 2.4	0.3 ± 0.4	96.1 ± 21.9	1.1 ± 3.3		79.0 ± 18.6	26.5 ± 25.2		113.7 ± 23.0	25.8 ± 25.4	
Motta et al, 1978[101]	6	47.0 ± 4.0	7.5 ± 6.3	73.0 ± 12.2	0.0 ± 0.0		–	–		–	–	
Weitzman et al, 1978[100]	1	67.0	0.5	96.7	4.1		–	–		–	–	
Summary	61	49.3 ± 9.9	19.0 ± 26.3	88.4 ± 25.7	0.5 ± 1.9	<0.001	63.8 ± 31.9	26.2 ± 29.2	<0.001	98.9 ± 36.0	21.6 ± 25.8	<0.001

Abbreviations: N, number; NREM, nonrapid eye movement sleep; REM, rapid eye movement sleep; Trach, tracheostomy.
[a] Mean (or percent) ± standard deviation. – denotes not reported.
[b] The apnea index is the average number of obstructive apneas per hour during sleep.
[c] The AHI is the average number of obstructive apneas and hyponeas per hour during sleep.
[d] P-value calculated via an extended t-test and evaluates pre- and posttracheostomy measures.

88/h before to 0.5/h after tracheostomy; $P<.001$) (see **Table 2**). However, patients may have persistent hypopneas with a surgical success rate of approximately 73% (see **Tables 2** and **3**). Rodman and Martin[92] reported persistent (although generally improved) obstructive apneas and oxygen desaturations in 3 morbidly obese patients after tracheostomy caused by kinking of the tracheostomy tube during sleep or external obstruction by the patient's own soft tissues. Haapaniemi and colleagues[86] reported that although obstructive apneas improved after tracheostomy (mean follow-up 5.1 years), most patients had persistent oxygen desaturations with many having oxygen dip indexes ($\geq4\%$) of ≥15/h. Fletcher and Brown[93] reported persistent REM-associated desaturations after tracheostomy in patients with OSA with concomitant chronic obstructive pulmonary disease. Despite improvements in obstructive apneas after tracheostomy, emergence or worsening of central apneas is frequently observed, although generally resolves within 3 to 6 months.[80,81,89,94–98]

Tracheostomy is effective at preventing OSA-related arrhythmias,[98–100] reducing pulmonary artery pressures,[80,81,101] and improving hypertension[81,88,100–103] and diabetes[102] in patients with OSA. Many (but not all)[86] studies have reported near complete resolution of nocturnal symptoms and daytime sleepiness.[80,81,84,90,91,96,100,101,103–106] A retrospective analysis by He and colleagues[107] suggested a mortality benefit of tracheostomy (0% vs 38% mortality at 8 years) compared with no OSA therapy. Partinen and colleagues[108,109] found similar mortality benefits (0% vs 11% at 5 years) after tracheostomy.

Unfortunately, tracheostomy has several problems including patient dissatisfaction (eg, psychosocial aspects), perioperative complications (eg, wound infection, tissue necrosis, bleeding), recurrent bronchitis, granulation tissue, trachea-innominate fistula formation, and stoma stenosis (often requiring surgical revision).[105,110–115] Perioperative mortality is higher in obese individuals than in nonobese individuals.[116] Permanent tracheostomy (either tube[111] or tube-free[117]) is currently used in highly select cases with severe OSA who are intolerant of CPAP (and poor candidates for other surgical procedures). A temporary tracheostomy is occasionally used before other OSA procedures (eg, uvulopalatopharyngoplasty, bariatric surgery) to protect the airway, particularly in morbidly obese subjects.[118]

Closure of a permanent tracheostomy (after resolution of OSA by other surgeries or weight loss[119]) may be associated with a relatively high complication rate ($\sim30\%$), especially when done with a 3-layer as opposed to a de-epithelialization technique.[120,121] In addition, long-term tracheostomy may cause pharyngeal tissue obstruction (eg, granulation tissue, tracheomalacia) that may predispose to OSA after closure.[122,123]

Procedures that Remove Soft Tissue

Laser-assisted uvulopalatoplasty (LAUP)

This office-based procedure (similar to uvulopalatopharyngoplasty, but omitting tonsillectomy) uses a CO_2 laser to shape the soft palate and is an effective surgical technique for snoring ($\sim90\%$ success), but has limited OSA efficacy (see **Table 3**).[124] Two randomized trials of LAUP found no significant change in the AHI after surgery compared with those randomized to no surgery.[125,126] A meta-analysis of these 2 studies found no statistically significant difference in daytime sleepiness (measured by the Epworth sleepiness scale) between surgery and control groups (mean difference −1.4; 95% confidence interval [CI] −5.0–2.2).[127] More worrisome is that LAUP may worsen OSA in up to 21% of patients.[128] LAUP is not approved by the American Academy of Sleep Medicine to treat OSA.[129] In addition, complications are common

Table 3
Comparison of surgical efficacy for OSA[a]

Study	Demographics			AHI[b]			Cure (%)[c]	Success (%)[c]	Ref.
	N	Studies	Age (y)	Before Surgery	After Surgery	% Change			
Bariatric surgery[f]	437	16	38.8 ± 14.9	53.3 ± 38.2	15.3 ± 18.7	−72.6 ± 60.6	44	–	338,339
GA	91	4	–	53.9	17.3	−67.8	–	62	134
HS	101	4	–	38.7	25.0	−33.0	–	50	134
HS and GA (or mortised genioplasty)	328	7	–	33.5	15.2	−58.0	–	55	134
LAUP	72	3	–	–	–	–	7	49	77
MMA	627	22	44.4 ± 9.4	63.9 ± 26.7	9.5 ± 10.7	−85.0 ± 18.2	43	86	266
Midline glossectomy	74	5	–	53.0	24.2	−54.4	–	50	134
Radiofrequency ablation (tongue)	394	11	–	37.0	23.4	−35.7	–	36	134
RME									
Children	88	3	7.1 ± 0.7	10.9 ± 4.7	0.8 ± 1.3	−91.0 ± 20.2	–	–	320
Adults[d]	10	1	27.0 ± 0.6	19.0 ± 1.3	7.0 ± 1.3	−63.2 ± 7.1	70	90	321
Tonsillectomy	1,079	23	6.5	18.6	4.9	−73.7	60	–	177,178
Tongue base suspension	77	6	–	29.0	16.3	−32.9	–	35	134
Tracheostomy[e]	33	2	47.2 ± 10.4	98.9 ± 36.0	26.2 ± 29.2	−79.2 ± 25.8	–	73	87,96
UPPP	992	37	48.1	60.0	–	−38.2	16	52	75,77
Multimodality surgery[g]	1,978	58	46.2	48.0	–	−60.3	–	66	74

Abbreviations: BMI, body mass index; GA, genioglossus advancement; HS, hyoid suspension; LAUP, laser-assisted uvulopalatoplasty; MMA, maxillomandibular advancement; N, number; RME, rapid maxillary expansion; UPPP, uvulopalatopharyngoplasty. – denotes not reported.
[a] Plus-minus values are mean (or percent) ± standard deviation. – denotes not reported.
[b] The AHI is the average number of apneas and hypopneas per hour during sleep.
[c] Surgical success defined as the percent of subjects with an AHI <20/h and a ≥50% reduction in the AHI after surgery. Surgical cure defined as an AHI <5/h after surgery. For tonsillectomy, surgical cure was defined as an AHI <1/h after surgery.
[d] Surgically assisted RME involved horizontal osteotomies.
[e] The AHI for tracheostomy reported during non-REM sleep only and included only obstructive apneas and hypopneas.
[f] A statistical significant reduction in BMI was noted at 18 months after bariatric surgery (pre-BMI 53.9 ± 15.7 vs post-BMI 37.8 ± 14.8 kg/m²; *P*<.001).
[g] Multimodality surgery refers to simultaneous nasal, palate, and/or base of tongue surgery for OSA.

including early postoperative pharyngeal edema,[130,131] with up to 59% complaining of persistent side effects (27% difficulty swallowing; 27% globus sensation in throat) after LAUP.[127]

Midline glossectomy

Surgical removal of the center portion of the tongue base (usually via laser) was proposed by Fujita and colleagues[132] and Woodson and Fujita[133] in 1991 for the treatment of OSA in patients with hyopharyngeal obstruction. A review of 5 case series (n = 74) showed a surgical success rate of approximately 50% (see **Table 3**).[134] Postoperative bleeding and pharyngeal edema requiring protective tracheostomy is not uncommon after surgery.[132,133]

Radiofrequency ablation of the tongue

Radiofrequency ablation uses a probe to precisely direct temperature-controlled radiofrequency energy to heat (between 60 and 90°C) and ablate target tissues without causing collateral damage to adjoining structures.[135] Radiofrequency treatment of the tongue base does not require general anesthesia, but usually requires multiple treatment sessions over several weeks, and is successful at eliminating snoring.[135–137] Eleven case series describing 394 patients with OSA (mean AHI 37/h) undergoing radiofrequency ablation of the tongue reported a surgical success rate of only 36% (see **Table 3**).[134] Statistically significant improvements in subjective daytime sleepiness and health-related quality of life were observed in most, but not all studies.[135,138–145] Radiofrequency ablation of the tongue is generally considered adjunctive (not primary) OSA treatment in select patients.[134]

Radiofrequency ablation of the turbinates (and other nasal procedures)

A relationship between nasal obstruction, mouth breathing and symptoms of OSA was first described in the 1800s.[146–150] Increased nasal resistance may result from septal deviation, turbinate hypertrophy, chronic nasal congestion, polyps, or collapsible valves. Various procedures include polypectomy, radiofrequency ablation of the turbinates, alar valve or rim reconstruction, and septoplasty (eg, straightening of the septum). Nasal surgery is generally not curative,[151,152] but can improve the AHI, and is often used in a multimodality surgical approach or to decrease CPAP pressure requirements.[153–155] In addition, surgical correction of nasal obstruction improves health-related quality of life in patients with OSA.[156]

Inferior turbinate enlargement is a frequent cause of nasal obstruction. Radiofrequency ablation is a highly successful surgical procedure producing volumetric inferior turbinate reduction. Radiofrequency ablation heats the hypertrophied turbinates causing scar tissue with resulting shrinkage over 1 to 3 weeks.[157] This procedure is generally performed in the outpatient setting with minimal discomfort beyond nasal stuffiness lasting 3 to 5 days.[158]

Radiofrequency volumetric soft palate tissue reduction (somnoplasty)

Somnoplasty involves directed radiofrequency energy to ablate and reduce soft tissues of the palate.[157,159–161] Decreased snoring occurs via scar-induced stabilization of the soft palate. Although symptom (eg, snoring) improvement after surgery is reported,[136,162] evidence for improvement of OSA is lacking.[163–165] A recent randomized placebo-controlled trial in patients with mild OSA found no statistically significant improvement in the AHI or symptoms after somnoplasty.[166]

Tonsillectomy

Tonsillectomy is one of the most common surgical procedures in children.[167,168] OSA is a frequent indication for tonsillectomy and is considered first-line therapy for children with OSA.[167,169] Surgical tonsillectomy techniques vary, but generally complete resection of the tonsils with adenoidectomy (if necessary) is preferred **(Fig. 1)**.[170] Partial intracapsular tonsillectomy (eg, tonsillotomy) has been found to reduce postoperative morbidity (eg, pain),[171–175] but postoperative objective measures of efficacy (eg, AHI reduction) are lacking.[176]

Tonsillectomy is curative (AHI <1/h) in 60% of pediatric cases of OSA (see **Table 3**).[177,178] Higher presurgery AHI and body mass index (BMI, calculated as weight in kilograms divided by the square of height in meters) are risk factors for residual disease after tonsillectomy.[179,180] In complicated cases of pediatric OSA (eg, morbid obesity, severe OSA), tonsillectomy is curative in 39% of children compared with 74% in uncomplicated cases.[178] Children with residual OSA after tonsillectomy may benefit from rapid maxillary expansion.[181] Tonsillectomy improves quality of life parameters (short- and long-term) in children with OSA,[182,183] with improvements in behavior scores[184] and sleep disturbances.[185,186]

Self-limited pain and swelling of the throat is common after tonsillectomy. Risks for postoperative complications include younger age (<24 months), increased severity of OSA, craniofacial abnormalities, obesity, poor functional status (eg, hypotonia, failure to thrive) and cor pulmonale.[182,187] Life-threatening complications are rare,[188] but postoperative respiratory failure requiring mechanical ventilation (usually transiently during postsurgery recovery) occurs in approximately 30% of children.[187,189] However, children left intubated electively after tonsillectomy have higher complication rates.[190] Hemorrhage, dehydration, and pulmonary edema occur in approximately 9% of cases.[191]

Uvulopalatopharyngoplasty

Fujita and colleagues[23] and Conway and colleagues[24] adapted Ikematsu's surgical snoring procedure[22] and reported his uvulopalatopharyngoplasty (UPPP) results for treating OSA in 1980. This operation enlarges the oropharyngeal airway lumen by

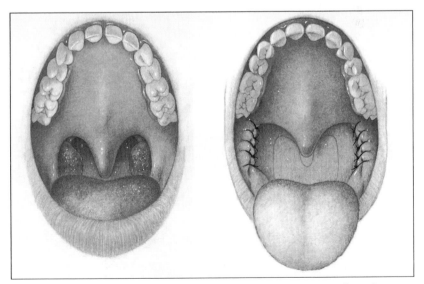

Fig. 1. Tonsillectomy. The primary treatment of OSA in children with tonsillar enlargement is tonsillectomy usually with concurrent adenoidectomy. To prevent collapse and improve OSA success, it is preferable that the lateral pharyngeal walls are sutured.

excising redundant tissues from the soft palate, tonsillar pillars, and uvula (**Fig. 2**). UPPP is currently the most widely performed OSA pharyngeal surgical technique in adults.[77] Several variations of the UPPP have been proposed including the methods of Fujita and colleagues,[23,192,193] Simmons and colleagues,[194] Fairbanks,[195] Dickson and Blokmanis,[196] Friedman and colleagues,[197] and Powell and colleagues[198] (uvulo-palatal flap surgery). Uvulopalatal flap surgery (**Fig. 3**) reduces the risk of nasopharyn-geal incompetence and is associated with less postoperative pain, but is contraindicated in patients with excessively long or bulky soft palates (or uvulas).[199–201] Woodson and Toohill[202] developed transpalatal advancement phar-yngoplasty, which combines a UPPP with removal of the posterior hard palate (via a curvilinear palatal incision), with subsequent advancement of the mucoperiosteal flap and suturing to the alveolar mucoperiosteum (**Fig. 4**). This technique is associated with a decrease in retropalatal collapsibility and an increase in the retropalatal airspace compared with traditional UPPP, and may provide higher surgical success and cure rates.[201,203]

There are no known randomized controlled trials of UPPP that assess pre- and post-surgery AHI,[74,204,205] and many studies do not report objective postsurgery sleep data.[206] One randomized trial found no statistically significant difference in the oxygen desaturation index between the surgery and conservative management groups.[204,207] UPPP is highly effective for eliminating snoring, with success rates between 70% and 90%.[193] However, several meta-analysis have reported surgical success rates for OSA between 40% and 60%, and a surgical cure rate (an AHI <5/h) of only 16%

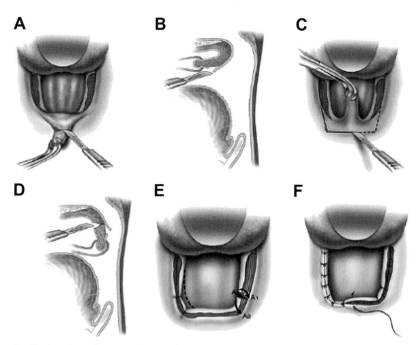

Fig. 2. Uvulopalatopharyngoplasty. This operation enlarges the oropharyngeal airway lumen by excising redundant tissues from the soft palate, tonsillar pillars, and uvula. Shown is Friedman's submucosal uvulopalatopharyngoplasty technique (*A–F*). (*Reproduced from* Friedman M, Schalch P. Surgery of the palate and oropharynx. Otolaryngol Clin N Am 2007;40:835; with permission from Elsevier.)

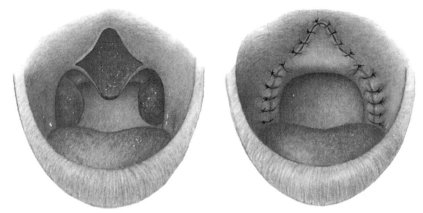

Fig. 3. Uvulopalatal flap. A modification of Fujita's uvulopalatopharyngoplasty involves retracting and advancing the uvula superiorly under the soft palate without removal.

(see **Table 3**).[74,75,134] A recent retrospective analysis of the Mayo Clinic experience found a similar UPPP cure rate of 24%.[208] Predictors of surgical cure in this analysis included younger age, lower preoperative BMI and AHI. Unfortunately, most patients with initial improvement in AHI after UPPP have recurrence within 5 years of therapy.[209] Fortunately, UPPP likely confers a mortality benefit in CPAP intolerant

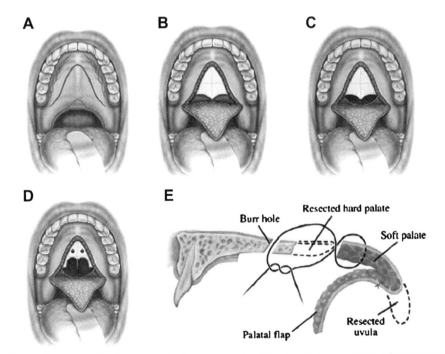

Fig. 4. Transpalatal advancement pharyngoplasty. Woodson's transpalatal advancement pharyngoplasty combines a uvulopalatopharyngoplasty with soft palate advancement. (*Reproduced from* Friedman M, Schalch P. Surgery of the palate and oropharynx. Otolaryngol Clin N Am 2007;40:840; with permission from Elsevier.)

patients (compared with no treatment), even when most patients do not obtain surgical cure.[210–212] However, because UPPP is likely to eliminate snoring but will often leave residual OSA causing silent apnea, all patients must have postoperative sleep studies to rule out persistent disease.

UPPP is generally more effective at reducing apneas than hypopneas,[75,193] and is most effective in patients with primarily oropharyngeal obstruction (as opposed to hypopharyngeal abnormalities).[70,193] However, using fiberoptic endoscopy to select patients with predominantly soft palate pharyngeal collapse during a Müller maneuver has shown variable improvement in surgical success (45%–85%).[213–216] Although the efficacy to cure OSA is suboptimal, UPPP may be useful in lowering positive airway pressure requirements, thus improving CPAP compliance in select patients.[217] However, UPPP may promote air leak during future CPAP therapy,[218,219] although a recent study disputes this finding.[220] Approximately 70% of patients are satisfied after UPPP.[221,222]

Early postoperative complications include wound dehiscence, hemorrhage, infection, and transient velopharyngeal incompetence (eg, nasal regurgitation and hypernasal speech).[195] Late postoperative complications include pharyngeal discomfort (eg, dryness, tightness), postnasal secretions, dysphagia, inability to initiate swallowing, odynophagia, nasopharyngeal stenosis, taste and speech disturbances, tongue numbness, and rarely permanent velopharyngeal incompetence. Up to 30% of patients complain of persistent although generally mild dysphagia.[223–226] A systematic review reported a serious complication rate of 2.5% with 30 deaths (~0.2% mortality) and persistent side effects in 58% (31% nasal regurgitation, 13% voice changes, 5% taste disturbances) of patients after UPPP.[127] Voice changes are generally mild.[227] A recent study noted that health-related quality of life measurements were better in patients with post-UPPP side effects compared with CPAP users (independent of compliance) with side effects.[228]

Procedures that Modify or Advance the Skeletal or Soft Tissue Structures

Genioglossus advancement

In the mid-1980s, Riley and colleagues[229,230] first described genioglossus muscle advancement (GA) to improve the posterior airspace (eg, base of tongue). Their initial technique (a modified horizontal mandibular osteotomy) was later improved in 1986 to include a limited inferior parasagittal mandibular osteotomy (**Fig. 5**).[230,231] Advancing the geniotubercle forward of the mandible positions the genioglossus and geniohyoid muscles anteriorly, thus enlarging the retrolinguinal space.[232] Variations of this procedure include mortised genioplasty, circle genioplasty, and standard genioplasty.[233,234] Four case series describing 91 patients with severe OSA (mean AHI 54/h) undergoing GA as sole treatment report a surgical success rate of 67% (range 39%–79%) (see **Table 3**).[134] GA is generally used within a multimodality approach to treat base of tongue obstructions.

Hyoid myotomy and suspension

In the mid-1980s, Riley and collagues[229,230,235] developed a hyoid suspension procedure to improve the posterior (retrolinguinal) airspace (**Fig. 6**). The hyoid bone is located in the anterior neck below the mandible and is involved in maintaining upper airway patency.[236,237] Several protocols have been described including hyoid to mandibular suspension (hypomandibular), hyoid to thyroid cartilage suspension (thyrohyoid), and hyoid expansion.[238] Hyoid suspension is generally used within a multimodality approach[238–240] with a surgical success rate (performed with previous or concurrent palate surgery) of approximately 50% (see **Table 3**).[134] However, there

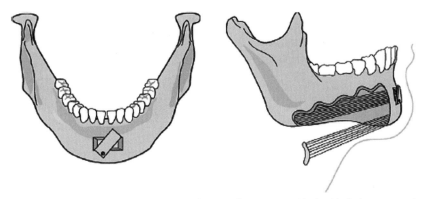

Fig. 5. Mandibular osteotomy with genioglossus advancement. Limited inferior parasagittal mandibular osteotomy (eg, a rectangular window in the symphyseal bone with advancement, rotation, and immobilization of the geniotubercle) with advancement of the genioglossus and geniohyoid muscles. (*Reproduced from* Li KL. Hypopharyngeal airway surgery. Otolaryngol Clin N Am 2007;40:848; with permission from Elsevier.)

are no reliable preoperative predictors for success with hyoid suspension following UPPP.[241] Furthermore, combining genioglossus advancement with hyoid suspension marginally improves surgical success (~55%) (see **Table 3**),[134] and 1 study of hyoid suspension with radiofrequency of the tongue reported a surgical success rate of only 49%.[242] Excessive daytime sleepiness generally improves after hyoid suspension, albeit inconsistently.[239,243–246]

Mandibular (or maxillary) distraction osteogenesis

Distraction osteogenesis (DO) of the mandible (and/or maxilla) involves bilateral segmental osteomies followed by gradual distraction (via an expandable intra- or extraoral device) with subsequent ossification and bone lengthening.[247] DO of the mandible effectively improves OSA in children with genetic craniofacial abnormalities.[248–251] One study of 5 otherwise normal adults with OSA reported a decrease in AHI from 49/h to 7/h after mandibular (or maxillary) DO.[247] However, this study

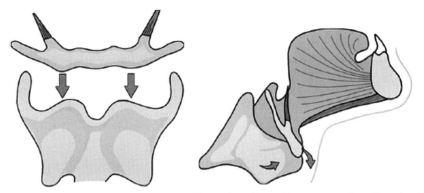

Fig. 6. Hyoid myotomy suspension. Hyoid to thyroid cartilage suspension (thyrohyoid) involves isolation of the hyoid bone that is advanced, sutured, and immobilized to the thyroid cartilage. (*Reproduced from* Li KL. Hypopharyngeal airway surgery. Otolaryngol Clin N Am 2007;40:848; with permission from Elsevier.)

reported several problems with DO including the technical difficulty of the procedure, a high risk of malocclusion, subsequent need for orthodontics because of limited control of the distractor vector, and poor patient satisfaction (eg, treatment required 4 months of stabilization via intraoral arch bars that inhibited mastication and speech).

Maxillomandibular advancement

In 1979, Kuo and colleagues[20] reported improvements in polysomnographic parameters and subjective sleepiness in 3 patients with OSA with retrognathia after mandibular osteotomy with advancement. Similar improvements in OSA parameters after mandibular advancement were noted by others.[21,252,253] However, by the mid-1980s, mandibular advancement alone was largely supplanted by combined maxillary and mandibular advancement to preserve the maxilla-mandibular relationship and from the recognition that the physiologic cause for OSA is often from concomitant mandibular and maxillary deficiency.[235,254] Mandibular osteotomy with advancement is currently relegated to the treatment of mandibular hypolasia in syndromic children with OSA.[255]

Maxillomandibular advancement (MMA) involves Le Fort I maxillary and bilateral sagittal ramus split mandibular osteomies with advancement of the maxilla and mandible followed by rigid fixation (**Fig. 7**).[256] Generally, the maxilla is advanced first, with the mandible advanced into occlusion. Combined MMA alleviates pharyngeal obstruction by expanding the skeletal framework that the tongue and other soft tissue

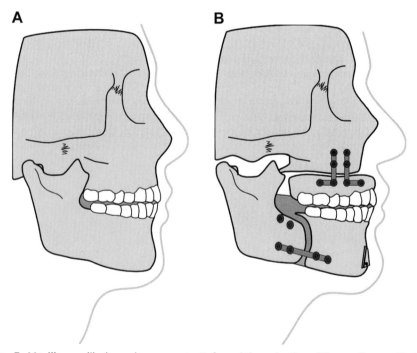

A   **B**

Fig. 7. Maxillomandibular advancement. Before (*A*) and after (*B*) maxillomandibular advancement surgery via a Le Fort I osteotomy (with rigid plate fixation) and bilateral sagittal split mandibular osteotomy (with bicortical screw fixation). (*Reproduced and modified from* Li KL. Hypopharyngeal airway surgery. Otolaryngol Clin N Am 2007;40:849; with permission from Elsevier.)

structures attach to resulting in reduced upper-airway restriction and collapsibility during inspiration.[257] Mandibular advancement advances the tongue and suprahyoid muscles.[258] Maxillary advancement pulls forward the velum and velopharyngeal muscles,[259] increases the nasopharyngeal and hypopharyngeal spaces,[260,261] and increases alar width with a concomitant decrease in nasal airway resistance.[262,263] Improvements in pharyngeal obstruction after MMA occur along the entire upper airway in the lateral and anteroposterior dimensions.[27,264]

MMA is the most effective craniofacial surgery (in adults) for the treatment of OSA.[76,265] A recent meta-analysis of 22 studies (627 subjects with OSA) determined that MMA is highly effective with a mean decrease in AHI from 64/h to 11/h ($P<.001$) with pooled surgical success and cure (AHI <5/h) rates of 86% and 43%, respectively (see **Table 3**).[266] Predictors of increased surgical success include younger age, lower preoperative AHI and BMI, and greater degree of maxillary advancement.[266] Furthermore, MMA maintains its efficacy at long-term follow-up.[267,268] Following MMA, most patients report improvements in health-related quality of life, depression, excessive daytime sleepiness, memory impairment, and hypertension.[267,269–279] Candidates for MMA include adults and adolescents (after the cranial sutures have completely ossified) with maxillomandibular insufficiency or those who have failed previous therapeutic interventions for OSA.[256,265] In addition, MMA is successful in patients with obesity or with severe OSA.[265]

MMA is generally safe with no reported deaths and a major complication rate of only 1.0% (mostly cardiac causes).[266] Between 0% and 15% of MMA patients experience mild surgical relapse without apparent symptoms or worsening of the AHI.[267,280–282] However, relapse is not associated with the degree of mandibular advancement.[281,283,284] Mild malocclusion occurs in up to 44% of patients and is generally treatable with prosthetics or minor occlusional equilibration.[267,285] Transient facial paresthesia (ie, inferior alveolar nerve neurosensory deficits) after MMA is common (~100%), although most cases (86%) resolve within 1 year.[266] Velopharyngeal insufficiency or mild speech and swallowing deficits are rarely reported after MMA.[272,280,286,287] Patients completing sequential phase I (UPPP) and phase II (MMA) surgery generally report less pain after MMA compared with phase I surgery.[287,288] The average hospitalization time is less than 1 week with most patients returning to work within 4 to 10 weeks after surgery.[275,288]

After MMA, most patients report a positive perception of facial aesthetics.[289] Li and colleagues[289,290] noted 6 months after surgery that 50% of patients report a younger facial appearance, 36% report a more attractive appearance, and only 9% report a less attractive facial appearance. In this same study, all patients (100%) reported satisfaction with the surgical outcome. Three other studies reported no patients (0%) were bothered by postoperative facial aesthetics.[272,274,286] Modified MMA techniques, particularly using counterclockwise rotation and pre- or postsurgical orthodontics, have been developed to prevent maxillary protrusion and improve aesthetics.[291]

Maxillomandibular expansion

Surgically assisted maxillomandibular expansion (MME; limited osteotomy at Le Fort I level and midline maxilla followed by expansion) may be an effective therapy for OSA in adults (**Fig. 8**).[292,293] One study (n = 6) reported improvements in excessive daytime sleepiness and OSA (AHI from 13/h to 5/h) at a mean follow-up of 18 months after an average mandibular and maxillary expansion of 9.5 and 10.3 mm, respectively.[293] The investigators concluded that nonobese adolescents or young adults with mild OSA and who require orthodontic treatment are ideal candidates for MME.

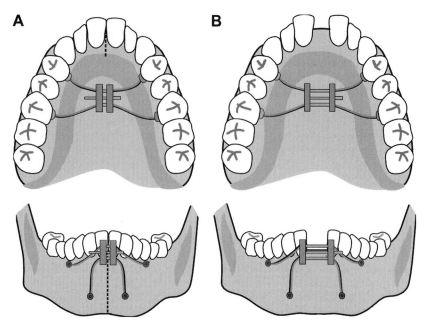

Fig. 8. Maxillomandibular expansion. Before (*A*) and after (*B*) surgically assisted maxillo-mandibular expansion with Le Fort I osteotomy and pterygomaxillary (midline) dysjunction followed by expansion using a orthodontic screwlike device.

Pillar palatal implants

This minimally invasive procedure involves inserting matchstick size rigid polyester implants via a hollow needle delivery tool into the soft palate.[294] Pillar implants improve snoring by stiffening the soft palate, but their effect on OSA is less clear and the long-term benefits on OSA are unknown.[295–298] In a prospective nonrandomized trial of 25 patients with mild-moderate OSA (mean AHI 16.2/h), the surgical success and cure rates were 40% and 28%, respectively.[296] Friedman and colleagues[295] in a randomized trial of 62 nonobese patients with mild-moderate OSA (mean AHI 23.5/h), found a statistically significant improvement in AHI after pillar implants (compared with placebo procedure), although the mean AHI after surgery was still within the moderate range (mean AHI 15.9/h) with a surgical success rate of 45%. Complications are rare, but include infrequent postinsertion extrusion.

Rapid maxillary expansion

In 1860, Angell[299] reported the first use of rapid maxillary expansion (RME) to correct a transverse maxillary deficiency. RME is currently a common orthodontic procedure to correct dental crowding and to ensure a normal mandibular-maxillary relationship.[300] RME expands the mid-palatal suture via a screw-type orthodontic appliance resulting in an increase in the upper transverse width.[300] RME induces normal tongue positioning via palatal widening and flattening, downward and forward displacement of the maxilla, widening of the nasal vault (with subsequent decreased resistance and improvement in nasal breathing) and transforms a class III to a class I prognathoid position.[301–312] After 2 to 4 weeks of expansion, a 2- to 6-month retention period is necessary while ossification between the expanded mid-palatal suture line is completed.[304] The suture line in prepubertal children is cartilaginous and easily separated, but horizontal osteotomy is often required in adults (whose suture line is generally ossified) before RME.[313]

Children without known OSA often report quieter nighttime breathing, reduced snoring, and improved sleep quality after RME.[303,314,315] In 1996, Palmisano and colleagues[316] reported the first use of RME to successfully treat OSA (AHI went from 22/h to 4/h) in a 22-year-old with maxillary constriction and a class I malocclusion. Subsequently, 3 studies evaluating RME in children with OSA (n = 88; mean expansion 6.2 ± 2.1 mm)[181,317–319] reported a mean decrease in AHI from 11/h to 0.8/h after RME ($P<.001$) with subjective improvements in snoring, excessive daytime sleepiness, and behavioral problems (see **Table 3**).[320] One study of 10 adults with OSA who received surgically assisted RME (mean expansion 12.1 mm) reported statistically significant improvements in AHI (19/h to 4/h; $P<.05$) with a 70% cure rate (AHI <5/h).[321]

SINGLE-STAGE MULTIMODALITY APPROACH

Pharyngeal surgeries are often combined to address airway obstruction(s) at multiple levels (eg, nose, palate, tonsils, hypopharynx). Multilevel surgery may improve surgical success compared with single-site therapy.[322–324] The most common single-stage multimodality procedure combines UPPP with a second procedure designed to improve the hypopharyngeal airway (eg, genioglossal advancement, hyoid suspension, base of tongue resection [uvulopalatopharyngoglossoplasty]). Lin and colleagues[74] in a meta-analysis of 58 studies emphasized the benefits of a multimodality approach reporting a surgical success rate of 66% (see **Table 3**).

Unfortunately, multimodality surgery does not always guarantee increased efficacy. A meta-analysis of hypopharyngeal surgery by Kezirian and Goldberg[134] concluded combination procedures such as genioglossus advancement with hyoid suspension or tongue radiofrequency treatment with tongue stabilization have lower surgical success rates and poorer AHI improvement compared with the same procedures performed alone.

STAGED SURGICAL PROTOCOL

The Riley-Powell-Stanford surgical protocol was developed to address the multilevel airway abnormalities that often contribute to OSA (**Fig. 9**).[325] Phase 1 consists of interventions directed at the site(s) of obstruction in the nasal, pharyngeal, or hyopharyngeal regions (eg, UPPP for oropharyngeal obstruction, genioglossus advancement for hypopharyngeal obstruction).[326] Approximately 6 months after surgery, repeat polysomnography is performed and patients who do not obtain surgical success (or cure), proceed to phase 2 surgery consisting of MMA.[327] The Stanford group reports a staged protocol surgical success rate of 95%.[325]

However, the appropriateness of the staged protocol has been questioned. Wagner and colleagues[274] noted that two-thirds of their MMA failures had previous phase 1 surgery (eg, UPPP). Others have proposed that MMA should be performed first with UPPP (or other palatal and hypopharyngeal surgeries) performed in those patients with residual OSA.[268] A review by the American Sleep Disorders Association found insufficient evidence to assess the efficacy of a staged verses primary MMA surgical approach.[75] A recent meta-analysis of MMA found that patients with previous UPPP before MMA were less likely to obtain surgical cure (25% vs 45%; $P = .002$) compared with those without previous surgery following MMA.[266] However, this finding was likely confounded by greater obesity and more severe OSA in patients with previous palatal surgery. The investigators concluded that, "further research is needed to identify

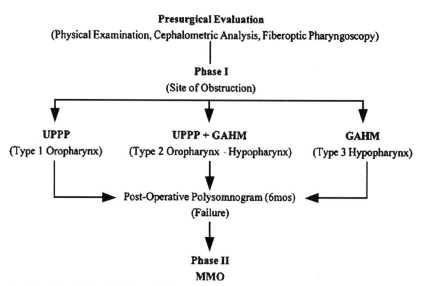

Presurgical Evaluation
(Physical Examination, Cephalometric Analysis, Fiberoptic Pharyngoscopy)

Phase I
(Site of Obstruction)

UPPP	UPPP + GAHM	GAHM
(Type 1 Oropharynx)	(Type 2 Oropharynx · Hypopharynx)	(Type 3 Hypopharynx)

Post-Operative Polysomnogram (6mos)
(Failure)

Phase II
MMO

Fig. 9. Riley-Powell-Stanford surgical staged protocol. (*Reproduced from* Riley RW, Powell ND, Li KK, et al. Surgery and obstructive sleep apnea: long-term clinical outcomes. Otolaryngol Head Neck Surg 2000;122:416; with permission from Mosby-Year Book, Inc.)

preoperative patient and clinical characteristics to select those patients who would benefit most from a staged versus primary MMA surgical approach."[266]

BARIATRIC SURGERY

Approximately 65% of adults in the United States are overweight (BMI >25 kg/m^2) and more than 30% are obese (BMI >30 kg/m^2).[328] Surgically induced weight loss was first performed in 1967[329] and is now a preferred weight reduction modality for morbidly obese individuals (BMI ≥40 kg/m^2) with more than 100,000 procedures performed annually in the United States.[330] Bariatric surgery is generally safe, results in marked and sustained weight loss, and is associated with improved mortality compared with conventional weight-loss strategies.[331–333] Procedures are classified as predominantly malabsorptive (eg, biliopancreatic diversion, duodenal switch, jejunoileal bypass), predominantly restrictive (eg, vertical banded gastroplasty, adjustable gastric banding, sleeve gastrectomy, intragastric balloon), or combined malabsorptive and restrictive (eg, Roux-en-Y gastric bypass, sleeve gastrectomy with duodenal switch).[333] Candidates for bariatric surgery should fulfill the 1991 National Institutes of Health guideline criteria that includes a BMI ≥40 kg/m^2, or a BMI ≥35 kg/m^2 with associated comorbidity (eg, OSA).[334,335]

Obesity is a leading cause of OSA with an estimated 40% prevalence in obese persons (BMI ≥30 kg/m^2).[336] A 10% increase in BMI results in a 32% increase in the AHI.[336] Mild to moderate weight reduction can improve sleep apnea and daytime sleepiness.[336,337] Two recent meta-analyses have evaluated the effectiveness of bariatric surgery to treat OSA.[338,339] Holty and colleagues[339] found OSA to be highly prevalent (79%) among bariatric candidates (of these 76% had moderate to severe disease), but exceedingly underdiagnosed (only 30% preoperatively). There were no identifiable presurgical symptoms or clinical findings predictive of polysomnographically confirmed OSA.[339] Greenberg and colleagues[338] noted that after surgically induced weight loss (BMI went from 55 to 38 kg/m^2), the AHI improved from 55 to 16/h (see **Table 3**). However, more than 50% of bariatric recipients with preoperative OSA have residual disease despite weight loss.[339] Predictors of greater AHI reduction (or OSA cure) included younger age, but not symptom improvement (eg, excessive daytime sleepiness) or the degree of BMI change.[338,339] In addition, initial improvements in AHI appeared to wane at follow-up despite maintained weight loss.[339]

SUMMARY

OSA is a prevalent condition associated with increased morbidity and mortality. Although CPAP is the preferred treatment, poor compliance is common. Fortunately, several surgical treatments exist to address a variety of pharyngeal abnormalities. Case series suggest that MMA has the highest surgical efficacy (86%) and cure rate (43%). Morbidly obese individuals may benefit from bariatric surgery, although less than 50% are cured after surgically induced weight loss. Soft palate surgical techniques are less successful, with UPPP having an OSA surgical success and cure rate of 50% and 16%, respectively. Patients may benefit from a multimodality surgical approach. In conclusion, individuals intolerant of CPAP may benefit from surgical therapies that address their particular airway obstruction(s). However, further research is needed to more thoroughly assess clinical outcomes (eg, quality of life, morbidity), better identify key preoperative patient and clinical characteristics that predict success, and confirm long-term effectiveness of surgical modalities to treat OSA.

ACKNOWLEDGMENTS

We thank Kasey K. Li, MD, DDS, for graciously providing the figures illustrating tonsillectomy, uvulopalatal flap, and maxillomandibular expansion procedures.

REFERENCES

1. Guilleminault C, Tilkian A, Dement WC. The sleep apnea syndromes. Annu Rev Med 1976;27:465–84.
2. Young T, Finn L, Peppard PE, et al. Sleep disordered breathing and mortality: eighteen-year follow-up of the Wisconsin sleep cohort. Sleep 2008;31(8):1071–8.
3. Duran J, Esnaola S, Rubio R, et al. Obstructive sleep apnea-hypopnea and related clinical features in a population-based sample of subjects aged 30 to 70 yr. Am J Respir Crit Care Med 2001;163(3 Pt 1):685–9.
4. Sogut A, Altin R, Uzun L, et al. Prevalence of obstructive sleep apnea syndrome and associated symptoms in 3–11-year-old Turkish children. Pediatr Pulmonol 2005;39(3):251–6.
5. Brunetti L, Rana S, Lospalluti ML, et al. Prevalence of obstructive sleep apnea syndrome in a cohort of 1,207 children of southern Italy. Chest 2001;120(6):1930–5.
6. Redline S, Tishler PV, Schluchter M, et al. Risk factors for sleep-disordered breathing in children. Associations with obesity, race, and respiratory problems. Am J Respir Crit Care Med 1999;159(5 Pt 1):1527–32.
7. Lumeng JC, Chervin RD, Lumeng JC, et al. Epidemiology of pediatric obstructive sleep apnea. Proc Am Thorac Soc 2008;5(2):242–52.
8. Young T, Peppard PE, Gottlieb DJ. Epidemiology of obstructive sleep apnea: a population health perspective. Am J Respir Crit Care Med 2002;165(9):1217–39.

9. Sullivan CE, Issa FG, Berthon-Jones M, et al. Reversal of obstructive sleep apnoea by continuous positive airway pressure applied through the nares. Lancet 1981;1(8225):862–5.

10. Indications and standards for use of nasal continuous positive airway pressure (CPAP) in sleep apnea syndromes. Am J Respir Crit Care Med 1994;150:1738–45.

11. Giles TL, Lasserson TJ, Smith BJ, et al. Continuous positive airways pressure for obstructive sleep apnoea in adults. Cochrane Database Syst Rev 2006;(3): CD001106.

12. Gay P, Weaver T, Loube D, et al. Evaluation of positive airway pressure treatment for sleep related breathing disorders in adults. Sleep 2006;29(3):381–401.

13. Jenkinson C, Davies RJ, Mullins R, et al. Comparison of therapeutic and subtherapeutic nasal continuous positive airway pressure for obstructive sleep apnoea: a randomised prospective parallel trial. Lancet 1999;353(9170):2100–5.

14. Weaver TE, Grunstein RR. Adherence to continuous positive airway pressure therapy: the challenge to effective treatment. Proc Am Thorac Soc 2008;5(2): 173–8.

15. Engleman HM, Wild MR. Improving CPAP use by patients with sleep apnoea/hypopnoea syndrome (SAHS). Sleep Med Rev 2003;7(1):81–99.

16. Campos-Rodriguez F, Pena-Grinan N, Reyes-Nunez N, et al. Mortality in obstructive sleep apnea-hypopnea patients treated with positive airway pressure. Chest 2005;128(2):624–33.

17. Yaggi HK, Concato J, Kernan WN, et al. Obstructive sleep apnea as a risk factor for stroke and death. N Engl J Med 2005;353(19):2034–41.

18. Rapoport DM, Sorkin B, Garay SM, et al. Reversal of the "Pickwickian syndrome" by long-term use of nocturnal nasal-airway pressure. N Engl J Med 1982; 307(15):931–3.

19. Kuhlo W, Doll E, Frank MC. [Successful management of Pickwickian Syndrome using long term tracheostomy]. Dtsch Med Wochenschr 1969;94(24):1286–90 [in German].

20. Kuo PC, West RA, Bloomquist DS, et al. The effect of mandibular osteotomy in three patients with hypersomnia sleep apnea. Oral Surg Oral Med Oral Pathol 1979;48(5):385–92.

21. Bear SE, Priest JH. Sleep apnea syndrome: correction with surgical advancement of the mandible. J Oral Surg 1980;38(7):543–9.

22. Ikematsu T. [Study of snoring. 4th report]. J Jpn Otol Rhinol Laryngol Soc 1964; 64:434–5 [in Japanese].

23. Fujita S, Conway W, Zorick F, et al. Surgical correction of anatomic abnormalities in obstructive sleep apnea syndrome: uvulopalatopharyngoplasty. Otolaryngol Head Neck Surg 1981;89(6):923–34.

24. Conway W, Fujita S, Zorick F, et al. Uvulo-palato-pharyngoplasty in treatment of upper airway sleep apnea [abstract]. Am Rev Respir Dis 1980;121(Suppl):121.

25. Johns FR, Strollo PJ Jr, Buckley M, et al. The influence of craniofacial structure on obstructive sleep apnea in young adults. J Oral Maxillofac Surg 1998;56(5): 596–602.

26. Rojewski TE, Schuller DE, Clark RW, et al. Videoendoscopic determination of the mechanism of obstruction in obstructive sleep apnea. Otolaryngol Head Neck Surg 1984;92(2):127–31.

27. Fairburn SC, Waite PD, Vilos G, et al. Three-dimensional changes in upper airways of patients with obstructive sleep apnea following maxillomandibular advancement. J Oral Maxillofac Surg 2007;65(1):6–12.

28. Suto Y, Matsuo T, Kato T, et al. Evaluation of the pharyngeal airway in patients with sleep apnea: value of ultrafast MR imaging. AJR Am J Roentgenol 1993; 160(2):311–4.

29. Nishino T. Physiological and pathophysiological implications of upper airway reflexes in humans. Jpn J Physiol 2000;50(1):3–14.

30. Pierce RJ, Worsnop CJ. Upper airway function and dysfunction in respiration. Clin Exp Pharmacol Physiol 1999;26(1):1–10.

31. Brouillette RT, Thach BT. A neuromuscular mechanism maintaining extrathoracic airway patency. J Appl Physiol 1979;46(4):772–9.

32. Remmers JE, deGroot WJ, Sauerland EK, et al. Pathogenesis of upper airway occlusion during sleep. J Appl Physiol 1978;44(6):931–8.

33. Petrof BJ, Hendricks JC, Pack AI. Does upper airway muscle injury trigger a vicious cycle in obstructive sleep apnea? A hypothesis. Sleep 1996;19(6): 465–71.

34. Schwab RJ, Gefter WB, Hoffman EA, et al. Dynamic upper airway imaging during awake respiration in normal subjects and patients with sleep disordered breathing. Am Rev Respir Dis 1993;148(5):1385–400.

35. Kushida CA, Efron B, Guilleminault C. A predictive morphometric model for the obstructive sleep apnea syndrome. Ann Intern Med 1997;127(8 Pt 1):581–7.

36. Schwab RJ, Gupta KB, Gefter WB, et al. Upper airway and soft tissue anatomy in normal subjects and patients with sleep-disordered breathing. Significance of the lateral pharyngeal walls. Am J Respir Crit Care Med 1995;152(5 Pt 1): 1673–89.

37. Rodenstein DO, Dooms G, Thomas Y, et al. Pharyngeal shape and dimensions in healthy subjects, snorers, and patients with obstructive sleep apnoea. Thorax 1990;45(10):722–7.

38. Lee SH, Choi JH, Shin C, et al. How does open-mouth breathing influence upper airway anatomy? Laryngoscope 2007;117(6):1102–6.

39. Chen W, Kushida CA. Nasal obstruction in sleep-disordered breathing. Otolaryngol Clin North Am 2003;36(3):437–60.

40. Konno A, Togawa K, Hoshino T. The effect of nasal obstruction in infancy and early childhood upon ventilation. Laryngoscope 1980;90(4):699–707.

41. Olsen KD, Kern EB, Westbrook PR. Sleep and breathing disturbance secondary to nasal obstruction. Otolaryngol Head Neck Surg 1981;89(5):804–10.

42. Zwillich CW, Pickett C, Hanson FN, et al. Disturbed sleep and prolonged apnea during nasal obstruction in normal men. Am Rev Respir Dis 1981;124(2): 158–60.

43. Rubin A, Phillipson E, Lavie P. The effects of airway anesthesia on breathing in sleep [abstract]. Chest 1983;84:337.

44. Patil SP, Schneider H, Marx JJ, et al. Neuromechanical control of upper airway patency during sleep. J Appl Physiol 2007;102(2):547–56.

45. Guilleminault C, Huang YS, Kirisoglu C, et al. Is obstructive sleep apnea syndrome a neurological disorder? A continuous positive airway pressure follow-up study. Ann Neurol 2005;58(6):880–7.

46. Kuna ST, Bedi DG, Ryckman C. Effect of nasal airway positive pressure on upper airway size and configuration. Am Rev Respir Dis 1988;138(4):969–75.

47. Edstrom L, Larsson H, Larsson L. Neurogenic effects on the palatopharyngeal muscle in patients with obstructive sleep apnoea: a muscle biopsy study. J Neurol Neurosurg Psychiatr 1992;55(10):916–20.

48. Woodson BT, Garancis JC, Toohill RJ. Histopathologic changes in snoring and obstructive sleep apnea syndrome. Laryngoscope 1991;101(12 Pt 1):1318–22.

49. McGinley BM, Schwartz AR, Schneider H, et al. Upper airway neuromuscular compensation during sleep is defective in obstructive sleep apnea. J Appl Physiol 2008;105(1):197–205.

50. Fregosi RF, Quan SF, Morgan WL, et al. Pharyngeal critical pressure in children with mild sleep-disordered breathing. J Appl Physiol 2006;101(3):734–9.

51. Marcus CL, Katz ES, Lutz J, et al. Upper airway dynamic responses in children with the obstructive sleep apnea syndrome. Pediatr Res 2005;57(1):99–107.

52. Troell RJ, Riley RW, Powell NB, et al. Surgical management of the hypopharyngeal airway in sleep disordered breathing. Otolaryngol Clin North Am 1998;31(6):979–1012.

53. Powell NB, Riley RW, Guilleminault C, et al. Obstructive sleep apnea, continuous positive airway pressure, and surgery. Arch Otolaryngol Head Neck Surg 1988;99(4):362–9.

54. Guilleminault C, Partinen M, Praud JP, et al. Morphometric facial changes and obstructive sleep apnea in adolescents. J Pediatr 1989;114(6):997–9.

55. Rondeau BH. Importance of diagnosing and treating orthodontic and orthopedic problems in children. Funct Orthod 2004;21(3):4.

56. Guilleminault C, Lee JH, Chan A, et al. Pediatric obstructive sleep apnea syndrome. Arch Pediatr Adolesc Med 2005;159(8):775–85.

57. Pirila K, Tahvanainen P, Huggare J, et al. Sleeping positions and dental arch dimensions in children with suspected obstructive sleep apnea syndrome. Eur J Oral Sci 1995;103(5):285–91.

58. Pirila-Parkkinen K, Pirttiniemi P, Nieminen P, et al. Dental arch morphology in children with sleep-disordered breathing. Eur J Orthod 2009;31(2):160–7.

59. Smith RM, Gonzalez C. The relationship between nasal obstruction and craniofacial growth. Pediatr Clin North Am 1989;36(6):1423–34.

60. Bresolin D, Shapiro PA, Shapiro GG, et al. Mouth breathing in allergic children: its relationship to dentofacial development. Am J Orthod Dentofacial Orthop 1983;83(4):334–40.

61. Subtelny JD. Oral respiration: facial maldevelopment and corrective dentofacial orthopedics. Angle Orthod 1980;50(3):147–64.

62. Kerr WJ, McWilliam JS, Linder-Aronson S. Mandibular form and position related to changed mode of breathing–a five-year longitudinal study. Angle Orthod 1989;59(2):91–6.

63. Vargervik K, Harvold EP. Experiments on the interaction between orofacial function and morphology. Ear Nose Throat J 1987;66(5):201–8.

64. Miller AJ, Vargervik K, Chierici G. Experimentally induced neuromuscular changes during and after nasal airway obstruction. Am J Orthod Dentofacial Orthop 1984;85(5):385–92.

65. Tomer BS, Harvold EP. Primate experiments on mandibular growth direction. Am J Orthod Dentofacial Orthop 1982;82(2):114–9.

66. Harvold EP, Tomer BS, Vargervik K, et al. Primate experiments on oral respiration. Am J Orthod Dentofacial Orthop 1981;79(4):359–72.

67. Harvold EP, Vargervik K, Chierici G. Primate experiments on oral sensation and dental malocclusions. Am J Orthod Dentofacial Orthop 1973;63(5):494–508.

68. Harvold EP, Chierici G, Vargervik K. Experiments on the development of dental malocclusions. Am J Orthod Dentofacial Orthop 1972;61(1):38–44.

69. Arens R, McDonough JM, Costarino AT, et al. Magnetic resonance imaging of the upper airway structure of children with obstructive sleep apnea syndrome. Am J Respir Crit Care Med 2001;164(4):698–703.

70. Riley R, Guilleminault C, Powell N, et al. Palatopharyngoplasty failure, cephalometric roentgenograms, and obstructive sleep apnea. Otolaryngol Head Neck Surg 1985;93(2):240–4.
71. Olszewska E, Sieskiewicz A, Rozycki J, et al. A comparison of cephalometric analysis using radiographs and craniofacial computed tomography in patients with obstructive sleep apnea syndrome: preliminary report. Eur Arch Otorhinolaryngol 2009;266(4):535–42.
72. Fujita S. Pharyngeal surgery for obstructive sleep apnea and snoring. In: Fairbanks DN, Fujita S, editors. Snoring and obstructive sleep apnea. 2nd edition. New York: Raven Press; 1994. p. 77–95.
73. Riley RW, Powell NB, Guilleminault C. Maxillary, mandibular, and hyoid advancement for treatment of obstructive sleep apnea: a review of 40 patients. J Oral Maxillofac Surg 1990;48(1):20–6.
74. Lin HC, Friedman M, Chang HW, et al. The efficacy of multilevel surgery of the upper airway in adults with obstructive sleep apnea/hypopnea syndrome. Laryngoscope 2008;118(5):902–8.
75. Sher AE, Schechtman KB, Piccirillo JF. The efficacy of surgical modifications of the upper airway in adults with obstructive sleep apnea syndrome. Sleep 1996; 19(2):156–77.
76. Li KK. Surgical management of obstructive sleep apnea. Clin Chest Med 2003; 24(2):365–70.
77. Elshaug AG, Moss JR, Southcott AM, et al. Redefining success in airway surgery for obstructive sleep apnea: a meta analysis and synthesis of the evidence. Sleep 2007;30(4):461–7.
78. Valero A, Alroy G. Hypoventilation in acquired micrognathia. Arch Intern Med 1965;115:307–9.
79. Lugarese E, Coccagna G, Mantovani M, et al. Effets de la tracheotomie dans les hypersomnies avec respiration periodique [Effects of tracheostomy in the hypersomnia with periodic breathing]. Rev Neurol (Paris) 1970;123:267–8 [in French].
80. Lugarese E, Coccagna G, Mantovani M, et al. Effects of tracheostomy in two cases of hypersomnia with periodic breathing. J Neurol Neurosurg Psychiatr 1973;36(1):15–26.
81. Guilleminault C, Simmons FB, Motta J, et al. Obstructive sleep apnea syndrome and tracheostomy. Long-term follow-up experience. Arch Intern Med 1981; 141(8):985–8.
82. Campanini A, De Vito A, Frassineti S, et al. Role of skin-lined tracheotomy in obstructive sleep apnoea syndrome: personal experience. Acta Otorhinolaryngol Ital 2004;24(2):68–74.
83. Katsantonis GP, Schweitzer PK, Branham GH, et al. Management of obstructive sleep apnea: comparison of various treatment modalities. Laryngoscope 1988; 98(3):304–9.
84. Borowiecki BD, Sassin JF. Surgical treatment of sleep apnea. Arch Otolaryngol Head Neck Surg 1983;109(8):508–12.
85. Stradling JR. Avoidance of tracheostomy in sleep apnoea syndrome. BMJ 1982; 285(6339):407–8.
86. Haapaniemi JJ, Laurikainen EA, Halme P, et al. Long-term results of tracheostomy for severe obstructive sleep apnea syndrome. ORL J Otorhinolaryngol Relat Spec 2001;63(3):131–6.
87. Kim SH, Eisele DW, Smith PL, et al. Evaluation of patients with sleep apnea after tracheotomy. Arch Otolaryngol Head Neck Surg 1998;124(9):996–1000.

88. Fletcher EC, Miller J, Schaaf JW, et al. Urinary catecholamines before and after tracheostomy in patients with obstructive sleep apnea and hypertension. Sleep 1987;10(1):35–44.
89. Guilleminault C, Cummiskey J. Progressive improvement of apnea index and ventilatory response to CO_2 after tracheostomy in obstructive sleep apnea syndrome. Am Rev Respir Dis 1982;126(1):14–20.
90. Sugita Y, Wakamatsu H, Teshima Y, et al. Therapeutic effects of tracheostomy in two cases of hypersomnia with respiratory disturbance during sleep. Folia Psychiatr Neurol Jpn 1980;34(1):17–25.
91. Imes NK, Orr WC, Smith RO, et al. Retrognathia and sleep apnea: a life-threatening condition masquerading as narcolepsy. JAMA 1977;237(15):1596–7.
92. Rodman DM, Martin RJ. Tracheostomy tube failure in obstructive sleep apnea. West J Med 1987;147(1):41–3.
93. Fletcher EC, Brown DL. Nocturnal oxyhemoglobin desaturation following tracheostomy for obstructive sleep apnea. Am J Med 1985;79(1):35–42.
94. Jin K, Okabe S, Chida K, et al. Tracheostomy can fatally exacerbate sleep-disordered breathing in multiple system atrophy. Neurology 2007;68(19):1618–21.
95. Fletcher EC. Recurrence of sleep apnea syndrome following tracheostomy. A shift from obstructive to central apnea. Chest 1989;96(1):205–9.
96. Weitzman ED, Kahn E, Pollak CP. Quantitative analysis of sleep and sleep apnea before and after tracheostomy in patients with the hypersomnia-sleep apnea syndrome. Sleep 1980;3(3-4):407–23.
97. Glenn WW, Gee JB, Cole DR, et al. Combined central alveolar hypoventilation and upper airway obstruction. Treatment by tracheostomy and diaphragm pacing. Am J Med 1978;64(1):50–60.
98. Tilkian AG, Guilleminault C, Schroeder JS, et al. Sleep-induced apnea syndrome. Prevalence of cardiac arrhythmias and their reversal after tracheostomy. Am J Med 1977;63(3):348–58.
99. Hastie SJ, Prowse K, Perks WH, et al. Obstructive sleep apnoea during pregnancy requiring tracheostomy. Aust N Z J Obstet Gynaecol 1989;29(3 Pt 2): 365–7.
100. Weitzman ED, Pollack CP, Borowiecki B. Hypersomnia-sleep apnea due to micrognathia. Reversal by tracheoplasty. Arch Neurol 1978;35(6):392–5.
101. Motta J, Guilleminault C, Schroeder JS, et al. Tracheostomy and hemodynamic changes in sleep-inducing apnea. Ann Intern Med 1978;89(4):454–8.
102. Bhimaraj A, Havaligi N, Ramachandran S. Rapid reduction of antihypertensive medications and insulin requirements after tracheostomy in a patient with severe obstructive sleep apnea syndrome. J Clin Sleep Med 2007;3(3):297–9.
103. Simmons FB, Guilleminault C, Dement WC, et al. Surgical management of airway obstructions during sleep. Laryngoscope 1977;87(3):326–38.
104. Van de Heyning PH, De Roeck J, Claes J, et al. [Tracheostomy in the sleep apnea syndrome]. Acta Otorhinolaryngol Belg 1984;38(5):489–502 [in French].
105. Conway WA, Victor LD, Magilligan DJ Jr, et al. Adverse effects of tracheostomy for sleep apnea. JAMA 1981;246(4):347–50.
106. Conway WA, Bower GC, Barnes ME. Hypersomnolence and intermittent upper airway obstruction. Occurrence caused by micrognathia. JAMA 1977;237(25): 2740–2.
107. He J, Kryger MH, Zorick FJ, et al. Mortality and apnea index in obstructive sleep apnea. Experience in 385 male patients. Chest 1988;94(1):9–14.
108. Partinen M, Jamieson A, Guilleminault C. Long-term outcome for obstructive sleep apnea syndrome patients. Mortality. Chest 1988;94(6):1200–4.

109. Partinen M, Guilleminault C. Daytime sleepiness and vascular morbidity at seven-year follow-up in obstructive sleep apnea patients. Chest 1990;97(1):27–32.
110. Thatcher GW, Maisel RH. The long-term evaluation of tracheostomy in the management of severe obstructive sleep apnea. Laryngoscope 2003;113(2): 201–4.
111. Fedok FG, Strauss M, Houck JR, et al. Further clinical experience with the silicone tracheal cannula in obstructive sleep apnea. Otolaryngol Head Neck Surg 1987;97(3):313–8.
112. Orsini MA, Conner GH, Cadieux RJ, et al. Clinical experience with the silicone tracheal cannula in obstructive sleep apnea. Otolaryngol Head Neck Surg 1984;92(2):132–5.
113. Gross ND, Cohen JI, Andersen PE, et al. 'Defatting' tracheotomy in morbidly obese patients. Laryngoscope 2002;112(11):1940–4.
114. Ashley MJ. Concerns of sleep apnea patients with tracheostomies. West J Nurs Res 1989;11(5):600–8.
115. Harmon JD, Morgan W, Chaudhary B. Sleep apnea: morbidity and mortality of surgical treatment. South Med J 1989;82(2):161–4.
116. Darrat I, Yaremchuk K. Early mortality rate of morbidly obese patients after tracheotomy. Laryngoscope 2008;118(12):2125–8.
117. Eliashar R, Goldfarb A, Gross M, et al. A permanent tube-free tracheostomy in a morbidly obese patient with severe obstructive sleep apnea syndrome. Isr Med Assoc J 2002;4(12):1156–7.
118. Campanini A, De Vito A, Frassineti S, et al. Temporary tracheotomy in the surgical treatment of obstructive sleep apnea syndrome: personal experience. Acta Otorhinolaryngol Ital 2003;23(6):474–8.
119. Charuzi I, Peiser J, Ovnat A, et al. Removal of tracheostomy in a morbidly obese sleep apneic patient after gastric bypass. Sleep 1986;9(3):449–50.
120. Mickelson SA, Rosenthal L. Closure of permanent tracheostomy in patients with sleep apnea: a comparison of two techniques. Otolaryngol Head Neck Surg 1997;116(1):36–40.
121. Hickey SA, Ford GR, Evans JN, et al. Tracheostomy closure in restrictive respiratory insufficiency. J Laryngol Otol 1990;104(11):883–6.
122. Law JH, Barnhart K, Rowlett W, et al. Increased frequency of obstructive airway abnormalities with long-term tracheostomy. Chest 1993;104(1):136–8.
123. Verse T, Pirsig W, Zimmermann E. [Obstructive sleep apnea in older patients after the closure of a tracheostoma]. Dtsch Med Wochenschr 2000;125(6): 137–41 [in German].
124. Verse T, Pirsig W. [Meta-analysis of laser-assisted uvulopalatopharyngoplasty. What is clinically relevant up to now?]. Laryngorhinootologie 2000;79(5): 273–84 [in German].
125. Larrosa F, Hernandez L, Morello A, et al. Laser-assisted uvulopalatoplasty for snoring: does it meet the expectations? Eur Respir J 2004;24(1):66–70.
126. Ferguson KA, Heighway K, Ruby RR. A randomized trial of laser-assisted uvulopalatoplasty in the treatment of mild obstructive sleep apnea. Am J Respir Crit Care Med 2003;167(1):15–9.
127. Franklin KA, Anttila H, Axelsson S, et al. Effects and side-effects of surgery for snoring and obstructive sleep apnea–a systematic review. Sleep 2009;32(1): 27–36.
128. Walker RP, Grigg-Damberger MM, Gopalsami C, et al. Laser-assisted uvulopalatoplasty for snoring and obstructive sleep apnea: results in 170 patients. Laryngoscope 1995;105(9 Pt 1):938–43.

129. Littner M, Hirshkowitz M, Davila D, et al. Practice parameters for the use of auto-titrating continuous positive airway pressure devices for titrating pressures and treating adult patients with obstructive sleep apnea syndrome. An American Academy of Sleep Medicine report. Sleep 2002;25(2):143–7.

130. Walker RP, Gopalsami C. Laser-assisted uvulopalatoplasty: postoperative complications. Laryngoscope 1996;106(7):834–8.

131. Terris DJ, Clerk AA, Norbash AM, et al. Characterization of postoperative edema following laser-assisted uvulopalatoplasty using MRI and polysomnography: implications for the outpatient treatment of obstructive sleep apnea syndrome. Laryngoscope 1996;106(2 Pt 1):124–8.

132. Fujita S, Woodson BT, Clark JL, et al. Laser midline glossectomy as a treatment for obstructive sleep apnea. Laryngoscope 1991;101(8):805–9.

133. Woodson BT, Fujita S. Clinical experience with lingualplasty as part of the treatment of severe obstructive sleep apnea. Otolaryngol Head Neck Surg 1992; 107(1):40–8.

134. Kezirian EJ, Goldberg AN. Hypopharyngeal surgery in obstructive sleep apnea: an evidence-based medicine review. Arch Otolaryngol Head Neck Surg 2006; 132(2):206–13.

135. Powell NB, Riley RW, Guilleminault C. Radiofrequency tongue base reduction in sleep-disordered breathing: a pilot study. Otolaryngol Head Neck Surg 1999; 120(5):656–64.

136. Stuck BA, Maurer JT, Hein G, et al. Radiofrequency surgery of the soft palate in the treatment of snoring: a review of the literature. Sleep 2004; 27(3):551–5.

137. Li KK, Powell NB, Riley RW, et al. Temperature-controlled radiofrequency tongue base reduction for sleep-disordered breathing: long-term outcomes. Otolaryngol Head Neck Surg 2002;127(3):230–4.

138. Stuck BA, Starzak K, Hein G, et al. Combined radiofrequency surgery of the tongue base and soft palate in obstructive sleep apnoea. Acta Otolaryngol 2004;124(7):827–32.

139. Fischer Y, Khan M, Mann WJ. Multilevel temperature-controlled radiofrequency therapy of soft palate, base of tongue, and tonsils in adults with obstructive sleep apnea. Laryngoscope 2003;113(10):1786–91.

140. Friedman M, Ibrahim H, Lee G, et al. Combined uvulopalatopharyngoplasty and radiofrequency tongue base reduction for treatment of obstructive sleep apnea/hypopnea syndrome. Otolaryngol Head Neck Surg 2003;129(6):611–21.

141. Riley RW, Powell NB, Li KK, et al. An adjunctive method of radiofrequency volumetric tissue reduction of the tongue for OSAS. Otolaryngol Head Neck Surg 2003;129(1):37–42.

142. Woodson BT, Steward DL, Weaver EM, et al. A randomized trial of temperature-controlled radiofrequency, continuous positive airway pressure, and placebo for obstructive sleep apnea syndrome. Otolaryngol Head Neck Surg 2003;128(6): 848–61.

143. Stuck BA, Maurer JT, Verse T, et al. Tongue base reduction with temperature-controlled radiofrequency volumetric tissue reduction for treatment of obstructive sleep apnea syndrome. Acta Otolaryngol 2002;122(5):531–6.

144. Stuck BA, Maurer JT, Hormann K. [Tongue base reduction with radiofrequency energy in sleep apnea]. HNO 2001;49(7):530–7 [in German].

145. Woodson BT, Nelson L, Mickelson S, et al. A multi-institutional study of radiofrequency volumetric tissue reduction for OSAS. Otolaryngol Head Neck Surg 2001;125(4):303–11.

146. Tomes CS. The bearing of the development of the jaws on irregularities. Dental Cosmos 1873;115:292–6.
147. Carpenter JE. Mental aberration and attending hypertrophic rhinitis with subacute otitus media. JAMA 1892;19:539–42.
148. Cline CL. The effects of intra-nasal obstruction on the general health. Med Surg Rep 1892;67:259–60.
149. Hill W. On some causes of backwardness and stupidity of children. BMJ 1889;2:711–2.
150. Wells WA. Some nervous and mental manifestations occurring in connection with nasal disease. Am J Med Sci 1898;116:677–92.
151. Koutsourelakis I, Georgoulopoulos G, Perraki E, et al. Randomised trial of nasal surgery for fixed nasal obstruction in obstructive sleep apnoea. Eur Respir J 2008;31(1):110–7.
152. Pirsig W, Verse T. Long-term results in the treatment of obstructive sleep apnea. Eur Arch Otorhinolaryngol 2000;257(10):570–7.
153. Powell NB, Zonato AI, Weaver EM, et al. Radiofrequency treatment of turbinate hypertrophy in subjects using continuous positive airway pressure: a randomized, double-blind, placebo-controlled clinical pilot trial. Laryngoscope 2001;111(10):1783–90.
154. Friedman M, Tanyeri H, Lim JW, et al. Effect of improved nasal breathing on obstructive sleep apnea. Otolaryngol Head Neck Surg 2000;122(1):71–4.
155. Olsen KD, Kern EB. Nasal influences on snoring and obstructive sleep apnea. Mayo Clin Proc 1990;65(8):1095–105.
156. Li HY, Lin Y, Chen NH, et al. Improvement in quality of life after nasal surgery alone for patients with obstructive sleep apnea and nasal obstruction. Arch Otolaryngol Head Neck Surg 2008;134(4):429–33.
157. Li KK, Powell NB, Riley RW, et al. Radiofrequency volumetric tissue reduction for treatment of turbinate hypertrophy: a pilot study. Otolaryngol Head Neck Surg 1998;119(6):569–73.
158. Kezirian EJ, Powell NB, Riley RW, et al. Incidence of complications in radiofrequency treatment of the upper airway. Laryngoscope 2005;115(7):1298–304.
159. Li KK, Powell NB, Riley RW, et al. Radiofrequency volumetric reduction of the palate: an extended follow-up study. Otolaryngol Head Neck Surg 2000;122(3):410–4.
160. Coleman SC, Smith TL. Midline radiofrequency tissue reduction of the palate for bothersome snoring and sleep-disordered breathing: a clinical trial. Otolaryngol Head Neck Surg 2000;122(3):387–94.
161. Powell NB, Riley RW, Troell RJ, et al. Radiofrequency volumetric tissue reduction of the palate in subjects with sleep-disordered breathing. Chest 1998;113(5):1163–74.
162. Stuck BA, Sauter A, Hormann K, et al. Radiofrequency surgery of the soft palate in the treatment of snoring. A placebo-controlled trial. Sleep 2005;28(7):847–50.
163. Hofmann T, Schwantzer G, Reckenzaun E, et al. Radiofrequency tissue volume reduction of the soft palate and UPPP in the treatment of snoring. Eur Arch Otorhinolaryngol 2006;263(2):164–70.
164. Blumen MB, Dahan S, Fleury B, et al. Radiofrequency ablation for the treatment of mild to moderate obstructive sleep apnea. Laryngoscope 2002;112(11):2086–92.
165. Brown DJ, Kerr P, Kryger M. Radiofrequency tissue reduction of the palate in patients with moderate sleep-disordered breathing. J Otolaryngol 2001;30(4):193–8.

166. Back LJ, Liukko T, Rantanen I, et al. Radiofrequency surgery of the soft palate in the treatment of mild obstructive sleep apnea is not effective as a single-stage procedure: a randomized single-blinded placebo-controlled trial. Laryngoscope 2009;119(8):1621–7.

167. Bluestone CD. Current indications for tonsillectomy and adenoidectomy. Ann Otol Rhinol Laryngol Suppl 1992;155:58–64.

168. Rosenfeld RM, Green RP. Tonsillectomy and adenoidectomy: changing trends. Ann Otol Rhinol Laryngol 1990;99(3 Pt 1):187–91.

169. Waters KA, Cheng AT. Adenotonsillectomy in the context of obstructive sleep apnoea. Paediatr Respir Rev 2009;10(1):25–31.

170. Krishna P, LaPage MJ, Hughes LF, et al. Current practice patterns in tonsillectomy and perioperative care. Int J Pediatr Otorhinolaryngol 2004;68(6):779–84.

171. Celenk F, Bayazit YA, Yilmaz M, et al. Tonsillar regrowth following partial tonsillectomy with radiofrequency. Int J Pediatr Otorhinolaryngol 2008;72(1):19–22.

172. Vlastos IM, Parpounas K, Economides J, et al. Tonsillectomy versus tonsillotomy performed with scissors in children with tonsillar hypertrophy. Int J Pediatr Otorhinolaryngol 2008;72(6):857–63.

173. Koltai PJ, Solares CA, Mascha EJ, et al. Intracapsular partial tonsillectomy for tonsillar hypertrophy in children. Laryngoscope 2002;112(8 Pt 2 Suppl 100): 17–9.

174. Densert O, Desai H, Eliasson A, et al. Tonsillotomy in children with tonsillar hypertrophy. Acta Otolaryngol 2001;121(7):854–8.

175. Hultcrantz E, Linder A, Markstrom A. Tonsillectomy or tonsillotomy?–A randomized study comparing postoperative pain and long-term effects. Int J Pediatr Otorhinolaryngol 1999;51(3):171–6.

176. Eviatar E, Kessler A, Shlamkovitch N, et al. Tonsillectomy vs. partial tonsillectomy for OSAS in children–10 years post-surgery follow-up. Int J Pediatr Otorhinolaryngol 2009;73(5):637–40.

177. Brietzke SE, Gallagher D. The effectiveness of tonsillectomy and adenoidectomy in the treatment of pediatric obstructive sleep apnea/hypopnea syndrome: a meta-analysis. Otolaryngol Head Neck Surg 2006;134(6): 979–84.

178. Friedman M, Wilson M, Lin HC, et al. Updated systematic review of tonsillectomy and adenoidectomy for treatment of pediatric obstructive sleep apnea/hypopnea syndrome. Otolaryngol Head Neck Surg 2009;140(6):800–8.

179. Mitchell RB, Kelly J. Outcome of adenotonsillectomy for obstructive sleep apnea in obese and normal-weight children. Otolaryngol Head Neck Surg 2007;137(1): 43–8.

180. O'Brien LM, Sitha S, Baur LA, et al. Obesity increases the risk for persisting obstructive sleep apnea after treatment in children. Int J Pediatr Otorhinolaryngol 2006;70(9):1555–60.

181. Guilleminault C, Quo S, Huynh NT, et al. Orthodontic expansion treatment and adenotonsillectomy in the treatment of obstructive sleep apnea in prepubertal children. Sleep 2008;31(7):953–7.

182. Ye J, Liu H, Zhang G, et al. Postoperative respiratory complications of adenotonsillectomy for obstructive sleep apnea syndrome in older children: prevalence, risk factors, and impact on clinical outcome. J Otolaryngol Head Neck Surg 2009;38(1):49–58.

183. Lima Junior JM, Silva VC, Freitas MR. Long term results in the life quality of children with obstructive sleep disorders submitted to adenoidectomy/adenotonsillectomy. Braz J Otorhinolaryngol 2008;74(5):718–24.

184. Goldstein NA, Fatima M, Campbell TF, et al. Child behavior and quality of life before and after tonsillectomy and adenoidectomy. Arch Otolaryngol Head Neck Surg 2002;128(7):770–5.

185. Mitchell RB, Kelly J. Behavioral changes in children with mild sleep-disordered breathing or obstructive sleep apnea after adenotonsillectomy. Laryngoscope 2007;117(9):1685–8.

186. Mitchell RB. Adenotonsillectomy for obstructive sleep apnea in children: outcome evaluated by pre- and postoperative polysomnography. Laryngoscope 2007;117(10):1844–54.

187. Rosen GM, Muckle RP, Mahowald MW, et al. Postoperative respiratory compromise in children with obstructive sleep apnea syndrome: can it be anticipated? Pediatrics 1994;93(5):784–8.

188. Richter GT, Bower CM. Cervical complications following routine tonsillectomy and adenoidectomy. Curr Opin Otolaryngol Head Neck Surg 2006;14(6): 375–80.

189. McColley SA, April MM, Carroll JL, et al. Respiratory compromise after adenotonsillectomy in children with obstructive sleep apnea. Arch Otolaryngol Head Neck Surg 1992;118(9):940–3.

190. Schroeder JW Jr, Anstead AS, Wong H. Complications in children who electively remain intubated after adenotonsillectomy for severe obstructive sleep apnea. Int J Pediatr Otorhinolaryngol 2009;73(8):1095–9.

191. Brigger MT, Brietzke SE. Outpatient tonsillectomy in children: a systematic review. Otolaryngol Head Neck Surg 2006;135(1):1–7.

192. Conway W, Fujita S, Zorick F, et al. Uvulopalatopharyngoplasty. One-year follow-up. Chest 1985;88(3):385–7.

193. Fujita S, Conway WA, Zorick FJ, et al. Evaluation of the effectiveness of uvulopalatopharyngoplasty. Laryngoscope 1985;95(1):70–4.

194. Simmons FB, Guilleminault C, Silvestri R. Snoring, and some obstructive sleep apnea, can be cured by oropharyngeal surgery. Arch Otolaryngol Head Neck Surg 1983;109(8):503–7.

195. Fairbanks DN. Uvulopalatopharyngoplasty complications and avoidance strategies. Otolaryngol Head Neck Surg 1990;102(3):239–45.

196. Dickson RI, Blokmanis A. Treatment of obstructive sleep apnea by uvulopalatopharyngoplasty. Laryngoscope 1987;97(9):1054–9.

197. Friedman M, Landsberg R, Tanyeri H. Submucosal uvulopalatopharnyoplasty. Op Tec Otolaryngol Head Neck Surg 2000;11:26–9.

198. Powell N, Riley R, Guilleminault C, et al. A reversible uvulopalatal flap for snoring and sleep apnea syndrome. Sleep 1996;19(7):593–9.

199. Li HY, Li KK, Chen NH, et al. Three-dimensional computed tomography and polysomnography findings after extended uvulopalatal flap surgery for obstructive sleep apnea. Am J Otolaryngol 2005;26(1):7–11.

200. Li HY, Chen NH, Shu YH, et al. Changes in quality of life and respiratory disturbance after extended uvulopalatal flap surgery in patients with obstructive sleep apnea. Arch Otolaryngol Head Neck Surg 2004;130(2):195–200.

201. Li HY, Li KK, Chen NH, et al. Modified uvulopalatopharyngoplasty: the extended uvulopalatal flap. Am J Otolaryngol 2003;24(5):311–6.

202. Woodson BT, Toohill RJ. Transpalatal advancement pharyngoplasty for obstructive sleep apnea. Laryngoscope 1993;103(3):269–76.

203. Shine NP, Lewis RH. Transpalatal advancement pharyngoplasty for obstructive sleep apnea syndrome: results and analysis of failures. Arch Otolaryngol Head Neck Surg 2009;135(5):434–8.

204. Sundaram S, Lim J, Lasserson TJ. Surgery for obstructive sleep apnoea. Cochrane Database Syst Rev 2005;(4):CD001004.

205. Conaway JR, Scherr SC, Conaway JR, et al. Multidisciplinary management of the airway in a trauma-induced brain injury patient. Sleep Breath 2004;8(3):165–70.

206. Megwalu UC, Piccirillo JF. Methodological and statistical problems in uvulopalatopharyngoplasty research: a follow-up study. Arch Otolaryngol Head Neck Surg 2008;134(8):805–9.

207. Lojander J, Maasilta P, Partinen M, et al. Nasal-CPAP, surgery, and conservative management for treatment of obstructive sleep apnea syndrome. A randomized study. Chest 1996;110(1):114–9.

208. Khan A, Ramar K, Maddirala S, et al. Uvulopalatopharyngoplasty in the management of obstructive sleep apnea: the Mayo Clinic experience. Mayo Clin Proc 2009;84(9):795–800.

209. Sher AE. Upper airway surgery for obstructive sleep apnea. Sleep Med Rev 2002;6(3):195–212.

210. Weaver EM, Maynard C, Yueh B. Survival of veterans with sleep apnea: continuous positive airway pressure versus surgery. Otolaryngol Head Neck Surg 2004;130(6):659–65.

211. Marti S, Sampol G, Munoz X, et al. Mortality in severe sleep apnoea/hypopnoea syndrome patients: impact of treatment. Eur Respir J 2002;20(6):1511–8.

212. Keenan SP, Burt H, Ryan CF, et al. Long-term survival of patients with obstructive sleep apnea treated by uvulopalatopharyngoplasty or nasal CPAP. Chest 1994;105(1):155–9.

213. Boot H, Poublon RM, Van Wegen R, et al. Uvulopalatopharyngoplasty for the obstructive sleep apnoea syndrome: value of polysomnography, Mueller manoeuvre and cephalometry in predicting surgical outcome. Clin Otolaryngol 1997;22(6):504–10.

214. Katsantonis GP, Maas CS, Walsh JK. The predictive efficacy of the Muller maneuver in uvulopalatopharyngoplasty. Laryngoscope 1989;99(7 Pt 1): 677–80.

215. Gereau SA, Sher AE, Glovinsky P, et al. Results of uvulopalatopharyngoplasty (UPPP) in patients selected by Mueller Maneuver [abstract]. Sleep Res 1986; 15(124).

216. Sher AE, Thorpy MJ, Shprintzen RJ, et al. Predictive value of Muller maneuver in selection of patients for uvulopalatopharyngoplasty. Laryngoscope 1985;95(12): 1483–7.

217. Chandrashekariah R, Shaman Z, Auckley D. Impact of upper airway surgery on CPAP compliance in difficult-to-manage obstructive sleep apnea. Arch Otolaryngol Head Neck Surg 2008;134(9):926–30.

218. Han F, Song W, Li J, et al. Influence of UPPP surgery on tolerance to subsequent continuous positive airway pressure in patients with OSAHS. Sleep Breath 2006; 10(1):37–42.

219. Mortimore IL, Bradley PA, Murray JA, et al. Uvulopalatopharyngoplasty may compromise nasal CPAP therapy in sleep apnea syndrome. Am J Respir Crit Care Med 1996;154(6 Pt 1):1759–62.

220. Friedman M, Soans R, Joseph N, et al. The effect of multilevel upper airway surgery on continuous positive airway pressure therapy in obstructive sleep apnea/hypopnea syndrome. Laryngoscope 2009;119(1):193–6.

221. Miljeteig H, Mateika S, Haight JS, et al. Subjective and objective assessment of uvulopalatopharyngoplasty for treatment of snoring and obstructive sleep apnea. Am J Respir Crit Care Med 1994;150(5 Pt 1):1286–90.

222. Macnab T, Blokmanis A, Dickson RI. Long-term results of uvulopalatopharyng-oplasty for snoring. J Otolaryngol 1992;21(5):350–4.
223. Jaghagen EL, Berggren D, Dahlqvist A, et al. Prediction and risk of dysphagia after uvulopalatopharyngoplasty and uvulopalatoplasty. Acta Otolaryngol 2004; 124(10):1197–203.
224. Lysdahl M, Haraldsson PO. Uvulopalatopharyngoplasty versus laser uvulopala-toplasty: prospective long-term follow-up of self-reported symptoms. Acta Oto-laryngol 2002;122(7):752–7.
225. Grontved AM, Karup P. Complaints and satisfaction after uvulopalatopharyngo-plasty. Acta Otolaryngol Suppl 2000;543:190–2.
226. Levring-Jaghagen E, Nilsson ME, Isberg A. Persisting dysphagia after uvulopa-latoplasty performed with steel scalpel. Laryngoscope 1999;109(1):86–90.
227. Kosztyla-Hojna B, Rogowski M, Olszewska E, et al. [Voice quality evaluation in patients with obstructive sleep apnea syndrome treated with uvulopalatophar-yngoplasty (UPPP)]. Pol Merkur Lekarski 2008;25(145):46–50 [in Polish].
228. Robinson S, Chia M, Carney AS, et al. Upper airway reconstructive surgery long-term quality-of-life outcomes compared with CPAP for adult obstructive sleep apnea. Otolaryngol Head Neck Surg Aug 2009;141(2):257–63.
229. Riley R, Guilleminault C, Powell N, et al. Mandibular osteotomy and hyoid bone advancement for obstructive sleep apnea: a case report. Sleep 1984;7(1): 79–82.
230. Riley RW, Powell NB, Guilleminault C. Inferior sagittal osteotomy of the mandible with hyoid myotomy-suspension: a new procedure for obstructive sleep apnea. Otolaryngol Head Neck Surg 1986;94(5):589–93.
231. Riley RW, Powell NB, Guilleminault C. Inferior mandibular osteotomy and hyoid myotomy suspension for obstructive sleep apnea: a review of 55 patients. J Oral Maxillofac Surg 1989;47(2):159–64.
232. Li KK, Riley RW, Powell NB, et al. Obstructive sleep apnea surgery: genioglos-sus advancement revisited. J Oral Maxillofac Surg 2001;59(10):1181–4.
233. Silverstein K, Costello BJ, Giannakpoulos H, et al. Genioglossus muscle attachments: an anatomic analysis and the implications for genioglossus advancement. Oral Surg Oral Med Oral Pathol Oral Radiol Endod 2000; 90(6):686–8.
234. Demian NM, Alford J, Takashima M. An alternative technique for genioglossus muscle advancement in phase I surgery in the treatment of obstructive sleep apnea. J Oral Maxillofac Surg 2009;67(10):2315–8.
235. Riley RW, Powell NB, Guilleminault C, et al. Maxillary, mandibular, and hyoid advancement: an alternative to tracheostomy in obstructive sleep apnea syndrome. Otolaryngol Head Neck Surg 1986;94(5):584–8.
236. Van de Graaff WB, Gottfried SB, Mitra J, et al. Respiratory function of hyoid muscles and hyoid arch. J Appl Physiol 1984;57(1):197–204.
237. Patton TJ, Thawley SE, Waters RC, et al. Expansion hyoidplasty: a potential surgical procedure designed for selected patients with obstructive sleep apnea syndrome. Experimental canine results. Laryngoscope 1983;93(11 Pt 1): 1387–96.
238. Riley RW, Powell NB, Guilleminault C. Obstructive sleep apnea and the hyoid: a revised surgical procedure. Otolaryngol Head Neck Surg 1994;111(6): 717–21.
239. Bowden MT, Kezirian EJ, Utley D, et al. Outcomes of hyoid suspension for the treatment of obstructive sleep apnea. Arch Otolaryngol Head Neck Surg 2005;131(5):440–5.

240. Baisch A, Maurer JT, Hormann K. The effect of hyoid suspension in a multilevel surgery concept for obstructive sleep apnea. Otolaryngol Head Neck Surg 2006;134(5):856–61.
241. Stuck BA, Neff W, Hormann K, et al. Anatomic changes after hyoid suspension for obstructive sleep apnea: an MRI study. Otolaryngol Head Neck Surg 2005; 133(3):397–402.
242. Verse T, Baisch A, Hormann K. [Multi-level surgery for obstructive sleep apnea. Preliminary objective results]. Laryngorhinootologie 2004;83(8):516–22 [in German].
243. Vilaseca I, Morello A, Montserrat JM, et al. Usefulness of uvulopalatopharyngo-plasty with genioglossus and hyoid advancement in the treatment of obstructive sleep apnea. Arch Otolaryngol Head Neck Surg 2002;128(4):435–40.
244. Neruntarat C. Genioglossus advancement and hyoid myotomy under local anesthesia. Otolaryngol Head Neck Surg 2003;129(1):85–91.
245. Neruntarat C. Genioglossus advancement and hyoid myotomy: short-term and long-term results. J Laryngol Otol 2003;117(6):482–6.
246. den Herder C, van Tinteren H, de Vries N, et al. Hyoidthyroidpexia: a surgical treatment for sleep apnea syndrome. Laryngoscope 2005;115(4):740–5.
247. Li KK, Powell NB, Riley RW, et al. Distraction osteogenesis in adult obstructive sleep apnea surgery: a preliminary report. J Oral Maxillofac Surg 2002;60(1): 6–10.
248. Morovic CG, Monasterio L. Distraction osteogenesis for obstructive apneas in patients with congenital craniofacial malformations. Plast Reconstr Surg 2000; 105(7):2324–30.
249. Williams JK, Maull D, Grayson BH, et al. Early decannulation with bilateral mandibular distraction for tracheostomy-dependent patients. Plast Reconstr Surg 1999;103(1):48–57.
250. Cohen SR, Ross DA, Burstein FD, et al. Skeletal expansion combined with soft-tissue reduction in the treatment of obstructive sleep apnea in children: physio-logic results. Otolaryngol Head Neck Surg 1998;119(5):476–85.
251. McCarthy JG, Schreiber J, Karp N, et al. Lengthening the human mandible by gradual distraction. Plast Reconstr Surg 1992;89(1):1–8.
252. Spire JP, Kuo PC, Campbell N. Maxillo-facial surgical approach: an introduction and review of mandibular advancement. Bull Eur Physiopathol Respir 1983; 19(6):604–6.
253. Powell N, Guilleminault C, Riley R, et al. Mandibular advancement and obstruc-tive sleep apnea syndrome. Bull Eur Physiopathol Respir 1983;19(6):607–10.
254. Jamieson A, Guilleminault C, Partinen M, et al. Obstructive sleep apneic patients have craniomandibular abnormalities. Sleep 1986;9(4):469–77.
255. Bell RB, Turvey TA. Skeletal advancement for the treatment of obstructive sleep apnea in children. Cleft Palate Craniofac J 2001;38(2):147–54.
256. Cao M, Li K, Guilleminault C. Maxillomandibular advancement surgery for obstructive sleep apnea treatment. Minerva Pneumol 2008;47:203–12.
257. Li KK, Guilleminault C, Riley RW, et al. Obstructive sleep apnea and maxilloman-dibular advancement: an assessment of airway changes using radiographic and nasopharyngoscopic examinations. J Oral Maxillofac Surg 2002;60(5): 526–30 [discussion: 531].
258. Wickwire NA, White RP Jr, Proffit WR. The effect of mandibular osteotomy on tongue position. J Oral Maxillofac Surg 1972;30(3):184–90.
259. Schendel SA, Oeschlaeger M, Wolford LM, et al. Velopharyngeal anatomy and maxillary advancement. J Maxillofac Surg 1979;7(2):116–24.

260. Frohberg U, Greco JM. [Maxillary osteotomy: an alternative treatment concept for obstructive sleep apnea syndrome]. Dtsch Z Mund Kiefer Gesichtschir 1990;14(5):343–7 [in German].

261. Greco JM, Frohberg U, Van Sickels JE. Cephalometric analysis of long-term airway space changes with maxillary osteotomies. Oral Surg Oral Med Oral Pathol 1990;70(5):552–4.

262. Walker DA, Turvey TA, Warren DW. Alterations in nasal respiration and nasal airway size following superior repositioning of the maxilla. J Oral Maxillofac Surg 1988;46(4):276–81.

263. Guenthner TA, Sather AH, Kern EB. The effect of Le Fort I maxillary impaction on nasal airway resistance. Am J Orthod Dentofacial Orthop Apr 1984;85(4): 308–15.

264. Yu CC, Hsiao HD, Lee LC, et al. Computational fluid dynamic study on obstructive sleep apnea syndrome treated with maxillomandibular advancement. J Craniofac Surg 2009;20(2):426–30.

265. Waite PD, Shettar SM. Maxillomandibular advancement surgery: a cure for obstructive sleep apnea syndrome. Oral Maxillofac Surg Clin North Am 1995; 7(2):327–36.

266. Holty JE, Guilleminault C. Maxillomandibular advancement for the treatment of obstructive sleep apnea: a systematic review and meta-analysis. Sleep Med Rev 2010. [Epub ahead of print].

267. Li K, Powell N, Riley R, et al. Long-term results of maxillomandibular advancement surgery. Sleep Breath 2000;4(3):137–9.

268. Conradt R, Hochban W, Brandenburg U, et al. Long-term follow-up after surgical treatment of obstructive sleep apnoea by maxillomandibular advancement. Eur Respir J 1997;10(1):123–8.

269. Lye KW, Waite PD, Meara D, et al. Quality of life evaluation of maxillomandibular advancement surgery for treatment of obstructive sleep apnea. J Oral Maxillofac Surg 2008;66(5):968–72.

270. Dekeister C, Lacassagne L, Tiberge M, et al. [Mandibular advancement surgery in patients with severe obstructive sleep apnea uncontrolled by continuous positive airway pressure. A retrospective review of 25 patients between 1998 and 2004]. Rev Mal Respir 2006;23(5 Pt 1):430–7 [in French].

271. Hoekema A, de Lange J, Stegenga B, et al. Oral appliances and maxillomandibular advancement surgery: an alternative treatment protocol for the obstructive sleep apnea-hypopnea syndrome. J Oral Maxillofac Surg 2006; 64(6):886–91.

272. Smatt Y, Ferri J. Retrospective study of 18 patients treated by maxillomandibular advancement with adjunctive procedures for obstructive sleep apnea syndrome. J Craniofac Surg 2005;16(5):770–7.

273. Goh YH, Lim KA. Modified maxillomandibular advancement for the treatment of obstructive sleep apnea: a preliminary report. Laryngoscope 2003;113(9): 1577–82.

274. Wagner I, Coiffier T, Sequert C, et al. [Surgical treatment of severe sleep apnea syndrome by maxillomandibular advancing or mental tranposition]. Ann Otolaryngol Chir Cervicofac 2000;117(3):137–46 [in French].

275. Prinsell JR. Maxillomandibular advancement surgery in a site-specific treatment approach for obstructive sleep apnea in 50 consecutive patients. Chest 1999; 116(6):1519–29.

276. Guilleminault C, Quera-Salva MA, Powell NB, et al. Maxillo-mandibular surgery for obstructive sleep apnoea. Eur Respir J 1989;2(7):604–12.

277. Conradt R, Hochban W, Heitmann J, et al. Sleep fragmentation and daytime vigilance in patients with OSA treated by surgical maxillomandibular advancement compared to CPAP therapy. J Sleep Res 1998;7(3):217–23.

278. Conradt R, Hochban W, Brandenburg U, et al. [nCPAP therapy and maxillary and mandibular osteotomy compared: attention during the day in obstructive sleep apnea]. Wien Med Wochenschr 1996;146(13–14):372–4 [in German].

279. Hochban W, Brandenburg U, Peter JH. Surgical treatment of obstructive sleep apnea by maxillomandibular advancement. Sleep 1994;17(7):624–9.

280. Hendler BH, Costello BJ, Silverstein K, et al. A protocol for uvulopalatopharyngoplasty, mortised genioplasty, and maxillomandibular advancement in patients with obstructive sleep apnea: an analysis of 40 cases. J Oral Maxillofac Surg 2001;59(8):892–7.

281. Nimkarn Y, Miles PG, Waite PD. Maxillomandibular advancement surgery in obstructive sleep apnea syndrome patients: long-term surgical stability. J Oral Maxillofac Surg 1995;53(12):1414–8.

282. Riley RW, Powell NB, Guilleminault C. Maxillofacial surgery and nasal CPAP. A comparison of treatment for obstructive sleep apnea syndrome. Chest 1990; 98(6):1421–5.

283. Miles PG, Nimkarn Y. Maxillomandibular advancement surgery in patients with obstructive sleep apnea: mandibular morphology and stability. Int J Adult Orthodon Orthognath Surg 1995;10(3):193–200.

284. Louis PJ, Waite PD, Austin RB. Long-term skeletal stability after rigid fixation of Le Fort I osteotomies with advancements. Int J Oral Maxillofac Surg 1993;22(2): 82–6.

285. Waite PD, Wooten V. Maxillomandibular advancement: a surgical treatment of obstructive sleep apnea. In: Bell WH, editor, Modern practice in orthognathic and reconstructive surgery, vol. 3. Philadelphia: WB Saunders; 1992. p. 2042–59.

286. Lu XF, Zhu M, He JD, et al. [Uvulopalatopharyngoplasty and maxillomandibular advancement for obese patients with obstructive sleep apnea hypopnea syndrome: a preliminary report]. Zhonghua Kou QiangYi Xue Za Zhi 2007; 42(4):199–202 [in Chinese].

287. Li KK, Riley RW, Powell NB, et al. Obstructive sleep apnea surgery: patient perspective and polysomnographic results. Otolaryngol Head Neck Surg 2000;123(5):572–5.

288. Bettega G, Pepin JL, Veale D, et al. Obstructive sleep apnea syndrome. Fifty-one consecutive patients treated by maxillofacial surgery. Am J Respir Crit Care Med 2000;162(2 Pt 1):641–9.

289. Li KK, Riley RW, Powell NB, et al. Patient's perception of the facial appearance after maxillomandibular advancement for obstructive sleep apnea syndrome. J Oral Maxillofac Surg 2001;59(4):377–80 [discussion: 380–1].

290. Li KK, Riley RW, Powell NB, et al. Maxillomandibular advancement for persistent obstructive sleep apnea after phase I surgery in patients without maxillomandibular deficiency. Laryngoscope 2000;110(10 Pt 1):1684–8.

291. Matsuo A, Nakai T, Toyoda J, et al. Good esthetic results after modified maxillomandibular advancement for obstructive sleep apnea syndrome. Sleep Biol Rhythms 2009;7:3–10.

292. Conley RS, Legan HL. Correction of severe obstructive sleep apnea with bimaxillary transverse distraction osteogenesis and maxillomandibular advancement. Am J Orthod Dentofacial Orthop 2006;129(2):283–92.

293. Guilleminault C, Li KK. Maxillomandibular expansion for the treatment of sleep-disordered breathing: preliminary result. Laryngoscope 2004;114(5):893–6.

294. Friedman M, Vidyasagar R, Bliznikas D, et al. Patient selection and efficacy of pillar implant technique for treatment of snoring and obstructive sleep apnea/hypopnea syndrome. Otolaryngol Head Neck Surg 2006;134(2):187–96.

295. Friedman M, Schalch P, Lin HC, et al. Palatal implants for the treatment of snoring and obstructive sleep apnea/hypopnea syndrome. Otolaryngol Head Neck Surg 2008;138(2):209–16.

296. Nordgard S, Stene BK, Skjostad KW. Soft palate implants for the treatment of mild to moderate obstructive sleep apnea. Otolaryngol Head Neck Surg 2006; 134(4):565–70.

297. Nordgard S, Stene BK, Skjostad KW, et al. Palatal implants for the treatment of snoring: long-term results. Otolaryngol Head Neck Surg 2006;134(4):558–64.

298. Maurer JT, Hein G, Verse T, et al. Long-term results of palatal implants for primary snoring. Otolaryngol Head Neck Surg 2005;133(4):573–8.

299. Angell EH. Treatment of irregularity of the permanent or adult teeth. Dental Cosmos 1860;1:540–4 [discussion: 599–600].

300. Lagravere MO, Heo G, Major PW, et al. Meta-analysis of immediate changes with rapid maxillary expansion treatment [comment]. J Am Dent Assoc 2006; 137(1):44–53.

301. Monini S, Malagola C, Villa MP, et al. Rapid maxillary expansion for the treatment of nasal obstruction in children younger than 12 years. Arch Otolaryngol Head Neck Surg 2009;135(1):22–7.

302. Basciftci FA, Mutlu N, Karaman AI, et al. Does the timing and method of rapid maxillary expansion have an effect on the changes in nasal dimensions? Angle Orthod 2002;72(2):118–23.

303. Gray LP. Results of 310 cases of rapid maxillary expansion selected for medical reasons. J Laryngol Otol 1975;89(6):601–14.

304. Timms DJ. Rapid maxillary expansion. Chicago: Quintessence Publishing; 1981.

305. Eysell. Uber die Verengung der Nasenhohle, bedingt durch Gaumenenge und Anomole Zahnstellung [Narrow oropharynx and abnormal dental position due to narrow nasal passages]. Dtsche Monat Zhk 1886;12:481 [in German].

306. White BC, Woodside DG, Cole P. The effect of rapid maxillary expansion on nasal airway resistance. J Otolaryngol 1989;18(4):137–43.

307. Timms DJ. Rapid maxillary expansion in the treatment of nasal obstruction and respiratory disease. Ear Nose Throat J 1987;66(6):242–7.

308. Warren DW, Hershey HG, Turvey TA, et al. The nasal airway following maxillary expansion. Am J Orthod Dentofacial Orthop 1987;91(2):111–6.

309. Timms DJ. The effect of rapid maxillary expansion on nasal airway resistance. Br J Orthod 1986;13(4):221–8.

310. Hershey HG, Stewart BL, Warren DW. Changes in nasal airway resistance associated with rapid maxillary expansion. Am J Orthod 1976;69(3):274–84.

311. Wertz RA. Changes in nasal airflow incident to rapid maxillary expansion. Angle Orthod 1968;38(1):1–11.

312. Linder-Aronson S, Aschan G. Nasal resistance to breathing and palatal height before and after expansion of the median palatine suture. Odontol Revy 1963; 14:254–70.

313. Woods M, Wiesenfeld D, Probert T. Surgically-assisted maxillary expansion. Aust Dent J 1997;42(1):38–42.

314. de Moura CP, Andrade D, Cunha LM, et al. Down syndrome: otolaryngological effects of rapid maxillary expansion. J Laryngol Otol 2008;122(12):1318–24.

315. Timms DJ. The reduction of nasal airway resistance by rapid maxillary expansion and its effect on respiratory disease. J Laryngol Otol 1984; 98(4):357–62.
316. Palmisano RG, Wilcox I, Sullivan CE, et al. Treatment of snoring and obstructive sleep apnoea by rapid maxillary expansion. Aust N Z J Med 1996;26(3):428–9.
317. Villa MP, Malagola C, Pagani J, et al. Rapid maxillary expansion in children with obstructive sleep apnea syndrome: 12-month follow-up. Sleep Med 2007;8(2): 128–34.
318. Pirelli P, Saponara M, Attanasio G, et al. Obstructive sleep apnoea syndrome (OSAS) and rhino-tubaric disfunction in children: therapeutic effects of RME therapy. Prog Orthod 2005;6(1):48–61.
319. Pirelli P, Saponara M, Guilleminault C. Rapid maxillary expansion in children with obstructive sleep apnea syndrome. Sleep 2004;27(4):761–6.
320. Holty JEC, Guilleminault C. Maxillo-mandibular expansion and advancement for the treatment of sleep-disordered breathing in children and adults. Semin Orthod, in press.
321. Cistulli PA, Palmisano RG, Poole MD. Treatment of obstructive sleep apnea syndrome by rapid maxillary expansion. Sleep 1998;21(8):831–5.
322. Friedman M, Lin HC, Gurpinar B, et al. Minimally invasive single-stage multilevel treatment for obstructive sleep apnea/hypopnea syndrome. Laryngoscope 2007;117(10):1859–63.
323. Verse T, Baisch A, Maurer JT, et al. Multilevel surgery for obstructive sleep apnea: short-term results. Otolaryngol Head Neck Surg 2006;134(4):571–7.
324. Li HY, Wang PC, Hsu CY, et al. Same-stage palatopharyngeal and hypopharyngeal surgery for severe obstructive sleep apnea. Acta Otolaryngol 2004; 124(7):820–6.
325. Riley RW, Powell NB, Guilleminault C. Obstructive sleep apnea syndrome: a review of 306 consecutively treated surgical patients. Otolaryngol Head Neck Surg 1993;108(2):117–25.
326. Li KK, Powell NB, Riley RW, et al. Overview of phase I surgery for obstructive sleep apnea syndrome. Ear Nose Throat J 1999;78(11):836–7.
327. Li KK, Riley RW, Powell NB, et al. Overview of phase II surgery for obstructive sleep apnea syndrome. Ear Nose Throat J 1999;78(11):851.
328. Flegal KM, Carrol MD, Ogden CL, et al. Prevalence and trends in obesity among US adults, 1999-2000. JAMA 2002;288:1723–7.
329. Brolin RE. Gastric bypass. Surg Clin North Am 1967;81(5):1077–95.
330. Santry HP, Gillen DL, Lauderdale DS. Trends in bariatric surgical procedures. JAMA 2005;294(15):1909–17.
331. Flum DR, Belle SH, King WC, et al. Perioperative safety in the longitudinal assessment of bariatric surgery. N Engl J Med 2009;361(5):445–54.
332. Sjostrom L, Narbro K, Sjostrom CD, et al. Effects of bariatric surgery on mortality in Swedish obese subjects. N Engl J Med 2007;357(8):741–52.
333. Buchwald H, Avidor Y, Braunwald E, et al. Bariatric surgery: a systematic review and meta-analysis. JAMA 2004;292(14):1724–37.
334. Gastrointestinal surgery for severe obesity: National Institutes of Health Consensus Development Conference Statement. Am J Clin Nutr 1992;55: 615S–9S.
335. Anonymous. Gastrointestinal surgery for severe obesity. NIH Consensus Statement Online 1991;9(1):1–20.
336. Peppard PE, Young T, Palta M, et al. Longitudinal study of moderate weight change and sleep-disordered breathing. JAMA 2000;284(23):3015–21.

337. Smith PL, Gold AR, Meyers DA, et al. Weight loss in mildly to moderately obese patients with obstructive sleep apnea. Ann Intern Med 1985;103(6 (Pt 1)):850–5.

338. Greenburg DL, Lettieri CJ, Eliasson AH. Effects of surgical weight loss on measures of obstructive sleep apnea: a meta-analysis. Am J Med 2009; 122(6):535–42.

339. Holty JE, Levesque BG, Schneider-Chafen J, et al. Obstructive sleep apnea is prevalent and persistent among patients undergoing bariatric surgery: a systematic review [abstract presentation]. Dig Dis Sci 2010.

Orthodontics and Obstructive Sleep Apnea in Children

Paola Pirelli, DDS[a,b,*], Maurizio Saponara, MD[c],
Chiara De Rosa, DDS[a], Ezio Fanucci, MD[d]

KEYWORDS

- Obstructive sleep apnea syndrome • Rapid maxillary expansion
- Nasal septum deviation • Polysomnography

The association between obstructive sleep apnea syndrome (OSAS), maxillofacial malformations, and malocclusions has attracted more attention in the recent past. In several reports, Guilleminault,[1–3] from the Stanford University Medical School, has underlined the importance of multidisciplinary collaboration in the treatment of breathing-related sleep disorders and has emphasized that children suffering from mild OSAS commonly present with airway obstruction related to nasal septum deviation associated with a narrow upper jaw. Also, he has mentioned that in children with obstructive sleep apnea (OSA), the role of craniofacial abnormalities and the impact of orthodontics have often been overlooked until now, despite their impact on public health. Treatment of OSA by rapid maxillary expansion (RME) was mentioned by Cistulli and colleagues.[4] At the third International Congress of Craniofacial and Maxillofacial Distraction Paris, France, June 2001, and the seventh World Congress on Sleep Apnea Helsinki, Finland, June 2003, Pirelli had several presentations on the potential role of RME in children with abnormal breathing during sleep, work that led to the first full report on the treatment of pediatric OSA by RME.[5] This report was based on a multidisciplinary collaboration, and it clearly showed that the contribution from different specialists could lead to effective therapy when considering the treatment of a disorder as complex as pediatric OSA. Particularly interesting were the correlations found between OSAS, malocclusion, and maxillofacial malformations. In fact, many patients with OSAS show craniofacial abnormalities in both jaws as well as alteration in the skeletal structure of the respiratory dynamic space.[3–6] Nasal septum alteration reduces airflow and increases resistance to nasal breathing.[6,7] Micrognathia and

[a] Department of Odontostomatological Sciences, University of Tor Vergata, Rome, Italy
[b] Via Tomacelli 103, Rome 00186, Italy
[c] Department of Neurology and Otolaryngology, University "La Sapienza", Rome, Italy
[d] Department of Diagnostic Imaging Interventional Radiology, University of Tor Vergata, Rome, Italy
* Corresponding author. Via Tomacelli 103, Rome 00186.
E-mail address: p.pirelli@gmail.com

Med Clin N Am 94 (2010) 517–529
doi:10.1016/j.mcna.2010.02.004
0025-7125/10/$ – see front matter © 2010 Elsevier Inc. All rights reserved.

medical.theclinics.com

nasal obstruction are among the risk factors for OSAS.[3–7] Maxillary impaired development results in a decrease in the size of the nasomaxillary complex and then of the nasopharyngeal airway dimension (as presented at the 81st congress of the European Orthodontic Society Amsterdam, The Netherlands, June 2005; "Therapeutic effects of R.M.E."). Nasal septum deviations are responsible not only for an asymmetric distribution of intranasal spaces but also for the internal structural alteration of the turbinates, more particularly the nasal inferior turbinate, which in turn causes a reduction of total airflow.[8–11] Considering that a significant number of children suffering from mild OSAS show an obstructive phenomenon with nasal septum deviation with or without turbinate hypertrophy, associated with a narrow upper jaw,[9] this report describes how rapid maxillary expansion may improve the patency of the nasal airway and to which extent it may improve pediatric OSA.

MATERIAL AND METHODS

Of a sample of 150 patients, the authors selected 60 children (38 males and 22 females) between 6 and 13 years of age (average 7.3 years) who were seen for oral breathing, snoring, and history of nocturnal apneas.

Selection criteria included no adenotonsillar hypertrophy, body mass index less than 24 kg/m^2, and malocclusion characterized by upper jaw contraction. Patients underwent an ear-nose-throat (ENT) visit with the following tests: audiometry, tympanometry with tubaric functionality maneuvers, active anterior rhinomanometry, nasal fibroscopy, and daytime sleepiness questionnaire. Polysomnography was performed with recording of 19 channels.

Sleep-wake states were based on electroencephalograms, electro-oculogram, electromyogram, electrocardiogram, body position, nasal and oral flow, thoracic and abdominal movement, snoring noise, and pulse oximetry. Polysomnograms were analyzed following the Rechtschaffen and Kales International Criteria for sleep-wake scoring and the American Academy for Sleep Medicine recommendation for the scoring and breathing events.[12] Abnormal events were considered present if longer than 2 breaths in duration. Events were classified as apnea or hypopnea based on air flow and as obstructive, mixed, or central based on thoracoabdominal movements and air flow. An orthognathodontic investigation was performed using radiographs that included not only the usual examination, that is, posteroanterior cephalographs and intraoral radiographs, but also CT scans. All the investigations, except CT Dentascan, were carried out (1) before the orthodontic therapy (pretreatment T0); (2) 1 month (T1) after therapy, with the device still in place; and (3) 4 months after the end of orthodontic treatment, which lasted 6 to 12 months. CT Dentascan was performed only before treatment (T0) and after about 20 to 30 days (at end of active expansion [T1]) with the device still in place.

To reduce radiation exposure, a low-dosage CT Dentascan protocol was used. The study was performed using the CT scanner Lightspeed Advantage (GE Medical System Milwaukee, WI, USA).

The experimental study was approved by the Human Care Committee, and all the patients signed an informed consent.

ORTHODONTIC EXAMINATION

The clinical orthodontic examination carried out on the basis of the authors' diagnostic criteria[13,14] gave the following results:

- Extraoral examination: presence of the typical facies of oral breathers characterized by (1) flattening of the middle-facial-third, (2) labial incompetence with hypotonia of the upper lip and with a resulting increase in the nasal-labial angle;

- Intraoral examination: presence in all cases of narrowness of the upper jaw with an ogival palate pattern resulting from a high and narrow palatal arch. This narrowness was clinically present in most of the treated cases with a malocclusion characterized by unilateral or bilateral crossbite and often by an anterior crossbite.

The narrowness of the upper jaw was diagnosed clinically and confirmed by cephalometric assessment according to Ricketts parameters in posteroanterior cephalograms.[15]

The following measurements were evaluated

For nasal cavity diameters: NC-CN
And for maxillary diameters: JL-JR.

For the assessment of the increase in the maxillary cross section, 2 planes were used: for nasal cavity width NC-CN and for maxillary width JL-JR (bilateral points located at the depth of the concavity of the lateral maxillary contour at the junction of the maxilla and zygomatic buttress).

In addition, the interincisive space A1-1A and the intermolar width A6-6A were measured.

RAPID MAXILLARY EXPANSION

The RME procedure, successfully performed for many years in clinical practice, uses an orthodontic fixed appliance with an expansion screw, anchored on selected teeth.[16] According to the phase of development of the teeth, the device is constructed using the first molars and permanent premolars as anchor teeth, whereas in the deciduous dentition, the second primary molars are selected, provided that they offer the stability required for appropriate treatment.

The device is made up of a central expansion screw with 4 arms: 2 front arms and 2 back arms of length 1.5 mm. Two types of screw are used: the Leone A0620/13 (Italy) and the Forestadent 1671326L (Germany); palatal split screw type "S" is used for especially narrow palates. The device must satisfy some fundamental construction criteria. The force is applied through the anchor teeth so as to act directly on the suture, without any undesired tipping of the teeth. This application produces a transpalatal force that exceeds physiologic levels that could produce orthodontic movement. At the same time, the midpalatal suture opens and orthopedic movement of the maxillae occurs.

Osteoid appears at the borders of the palatal processes, and a normal mineralized suture reforms after 3 to 4 months.[16–21] Valid treatment is possible only on proceeding as outlined earlier as the maxillary expansion must not be due to dental arch tipping but due to an actual increase in the palatal transversal diameters. This increase can be achieved only through changes induced in the midpalatal suture. The device must not be bulky but must be strong and fitting well on the anchor teeth; the expansion screw must be placed as high as possible in the palate. The effectiveness of this maneuver depends also on the amount of force applied and on the duration of application of the force.

ACTIVATION SYSTEM

The screw activation system the authors use works as follows[17,18]:

- On the first day, morning and evening, 3 consecutive activations are applied at 10-minute intervals.
- From the second day onwards, only 1 activation is applied every morning and evening.

The comparison of an occlusal intraoral radiograph obtained at T0 with another one at 3 days from the beginning of activation allows us to verify the opening of the mid-palatal suture and thus to continue expansion safely. Active expansion ranges from 10 to 20 days according to individual needs.

As in general practice, the device was well tolerated by all the patients in the presented study. All patients and their parents had been previously briefed on the behavior, diet, and oral hygiene needed to be followed for this particular device to avoid any complication that could interfere with the expansion maneuver.

STATISTICAL ANALYSIS

Data were analyzed with the statistical package for the social sciences program. The Wilcoxon signed rank test was used on data obtained before and after the study to assess changes caused by the procedure. The Wilcoxon signed rank test examines information on the differences and on the magnitude of difference between the 2 studied parameters (before and after treatment); it is the most powerful "sign test."

RESULTS
Orthopedic/Orthodontic Results

All the changes induced by RME on the upper jaw and adjacent structures were analyzed by posteroanterior cephalometric evaluation in T0, T1, and T2 and by CT Dentascan at T0 and T1. This evaluation is the most reliable way to assess the increase in the maxillary cross section. In fact, studies assessing the increase in upper dental arch width on cast models can be influenced by dental tipping that can show increases not actually corresponding to skeletal changes.

The Ricketts parameters were adopted for the posteroanterior cephalometric evaluation (**Fig. 1**).[5] In all treated cases, an opening of the midpalatal suture was obtained; the result was confirmed by intraoral occlusal radiographs (**Fig. 2**), posteroanterior cephalograms (**Fig. 3**), and CT Dentascan The evaluation of the variations of the maxillary width shows an increase, confirming that the RME maneuver directly influences the skeleton with the expansion of the midpalatal suture (**Fig. 4**). This maneuver is responsible for the expansion of both maxillas, with an average cross-sectional increase (JL-JR) of 5.91 ± 0.7 mm. The study of the upper intermolar distance (A6-6A) shows an average increase of 8.18 ± 0.3 mm. The interincisive space (A1-1A),

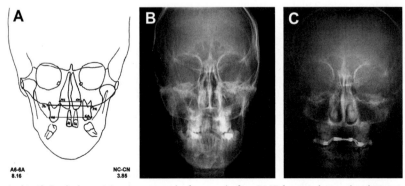

Fig. 1. (*A–C*) Cephalometric assessment before and after RME (mean data values). Anatomic changes in whole sample: all cross-sectional diameters increased at intermaxillar and inter-molar level. Nasal cavities and interincisive spaces increased in width.

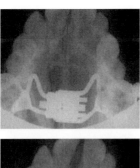

PRE R.M.E

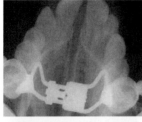

POST R.M.E. (1 WEEK)

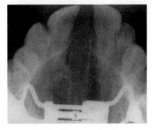

POST R.M.E. (3 WEEKS)

Fig. 2. Intraoral radiograph before and after RME.

hallmark of the midpalatal suture opening, was present in all treated cases, with an average opening of 4.72 $\pm$ 0.2 mm. This space gradually disappears, possibly because of transseptal fiber pull, which brings the fibers together. The increase in maxillary cross section is also shown by the study of the nasal cavities (NC-CN) that are widened by the maneuver with an average increase of the pyriform opening of 3.85 $\pm$ 0.3mm.

Results of ENT Examination

During the first (baseline) examination (T0) the selected sample reported the following results:

- Pharyngoscopy: 42 patients had previously had adenotonsillectomy surgery; there were normotrophic palatal tonsils in 18 cases.
- Posterior rhinoscopy with nasal fibroscopy: in all 60 cases, no significant adenoid lymphatic tissue or other obstructive causes were noted.
- Anterior rhinoscopy: nasal septum deviation with hypertrophy of the inferior turbinates was present in 41 cases, and 19 cases had normal inferior nasal turbinates.
- Active anterior rhinometry: that is, based on a nasal resistance value greater than 1.8 at a pressure of 75 Pa with a unilateral impairment that was considered as pathologic in another 10 cases.
- Allergological tests with prick test: negative outcome for major permanent and seasonal allergens in all subjects.

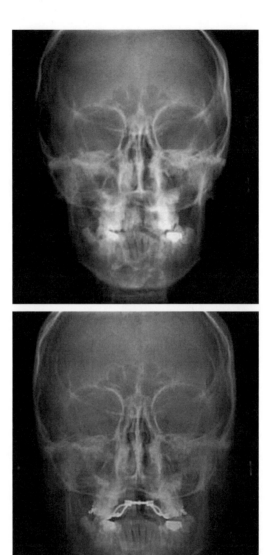

Fig. 3. Case of teleradiograph in posteroanterior view taken pre-RME (*top*) and post-RME (*bottom*).

- Audiometric tests: 14 patients showed moderate conductive hearing loss (15–30 dB HL), unilateral in 5 cases, bilateral in 9 cases.
- Tympanometric tests with tubaric functionality maneuvers: type C curve with tubaric deficit (compliance at pressure values <100 mm H_2O) was found in 16 children.

POLYSOMNOGRAPHY

Baseline: the apnea-hypopnea index (AHI) values of 60 patients ranged from 6.1 to 22.4 events per hour (average 16.3) (normal value<5). Patients were subdivided into

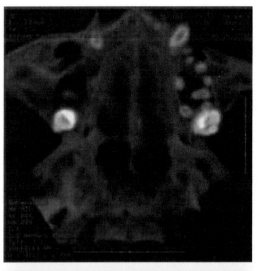

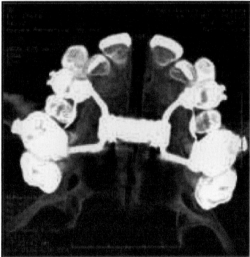

Fig. 4. CT volume rendering of maxilla pre-RME (*top*) and post-RME (*bottom*).

3 groups: group A had AHI values from 5 to 10, average 8.3 (16 cases); group B had AHI values between 11 and 15, average 12.88 (35 cases); group C had AHI values between 16 and 22.4, average 19 (9 cases) (**Table 1**).

After 4 months of orthodontic treatment with the device still in place (T1) nasal functional and polysomnographic tests showed the following:

- Out of the 36 cases with bilateral nose-breathing deficit, 28 went back to normal; in 8 cases the deficit was unilateral, and in 2 cases the deficit had improved but was still present; all of the 10 cases of unilateral deficit were within physiologic limits.
- Audiometric tests, tympanometry, and tubaric functionality tests: 7 of the 14 patients with tubaric disease healed without associated medical therapy, and 7 patients underwent mucolytic and/or cortisone therapy.

Table 1 Polysomnographic data in 60 children			
	T0	T1	T2
Obstructive AHI	Range, 6.1–22.4 Average, 16.3 ± 2.5	Range, 0–9.1 Average, 8.3 ± 2.3	Range, 0–26 Average, 0.8 ± 1.3
Nadir SPo₂ (%)	77.9 ± 8.4	90.2 ± 5.7	95.4 ± 1.4
Duration of Longest Obstructive Apneas	39.8 ± 17.2	24.3 ± 12.3	12.1 ± 6.5
Duration of Desaturation (S302<92%) ass% TST	18.5 ± 3.2	5.8 ± 1.3	1.3 ± 1.4
Sleep Efficiency (%)	88.5 ± 9.1	88.9 ± 5.7	89.8 ± 8.5

Note the significant improvement in all the functional parameters achieved at T2. All data are displayed as mean ± standard deviation.

Abbreviations: TST, total sleep time; T0, before any orthodontic therapy; T1, after 4 weeks with the device; T2, 4 months after the end of the orthodontic treatment.

- Polysomnography (**Figs. 5** and **6**): groups A and B present a normalization of recording, with AHI less than 5. In group C, 5 cases had an AHI less than 5, and in the last 4 cases, a significant improvement with AHI between 6.6 and 8.4 events per hour was noted.

Four months after end of the orthodontic treatment (T2), all tests showing a normalization of functional examinations were confirmed.

- Active anterior rhinometry: the 8 cases with residual unilateral deficit showed normal results; the 2 cases of group C with bilateral deficit continued to improve although physiologic levels were not reached.
- Polysomnography: the cases of group C with residual abnormal breathing events (AHI<5) were also normalized (see **Table 1**).

STATISTICAL FINDINGS

The baseline rhinomanometric data showed a statistically significant difference with respect to those measured at 2 and 4 months (Wilcoxon $Z = -4.86$, $P = .000$; Wilcoxon $Z = -5.39$, $P = .000$, respectively). The difference between rhinomanometric data at 2 and 4 months was also statistically significant (Wilcoxon $Z = -4.86$, $P = .000$).

The difference between baseline AHI and that at 2 and 4 months was also statistically significant (Wilcoxon $Z = -4.0$, $P = .000$; Wilcoxon $Z = -5.15$, $P = .000$, respectively). The difference between AHI at 2 and 4 months was also statistically significant (Wilcoxon $Z = -2.0$, $P = .046$).

DISCUSSION

The results obtained on the 60 patients show that the RME therapy widens nasal fossa and releases the septum, thus restoring a normal nasal airflow with disappearance of obstructive sleep-disordered breathing.

The improvement can be clearly linked to the skeletal expansion caused by the maneuver performed on the suture.

CT images before and after RME therapy confirm that the expansion occurs not only in the maxillary arch but also in the nasal cavity (**Fig. 7**): the widening of the nasal fossa and the septal release restore normal airflow. This anatomic change brings about an increased patency of the upper airway. This patency is the basis for the positive

Patient Information pre- RME
Name :   C.G. IN t0
Sex   :   M
Age   :   8 years
Date of study: 20/10/03 at 20.09.35
Duration (TSIT): 645 Min   Acquisition: 984

Apnea/ Hypopnea

	Number	Mean (sec)	Max (sec)	Index #/hr (TSIT)
Central	7	15.3	20.5	0.7
Obst	8	15.3	20.5	0.7
Mixed	3	14.8	17.5	0.3
Hypop	107	25.2	60	10
Total	125	23.7	60	11.6

Oximetry

<50% (min)	0
<60% (min)	0
<70% (min)	0
<75% (min)	0
<80% (min)	0
<85% (min)	0
<90% (min)	0
<95% (min)	5
Average (%)	98
Desat Index (#hr TSIT)	6.5

Body position

	Supine	Non- Supine
Time (min)	550.4	94.6
CA (#)	7	0
OA (#)	7	1
MA (#)	3	0
HYP (#)	97	10
Index (#/hr)	12.4	7
Desats (#)	61	8

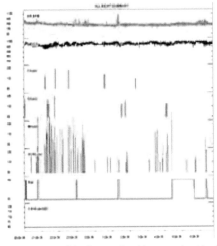

Fig. 5. Example of polysomnographic sheet raised by a patient before RME therapy (T0). The AHI value was 11.6 (normal value<5).

Patient Information

Name :   C.G. T1
Sex   :   M
Age   :   08 years
Date of study: 22/11/03 at 20.24.03
Duration (TSIT): 645 Min   Acquisition : 356

Apnea / Hypopnea

	Number	Mean (sec)	Max (sec)	Index #/hr (TSIT)
Central	0	0	0	0
Obst	0	0	0	0
Mixed	0	0	0	0
Hypop	12	26.8	58.5	1.1
Total	12	26.8	58.5	1.1

Oximetry

<50% (min)	0
<60% (min)	0
<70% (min)	0
<75% (min)	0
<80% (min)	0
<85% (min)	0
<90% (min)	0
<95% (min)	0.5
Average (%)	99
Desat Index (#hr TSIT)	1.1

Body position

	Supine	Non- Supine
Time (min)	150.5	494.5
CA (#)	0	0
OA (#)	0	0
MA (#)	0	0
HYP (#)	0	12
Index (#/hr)	0	1.5
Desats (#)	0	12

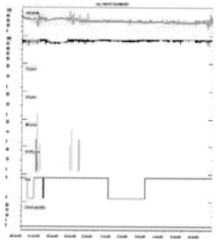

Fig. 6. Example of polysomnographic sheet raised by the same patient as in Fig 4 after 4 weeks of RME therapy (T1). Note the AHI value at 1.1.

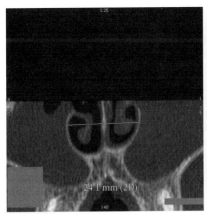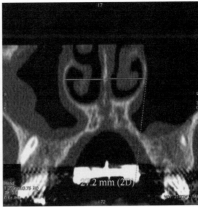

Fig. 7. TC Dentascan of nasal cavity increase before and after RME.

effects induced by the maneuver, and it acts on air exchange, with a net improvement of breathing disorders during sleep.

RME is a therapeutic procedure that the authors successfully performed for many years to obtain a skeletal expansion of the upper jaw. The anatomic criteria of this technique consist in the application of orthopedic forces, through particular procedures, on the midpalatal suture. This suture is mainly made up of compact bone laterally and fibrous tissue with fibroblasts, collagen fibers, and vessels centrally.[20–22] Bone distraction is possible because of the very biology of the bone and can be achieved by applying heavy forces through the orthodontic device anchored onto the teeth. Bone distraction at the suture level causes an actual widening of the maxilla, increasing its cross section as well as the anatomic space of the nasal cavity. Radiographic findings clearly show how the RME maneuver separates the nasal and palatal bones. A substantial increase is reported at the cross-sectional level, with a relevant improvement in nasal airflow. Increasing of upper jaw cross section also clearly affects the nasal cavities, and it is a true anatomic change that brings about an increased patency of the upper airways. This increase is also the basis for the positive effects induced by the RME maneuver on the respiratory function. Associated orthodontic movements can also indirectly improve the oropharyngeal space by modifying the resting posture of the tongue.

Beginning in 1984, Timms[19,23,24] has published several articles documenting the subjective and objective improvement of nasal resistance in 10-to-20-year-old subjects using rhinometry. However, he never made the connection between his findings and OSAS. Kurol and colleagues[25] also reported improvement of nasal resistance in 10 prospectively studied children, aged 8 to 13 years, treated with RME. Warren and colleagues[26] who performed a prospective study on 16 children aged 10 to 14 years demonstrated improvement in 45% of cases. Probably RME would not be as successful in isolation in presence of adenotonsillar hypertrophy, and for this reason, children with enlarged adenoids and tonsils were not included in the authors' study.

Moreover, abnormal nasal resistance affects not only the maxilla but also the mandible. Despite the change in tongue position with RME, the gain may not be sufficient. The width of the mandible should be considered when RME is performed, because upper and lower teeth must be in apposition. Combined treatment on the maxilla and mandible, as recently presented by Guilleminault and Li,[27] may be necessary. Correction of upper jaw narrowness in children not only can resolve all OSAS cases but also may help avoid septoplasty in the adult by widening nasal cavities and straightening the septum.

The authors suggest careful evaluation of the maxillary skeleton base status as a possible common cause of OSAS and recommend resorting to RME therapy.

Orthodontists may play an important role in the interdisciplinary treatment of OSAS because a high percentage of patients with OSAS suffer from maxillary narrowness as the authors showed at the 17th Annual Meeting of American Academy of Dental Sleep Medicine (Baltimore, Maryland, USA, June 2008). In young patients, RME treatment can be effective and can have a favorable orthopedic role in modifying facial bony structures and in conditioning further developmental processes positively.[28] The authors' experience shows that RME treatment has a positive effect on children affected by chronic snoring and OSA. By changing the anatomic structures, RME brings a functional improvement. It is always important to assess the condition of the upper jaw to consider RME therapy in the multidisciplinary treatment of OSAS in children.

REFERENCES

1. Guilleminault C, Khramtsov A. Upper airway resistance syndrome in children: a clinical review [review]. Semin Pediatr Neurol 2001;8(4):207–15.
2. Guilleminault C, Li KK, Khramtsov A, et al. Sleep disordered breathing: surgical outcomes in prepubertal children. Laryngoscope 2004;114(1):132–7.
3. Guilleminault C, Partinen M, Praud JP, et al. Morphometric facial changes and obstructive sleep apnea in adolescents. J Pediatr 1989;114(6):997–9.
4. Cistulli PA, Palmisano RG, Poole MD. Treatment of obstructive sleep apnea syndrome by rapid maxillary expansion. Sleep 1998;21:831–5.
5. Pirelli P, Saponara M, Guilleminault C. Rapid maxillary expansion in children with obstructive sleep apnea syndrome. Sleep 2004;27(4):761–6.
6. Harvold EP, Tomer BS, Vargervik K, et al. Primate experiments on oral respiration. Am J Orthod 1981;79(4):359 72.
7. Miller AJ, Vargervik K, Chierici G. Sequential neuromuscular changes on rhesus monkeys during the initial adaptation to oral respiration. Am J Orthod 1982;81(2):99–107.
8. Rubin RM. Effects of nasal airway obstruction on facial growth. Ear Nose Throat J 1987;66(5):212–9.
9. Pirelli P, Saponara M, Attanasio G. Obstructive sleep apnea syndrome (OSAS) and rhinotubaric disfunction in children: therapeutic effects of RME therapy. Prog Orthod 2005;6(1):48–61.
10. Linder-Aronson S. Dimensions of face and palate in nose breathers and habitual mouth breathers. Odontol Revy 1969;14:187–200.
11. Pirelli P. Respirazione orale e sviluppo cranio facciale: importanza dell'approccio interdisciplinare [Oral breathing and cranio-facial development: role of the multidisciplinary approach]. Mondo Ortod 1996;21:265–75 [in Italian].
12. Sleep-related breathing disorders in adults: recommendations for syndrome definition and measurement techniques in clinical research. The Report of an American Academy of Sleep Medicine Task Force. Sleep 1999;22:667–89.
13. Di Malta E. Basi Anatomo-Fisiologiche delle III Classi. Terapia Ortopedica. Bologna (Italy): Edizioni Martina; 1992.
14. Gianni E. La nuova Ortognatodonzia. Padova (Italy): Piccin; 1980.
15. Langlade M. Cefalometria Ortodontica. Milano (Italy): Scienza e Tecnica Dentistica; 1979.

16. Pirelli P. Suture craniofacciali e ortognatodonzia: applicazioni cliniche [Cranio-facial sutures and orthodontics: clinical applications]. Mondo Ortod 1996;21: 339–50 [in Italian].

17. Pirelli P, Giancotti A, Pirelli M. ERM: effetti strutturali e ripercussioni sul setto nasale [R.M.E. anatomical effects and responses of the nasal septum]. Mondo Ortod 1996;21:351–60 [in Italian].

18. Pirelli P, Marullo M, Casagrande M, et al. Espansione rapida del mascellare: effetti sulla funzionalità respiratoria ed uditiva [Rapid maxillary expansion: effects on the respiratory and auditive function]. Mondo Ortod 1995;20:129–35 [in Italian].

19. Timms DJ. The effect of rapid maxillary expansion on nasal airway resistance. Br J Orthod 1986;13(4):221–8.

20. Pirelli P, Arcuri C, Cocchia D, et al. Considerazioni sulla sinostosi della sutura mesiopalatina dell'uomo: studio istologico [Considerations on the synostosis of the human midpalatal suture: histological investigation]. Ortognatodonzia Italiana 1993;2(1):111–5 [in Italian].

21. Pirelli P, Botti F, Ragazzoni E, et al. Light microscopic investigation of the human midpalatal suture. Ital J Anat Embryol 1999;104(1):11–8.

22. Pirelli P, Botti F, Arcuri C, et al. New morphologic data on the human palatal suture [abstract]. Acts 72°Congress-Eur Orthod Soc Brighton; 1996.

23. Timms DJ. The reduction of nasal airway resistance by rapid maxillary expansion and its effect on respiratory disease. J Laryngol Otol 1984;98(4):357–62.

24. Timms DJ. Rapid maxillary expansion in the treatment of nocturnal enuresis. Angle Orthod 1990;60(3):229–33 [discussion: 234].

25. Kurol J, Modin H, Bjerkhoel A. Orthodontic maxillary expansion and its effect on nocturnal enuresis. Angle Orthod 1998;68(3):225–32.

26. Warren DW, Hershey HG, Turvey TA, et al. The nasal airway following maxillary expansion. Am J Orthod Dentofacial Orthop 1987;91(2):111–6.

27. Guilleminault C, Li KK. Maxillomandibular expansion for the treatment of sleep-disordered breathing: preliminary result. Laryngoscope 2004;11(5):893–6.

28. Darendelirer MA, Lam LC, Pirelli P, et al. Dentofacial orthopedics. In: Lavigne GJ, Cistulli PA, Smith MT, editors. Sleep medicine for dentists. Canada: Quintessence books; 2009. p. 85–91, chapter 11.

Sleepy Driving

Nelson B. Powell, DDS, MD[a,b,]*, Jason K.M. Chau, MD, MPH, FRCS(C)[c]

KEYWORDS
- Sleepiness • Drowsiness • Alcohol • Driving
- Accidents • Sleep apnea

SLEEPINESS AND DRIVING: A BRIEF REVIEW

Although the exact neurophysiologic mechanisms of sleep remain to be elucidated, there is ample scientific evidence identifying that adequate sleep is essential for healthy daily functioning and general well being.[1] Insufficient sleep may cause decrements in health and quality of life. Acute and chronic sleepiness is pervasive in our society and is generally the result of volitional insufficient sleep (sleep dept), or is secondary to an underlying sleep disorder such as obstructive sleep apnea (OSA) syndrome, narcolepsy, or insomnia.[2–6]

Regardless of the causes of sleepiness, driving while drowsy, tired, sleepy, or fatigued can result in human-error–related accidents and injuries due to decrements in neurobehavioral functions. These decrements may negatively affect reaction times and vigilance to such a degree to cause a motor vehicle accident.[7] Due to the large number of drivers on the United States highways, human-error accidents caused by sleepiness are of grave concern for public health and safety.[8–13] The National Transportation Safety Board (NTSB) reported in 2004 that there were 291 million individuals in the United States. Approximately 191 million were licensed to drive and of these about 42,000 die yearly in traffic-related accidents.[14] The National Sleep Foundation (NSF) "Sleep in America Poll" found that 51% of adult drivers polled admitted to driving drowsy and 17% reported falling asleep at the wheel in the previous year.[15] The prevalence of sleepiness in our society has been reported to be as high as 33%.[3,16] Hence, there is an immense pool of sleepy driving subjects, many of whom ignore or are oblivious to the signs of sleepiness and continue to drive. Some of the most common unambiguous behavioral signs of sleepy driving are: single or

The authors have no financial disclosures or conflicts of interest with any person or company to report.

a Department of Otolaryngology Head and Neck Surgery, Stanford University School of Medicine, Palo Alto, Stanford, CA 94305, USA
b Department of Psychiatry and Behavioral Science, Stanford University Sleep and Research Center, Stanford University School of Medicine, Palo Alto, Stanford, CA 94305, USA
c Department of Otolaryngology-Head and Neck Surgery, University of Manitoba, GB421 820 Sherbrook Street, Winnipeg, Manitoba R3A 1R9, Canada
* Corresponding author. 750 Welch Road, Suite 317, Palo Alto, CA 94304.
E-mail address: nelsonpowell@sbcglobal.net

Med Clin N Am 94 (2010) 531–540
doi:10.1016/j.mcna.2010.02.002
0025-7125/10/$ – see front matter © 2010 Elsevier Inc. All rights reserved.

repetitive head drops (called microsleeps = lapses of ≥ 500 ms), heavy eyelids with frequent eye closures, and yawning. These signs are often ignored by the driver and as a result a sleepy accident could occur. It has been reported that subjects who fell asleep while driving usually knew they were experiencing fitful levels of sleepiness beforehand.[17] However, sleepy drivers are generally unable to predict when their sleep impairment has escalated to a point where sleep will overtake them without notice.[18] Unfortunately, at present there is no objective method to evaluate an unfit driver due to sleepiness alone.

BRIEF HISTORY OF SLEEPINESS

The peer-review literature is replete with years of data collection on the dangers of sleepy driving.[19–21] Many of these investigations suggest countermeasures and educational programs for drivers.[22–24] This approach has merit, but has not been widely implemented and unfortunately sleepy driving behavior still persists at high levels.[15] Hundreds of government and medical investigations concerning sleepiness and driving have been published, yet they have either not reached the public and health care providers or they have not been given adequate attention. Therefore, a disconnect exists between the published information available and the level of understanding among the population as a whole. In fact the public's understanding of sleep in general lags far behind the advances reported in the scientific literature. This gap needs to be improved.

What Was Previously Accomplished?

To emphasize that much has been uncovered about sleepiness, a literature search of Medline (PubMed) and Ovid databases was conducted. Key words used in the search strategy included: drowsiness, sleepiness and accidents, drowsiness and accidents, drowsiness and driving, sleepiness and driving. Non-English articles that had an abstract in English were included in the overall number count. Peer-reviewed articles dating from the early 1920s (Ovid) through the present day were included in the survey (PubMed goes back only to 1950) (**Fig. 1**). Two early examples are presented so the reader can fully appreciate that investigations of sleepiness have been around for many years. In 1921, McComas[25] reported on the effect of altitude on a subject flying in an airplane at up to 20,000 feet. Although not a driving experience per se, he examined lowered oxygen tensions as related to human motor mechanism activity, impaired vision, early fatigue, and coordination disturbances. The subject underwent 50 tests each at 4 different altitudes. The outcomes suggested that there were alterations of higher brain functions along with drowsiness and irritability. In 1938 Mayer[26] reported on the human factor in the prevention of (French) traffic accidents. He noted in part that 77% of traffic accidents were due to psychological factors secondary to a lack of attention, fatigue, drowsiness, and/or imprudence.

What Have We Now Accomplished?

An excellent review article by Ellen and colleagues[27] reported on motor vehicle crash risks in sleep apnea. The objective was to determine if drivers with sleep apnea have an increased risk of motor vehicle accidents and if sleep apnea severity and excessive daytime sleepiness (EDS) could affect driving risks. Forty-one evidence-based medicine studies of noncommercial drivers with sleep apnea were identified. A 2- to 3-times greater crash rate was identified in this group at a statistically significant level. Commercial drivers had comparatively smaller crash rates. Approximately 50% of the studies included in the review showed an increased risk for crashes with increased

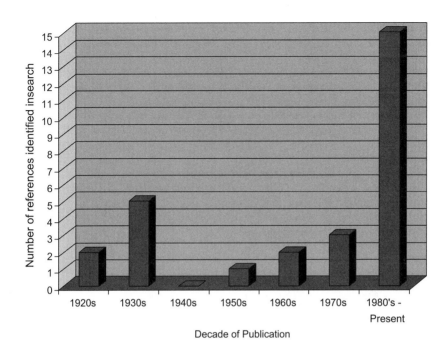

Fig. 1. November 2009 search results of Ovid and PubMed databases using the key words "drowsiness," "sleepiness," "drowsiness AND accidents," "sleepiness AND accidents," "drowsiness AND driving," and "sleepiness AND driving." The numbers of articles identified for a given decade are given on the Y-axis and their decade of publication on the X-axis. After 1980, more than 10,000 references were identified.

OSA severity, whereas the remaining 50% did not show this finding. Treatment of OSA was consistent with improvement of driver performance across all studies.

The Problem

Contrast the early research above to the current standards below and, although there is more sophisticated methodology today, the goals remain very similar. Sleepiness and drowsiness in America has been recognized for nearly 90 years but unfortunately very little has changed regarding its prevalence and impact on public health. The issue that has not been emphasized is the peripheral damage due to sleepy drivers. One might ask why it has taken so long for government and courts to act to protect the public. It seems unreasonable that sleep issues have been acknowledged for so many years, yet we are still without a universal mandate that drivers be accountable for the risks they take in driving sleepy.

Maggie's Law

A good example of the judicial system's failure or reluctance to acknowledge peripheral damage is the death of 20-year-old student Maggie McDonald in 1997. She was killed when a sleepy driver struck her automobile head on. The first trial of the driver ended in a deadlock. In the next trial, the driver received a suspended jail sentence and a $200 fine because at that time it was not against the law to fall asleep while driving. This remedy was totally unacceptable but did demonstrate how little education government and courts had concerning sleepiness and sleepy drivers. However, the family persisted in attaining justice and eventually the New Jersey Legislature enacted "Maggie's Law." The law was the first of its kind, making it illegal to drive while sleep-impaired in the state of New Jersey.[28,29] Should death occur, the law allows for a conviction of vehicular homicide if driving while sleep-deprived. Keep in mind that this outcome was not initiated due to pressure from sleep education specialists, or by concerned law enforcement, government, or public health officials, but through the dedication of Maggie McDonnell's family.

Despite the expected impact of Maggie's Law, there is still a lack of education about the significant dangers of driving while tired, drowsy, sleepy, or fatigued. However, a positive outcome of the New Jersey statute was that it placed employers at risk of corporate liability for drowsy driving accidents if employees were required to work excessively long hours, such as seen in commercial driving and medical training.[30–32] Fortunately, there are many US states that now have legislative bills pending or passed that address drowsy driving issues.[29]

THE NATIONAL COMMISSION ON SLEEP

An important positive step for sleep was accomplished in 1992 by William Dement, who was the Director of the National Commission on Sleep Disorders Research.[33] A report from this commission was submitted to the US Congress and cited that 40 million Americans were chronically affected by various sleep disorders and that an additional 20 to 30 million experience some sort of intermittent sleep-related problem. The report projected that by 2010, 79 million Americans would have difficulty falling asleep and nearly 40 million would experience debilitating EDS. By 2050, this was expected to increase to 100 million and 50 million, respectively. The report's projections for 2010 have been verified, at least in part, in a recent report by the Institute of Medicine[34] identifying that 50 to 70 million Americans have chronic sleep and wakefulness disorders. The burden of sleepiness that includes sleepy driving clearly continues to grow despite substantial and long-standing scientific evidence advocating the benefit of education and treatment. The problem will continue to grow unless the medical community, government officials, and society as a whole take responsibility and personal accountability for their role in the problem.

ALCOHOL VERSUS SLEEPY DRIVING: A COMPARATIVE MODEL

What may facilitate a better understanding of the potential risks of sleepy driving is the comparative model of driving under the influence of alcohol. Alcohol-related driving accidents have been a major focus of Mothers Against Drunk Driving (MADD), who intervened with national educational goals to reduce drunk-driving fatalities. Their strategy changed the national thinking over a 15-year period, which resulted in an enormous decrease in drunk-driving deaths.[35] We can learn from the experiences of this group because they have made significant strides in a short period of time. Sleepy drivers and drunk drivers exhibit a common finding, which is slowing of "reaction time" in a dose-response manner.[36] There are other commonalities they may share, such as decrements in neurocognitive functions and vigilance.[37,38] Peer-reviewed literature supports the fact that driving sleepy is the same as driving drunk.[19] This association brings attention to both dangerous activities (alcohol or sleepiness) separately or in combination. The specific outcomes of driving sleepy, driving drunk, or a combination of both is presented by knowledgeable researchers in this field. There are many excellent articles on this subject. Hence, only a limited number are presented here.

Dinges and Kribbs[36] reported that effects on simple reaction time effects are seen if alcohol and sleepiness are combined secondary to acceleration of habituation. These investigators showed that increasing alcohol levels or minimal sleep, or a combination of both could cause gross errors in judgment and attentiveness during driving. The importance of an adequate reaction time while driving could be life saving for the driver and others involved.

As a brief reminder, at a speed of 60 miles per hour an automobile will have traveled 88 ft in 1 second. It is not uncommon for sleepy drivers to have one-half to 1-second reaction time or more. A reaction time equal to or longer than 500 ms is defined as a "lapse." Lapses are extremely dangerous to any driver that is sleepy or under the influence of drugs or alcohol.

Dawson and Reid[39] reported that 17 hours of sleep deprivation (wakefulness) produces cognitive psychomotor performance (CPP) at a level that was equivalent to the performance impairments seen in blood alcohol concentrations (BAC) of 0.05%. At 24 hours of wakefulness CPP performance decreased to the same level as the performance of a BAC of 0.10%, which is well over the legal driving limit in many states.

Falleti and colleagues[40] examined cognitive impairment over 24 hours of sustained wakefulness and BAC of 0.05%, and found that fatigue from sleep caused more impairment than alcohol.

Roehrs and colleagues[41] examined dose-related sedative effects from sleep loss to those of ethanol. Sleep loss was 2.7 times more potent than ethanol in grams per kilogram in sedative effects. In addition, sleep loss reduced measures of the Multiple Sleep Latency Test (MSLT).

Roehrs and colleagues[42] also evaluated sleepiness with low-dose alcohol for simulated driving and divided performance attention, reporting on sleepiness and alcohol in simulated driving. The results showed that sleepiness and low-dose ethanol together impaired simulated driving. The investigators suggested it was possible that low breath ethanol concentrations (BEC) beyond the point of zero BEC could explain the incidence of driving accidents because sleepiness was also present.

Haraldsson and Akerstedt[43] reported from Sweden that drowsiness is a greater traffic hazard than alcohol and that drowsy driving is an underestimated risk factor in official statistics, as 15% to 30% of traffic accidents are related to drowsiness. Accidents while drowsy result in 3 times as many fatalities.

Powell and colleagues[44] reported on reaction time (RT) performance in OSA and alcohol-impaired controls. RTs were selected as a metric for evaluation because it is well known that RT is altered in unsafe alcohol consumption and sleepiness. This prospective study of a comparative model assessed alcohol-challenged normal subjects and subjects with OSA. Eighty healthy subjects performed 4 RT time trials using a validated psychomotor vigilance test (PVT) during which time breath alcohol concentrations (BrACs) were incrementally elevated to 0.08 g/dL or greater. The same PVT test was done on 113 subjects with OSA without alcohol. The OSA subjects had a mean respiratory disturbance index (RDI) of 29.2 events per hour of sleep. The findings of this study demonstrated that subjects with a mean age of 47 years with mild to moderate OSA had a worse RT test performance than healthy nonsleepy subjects with a mean age of 29 years and a BrAC that was illegally high for driving motor vehicles in the state of California.

Williamson and Feyer[45] compared the effects on performance of sleep deprivation and alcohol. Sleep deprivation of 17 to 19 hours showed that performance was equivalent or worse than a BAC of 0.05%. Response actions were 50% slower and accuracy was also lower than in those subjects with alcohol. This result suggested that sleep deprivation could compromise driving performance.

Powell and colleagues[19] continued to evaluate the comparative risks of drowsy driving and alcohol-impaired performances during a real-time study on track driving experience. This investigation was the first to include actual driving of a motor vehicle with the intention of assessing alcohol versus sleepiness while driving. This prospective cohort study included 16 healthy matched adult subjects with 50% being women. Two groups were identified: sleep-deprived and alcohol-challenged. The sleep-deprived group was further subdivided into an acute deprivation group and a chronic deprivation group. The acute group was sleep deprived for 24 hours (one night without sleep). The other subdivided group comprised chronic subjects, who slept 2 hours less than their usual sleep periods for 7 days. All subjects underwent baseline RT testing with a PVT device.

Each subject then drove on a closed course set up to test performance at the General Motors test track in Mesa, Arizona. Baseline data from that drive were collected for comparison with the final performance results for each subject (sleep-deprived and alcohol groups). Seven days later at the same time period as the baseline testing, the entire sequence was repeated for sleep deprivation or alcohol intake. The outcomes showed that there were no significant between-group differences in sleep-depravation or alcohol-intake groups before and after intervention for all 11 RT (PVT) tests. The magnitude of change was almost identical in both groups, even in light of the mean BAC of 0.089 g/dL in the alcohol group. On-track driving performance had similar results with a $P = .724$ when change scores for between groups were evaluated (baseline and at final driving). The overall outcome of the study could not be generalized because the subject numbers were small. However, the model suggests that there is a potential risk of driving sleepy that is at least as dangerous as driving illegally under the influence of alcohol.

The question is whether the general public is aware of these and the many other scientific investigations on driving sleepy, and whether without educational intervention they can be expected to make the correlation that driving sleepy is the same as driving drunk?

SLEEPY DRIVING ACCIDENT RISKS

The National Highway Traffic Safety Administration (NHTSA) and the National Center on Sleep Disorders Research (NCSDR) sponsored an expert panel on driver fatigue and sleepiness chaired by Strohl and colleagues.[24] This panel was a comprehensive effort to review the drowsy driving that has led to thousands of automobile accidents yearly. There were 7 sections from the introduction to the expert panel's recommendations. At completion, the panel suggested that there should be a focus on education concerning "drowsy driving," which included: education of young males, effective countermeasures, raising public awareness, educating shift workers, and education from other sectors. This study also covered crash characteristics and risks for drowsy driving crashes. The crash characteristics are summarized as follows: problems occur during late night and early morning, crashes are usually serious, single vehicle crash, occurs on high-speed roadway, no attempt to avoid crash, and the driver is alone. Population groups at the highest risk have been created based on crash reports. Three population groups exist: young males age 16 to 29, shift workers, and untreated sleep disorders. The risks of drowsy driving crashes are limited to inferential findings because there is presently no objective methodology for a clear-cut assessment of an individual's level of sleepiness. However, the important educational metrics are: sleep loss, driving patterns especially from midnight to 6 AM, driving excessive miles yearly or hours a day, and driving longer without a break. Risk factors also include the use of sedative medications, unrecognized or untreated OSA, and alcohol usage. Many of these factors have cumulative effects.

Powell and colleagues[46] reported on sleepy driver near misses that may predict accident risks in a prospective cross-sectional study using an Internet survey with Dateline NBC News. The results from 35,217 subjects (88% of the sample of 39,825) are as follows: the risk of 1 accident increased from 23.2% if there were no near misses to a high of 44.5% in those with 4 or more near-miss sleepy accidents over a 3-year period. The Epworth Sleepiness Scale (ESS) had an independent association with a near miss or an accident. An increase of 1 unit of ESS score (of a maximum of 24) was associated with having a 4.4% increase of being involved in at least 1 accident ($P<.0001$). There was a dose response between sleepy near misses and an actual accident. Hence, sleepy near-miss accidents may be a precursor of an actual driving accident.

Accidents and Injuries

Shortly after the aforementioned NCSDR/NHTSA report by Strohl and colleagues,[24] Powell and colleagues[9] published findings on sleepy driving accidents and injury. This investigation evaluated the associated risk of driving sleepy with predictors of driving accidents and injury secondary to sleepiness. The study was a cross-sectional Internet-linked survey during a Dateline NBC news program on sleepy driving. An online national driving test used a 15-question quiz and from that quiz, subjects could voluntarily move on to a more detailed questionnaire of 64 questions. These questions were designed to elicit data on driving habits, sleepiness, accidents, and injuries during the last 3 years. Responses from 10,870 drivers were evaluated. Demographic characteristics were recorded. The ESS baseline score was 7.4 ± 4.2 for drivers without accidents and ranged to 12.7 ± 7.2 for drivers with 4 or more accidents $P<.0001$. Twenty-three percent of all respondents had 1 or more accident in a 3-year period. Among respondents who reported 4 or more accidents, a marked association was seen for the most recent accident to include injury ($P<.0001$). Sleep disorders were reported in 22.5% of all respondents, and in drivers that had more than 3 accidents the prevalence was higher, at 35% ($P = .002$). Six independent predictors of accidents were identified based on a stepwise ordered multiple logistic regression analysis, which kept the variable if the adjusted P value was less than 0.01. These 6 predictors were age, not married, ESS, annual miles driven, percentage driving at night, and consulted a medical professional because tired.

Connor and colleagues[47] from the University of Auckland, New Zealand designed a case study to evaluate whether sleepy driving causes crash injuries. This population-based control study included 571 drivers who were involved in crashes. At least one subject per driver was injured or killed in the crash. Acute sleepy driving increased the risk of crashing where a subject in the car was either injured or killed. There was no increase in risk associated with measures of chronic sleepiness.

SUMMARY

Acute and chronic sleepiness are pervasive in modern society, and are generally the result of volitional insufficient sleep or are secondary to an underlying sleep disorder. However, regardless of the cause of sleepiness, the outcome can cause human-error–related accidents and injuries due to decrements in neurobehavioral functions. These decrements may negatively affect RTs and vigilance to such a degree as to cause a motor vehicle accident and possible injury or death. The prevalence of sleepiness in our society has been reported to be as high as 33% and therefore there is an immense pool of sleepy driving subjects, many of whom ignore or are oblivious to the signs of sleepiness and persist to drive. We know from the large number of peer-review investigations that driving sleepy is the same as driving drunk. Unfortunately, we presently have no reasonable objective method to evaluate an unfit driver due to sleepiness alone. This may be, in large part, why efforts to teach the public about the dangers of sleepy driving have been relatively unsuccessful.

The risks of sleepy driving have very few legal sanctions and presently no objective testing methods. The scientific effort over numerous decades to better understand sleepiness and driving has also evaluated sleepiness risks in fields that require constant vigilance, for example, airlines, nuclear power, railroads, and medicine. We are still waiting for a method to assist in monitoring the levels of sleepiness and vigilance of motor vehicle drivers. This method should objectively assess sleepiness in much the same way as a breath or blood alcohol test evaluates alcohol levels.

Education, however, remains a critical element if change is to occur. Information about sleepiness and driving is readily available in the scientific literature, but it is not reaching the public in a way that they can relate to on a personal basis. Everyone who tests for a driver's license, in every state of the Union and every country of the world, should be able to answer basic questions about the signs of sleepiness and about the risks of driving sleepy. A point to consider is that if the medical literature contained data about a previously ignored disease that was now known to kill thousands of people each year, the news outlets would spread the word overnight. The dangers of sleepy driving need to receive similar, sustained attention.

REFERENCES

1. Ohayon MM, Caulet M, Philip P, et al. How sleep and mental disorders are related to complaints of daytime sleepiness. Arch Intern Med 1997;157:2645–52.
2. Hublin C, Kaprio J, Partinen M, et al. Insufficient sleep—a population-based study in adults. Sleep 2001;24:392–400.
3. Bonnet M, Arand D. We are chronically sleep deprived. Sleep 1995;18:908–11.
4. Young T, Palta M, Dempsey J, et al. The occurrence of sleep disordered breathing among middle-aged adults. N Engl J Med 1993;328:1230–5.
5. Engleman H, Douglas N. Sleep-4: sleepiness, cognitive function, and quality of life in obstructive sleep apnoea/hypopnea syndrome. Thorax 2004;59:618–22.
6. Durmer JS, Dinges DF. Neurocognitive consequences of sleep deprivation. Semin Neurol 2005;25(1):117–29.
7. Young T, Blustein J, Finn L, et al. Sleep-disordered breathing and motor vehicle accidents in a population-based sample of employed adults. Sleep 1997;20(8):608–13.
8. Horne J, Reyner L. Vehicle accidents related to sleep: a review. Occup Environ Med 1999;56:289–94.
9. Powell N, Schechtman K, Riley R, et al. Sleepy driving: accidents and injury. Otolaryngol Head Neck Surg 2002;126:217–27.
10. George C, Smiley A. Sleep apnea and automobile crashes. Sleep 1999;22(6):790–5.
11. Lyznicki J, Doege T, Davis R, et al. Sleepiness, driving, and motor vehicle crashes. JAMA 1998;279:1908–13.
12. Maycock G. Sleepiness and driving: the experience of heavy goods vehicle drivers in the UK. J Sleep Res 1997;6:238–44.

13. Masa J, Rubio M, Findley L. Habitually sleepy drivers have a high frequency of automobile crashes associated with respiratory disorders during sleep. Am J Respir Crit Care Med 2000;162:1407–12.
14. National Transportation Safety Board [Internet]. Highway special investigation report medical oversight of noncommercial drivers. NTSB Number SIR-04/01. NTIS Number PB2004-917002. PDF Document. Available at: http://www.ntsb. gov/publictn/2004/SIR0401.htm. Accessed November 16, 2004.
15. Drobnich D. A National Sleep Foundation's conference summary: the National Summit to prevent drowsy driving and a new call to action. Ind Health 2005; 43:197–200.
16. Ohayon M. Prevalence and correlates of nonrestorative sleep complaints. Arch Intern Med 2005;165:35–41.
17. Reyner L, Horne J. Falling asleep whilst driving: are drivers aware of prior sleepiness? Int J Legal Med 1998;111:120–3.
18. Dinges D, Mallis M. Managing fatigue by drowsiness detection. In: Hartley L, editor. Managing fatigue in transportation: Proceedings of the 3rd Fatigue in Transportation Conference, Fremantle, Western Australia, 1998. Western Australia: Institute for Research in Safety and Transport Murdoch University; 1998. p. 209–18.
19. Powell N, Schechtman K, Riley R, et al. The road to danger: the comparative risks of driving while sleepy. Laryngoscope 2001;111:887–93.
20. Akerstedt T, Kecklund G, Hörte L. Night driving, season, and the risk of highway accidents. Sleep 2001;24:401–6.
21. Pack AI, Pack AM, Rodgman E, et al. Characteristics of crashes attributed to the driver having fallen asleep. Accid Anal Prev 1995;27:769–75.
22. Stutts J, Wilkins J, Vaughn B. Why do people have drowsy driving crashes? Input from drivers who just did. Washington, DC: University of North Carolina School of Medicine for AAA Foundation for Traffic Safety; 1999.
23. Strohl K, Bonnie R, Findley L, et al. Sleep apnea, sleepiness, and driving risk. Am J Respir Crit Care Med 1994;150:1463–73.
24. Strohl K, Blatt J, Council F, et al. Drowsy driving and automobile crashes. Washington, DC: National Highway Traffic Safety Administration; 2001. Available at: http://www.nhtsa.dot.gov/PEOPLE/INJURY/drowsy_driving1/drowsy.html.
25. McComas HC. In: Controlling the airplane at twenty thousand feet, vol. 12. New York: Scientific Monthly; 1921. p. 36–46.
26. Mayer M. Report on human factor in the prevention of traffic accidents (French). International management congress, Washington (personal-general papers). 1938; p. 97–101.
27. Ellen RL, Marshal SC, Palayew M, et al. Systematic review of motor vehicle crash risk in persons with sleep apnea. J Clin Sleep Med 2006;2(2):193–200.
28. New Jersey Legislature. Available at: http://www.njleg.state.nj.us/2002/Bills/A1500/1347_R2.HTM. Accessed February 10, 2003.
29. National Sleep Foundation. NSF statement regarding Maggie's law—nation's first law aimed at drowsy driving, May 2007.
30. Philip P, Taillarad J, Leger D, et al. Work and rest sleep schedules of 227 European truck drivers. Sleep Med 2002;3:507–11.
31. Barger L, Cade B, Ayas N, et al. Extended work shifts and the risk of motor vehicle crashes among interns. N Engl J Med 2005;352:125–34.
32. Pack AI, Maislin G, Staley B, et al. Impaired performance in commercial drivers role of sleep apnea and short sleep duration. Am J Respir Crit Care Med 2006; 174:446–54.
33. National Commission on Sleep Disorders Research. Report of the National Commission on Sleep Disorders Research. Washington, DC: Superintendent of

Documents, US Government Printing Office; 1992. Department of Health and Human Services Publication 92.

34. Institute of Medicine. Sleep disorders and sleep deprivation: an unmet public health problem. Washington, DC: National Academies Press; 2006.

35. National Highway Traffic Administration. Traffic safety facts 2007 data: alcohol impaired driving. DOT HS 810 985. PDF.2008. Washington, DC: National Highway Traffic Administration.

36. Dinges DF, Kribbs NB. Comparison of the effects of alcohol and sleepiness on simple reaction time performance: enhanced habituation as a common process. Alcohol Drugs Driving 1990;5(4):329–39.

37. Kribbs NB, Dinges DF. Vigilance decrements and sleepiness. In: Hash JR, Ogilvie RD, editors. Sleep onset mechanisms. Washington, DC: American Psychological Association; 1994. p. 113–25.

38. Nicholson ME, Wang M, Collins O, et al. Variability in behavioral impairment involved in the rising and falling BAC curve. J Stud Alcohol 1992;53(4):349–56.

39. Dawson D, Reid K. Fatigue, alcohol and performance impairment. Nature 1997; 388:235.

40. Falleti MG, Maruff P, Collie A, et al. Qualitative similarities in cognitive impairment associated with 24 h of sustained wakefulness and a blood alcohol concentration of 0.05%. J Sleep Res 2003;12:265–74.

41. Roehrs T, Burduvali E, Monahoom MA, et al. Ethanol and sleep loss: a "dose" comparison of impairing effects. Sleep 2003;26(8):981–5.

42. Roehrs T, Beare D, Zorick F, et al. Sleepiness and ethanol effects on simulated driving. Alcohol Clin Exp Res 1994;18(1):154–8.

43. Haraldsson PO, Akerstedt T. [Drowsiness-greater traffic hazard than alcohol. Causes, risks and treatment]. Lakartidningen 2001;98(25):3018–23 [in Swedish].

44. Powell NB, Riley RW, Schechtman KB, et al. A comparative model: reaction time performance in sleep-disordered breathing versus alcohol-impaired controls. Laryngoscope 1999;109:1648–54.

45. Williamson AM, Feyer AM. Moderate sleep deprivation produces impairments in cognitive and motor performance equivalent to legally prescribed levels of alcohol intoxication. Occup Environ Med 2000;57:649–55.

46. Powell NB, Schechtman KB, Riley RW, et al. Sleepy driver near-misses may predict accident risks. Sleep 2007;30(3):331–42.

47. Connor J, Norton R, Ameratunga S, et al. Driver sleepiness and risk of serious injury to car occupants: population based case control study. BMJ 2002;324: 1125.

Advances in Narcolepsy

Michelle Cao, DO[a,b,*]

KEYWORDS

- Narcolepsy • Cataplexy • Excessive daytime sleepiness
- Sodium oxybate • Modafinil • Hypocretin

Narcolepsy with cataplexy affects 1 in 2000 individuals, with prevalence close to 0.04%. It is a chronic neurologic sleep disorder characterized by excessive daytime sleepiness (EDS), cataplexy, disturbed nocturnal sleep, and manifestations related to rapid eye movement (REM) sleep, such as sleep paralysis and hypnopompic/hypnagogic hallucinations. Sporadic and familial forms of narcolepsy exist in humans. The sporadic form is predominant (95%).[1] Impairment of hypocretin neurotransmission is central to the pathology of narcolepsy. The discovery of hypocretin genes (ie, hypocretin and hypocretin receptor genes) in animals and postnatal selective hypocretin ligand deficiency in humans has allowed for ongoing research into the pathophysiology of this disease and new treatment options. Understanding of narcolepsy has evolved over the past decade; new insights into the pathophysiology of the disease, treatments for cataplexy and EDS, and investigational treatment modalities are reviewed.

CLINICAL CHARACTERISTICS

The second edition of the *International Classification of Sleep Disorders* (ICSD-2) [2] includes 2 entities: narcolepsy with cataplexy and narcolepsy without cataplexy. The classic tetrad for narcolepsy includes EDS, cataplexy, sleep paralysis, and hypnagogic hallucinations. All 4 symptoms may not be present in a patient. EDS, sleep paralysis, and hypnagogic/hypnopompic hallucinations can also occur in individuals who are severely sleep deprived; only cataplexy is unique to narcolepsy. Briefly, these characteristic symptoms are reviewed.

EDS and cataplexy are considered the primary symptoms of narcolepsy. Narcoleptics typically describe feeling sleep deprived and complain of chronic daytime fatigue.

[a] Division of Sleep Medicine, Stanford University School of Medicine, 300 Pasteur Drive, Stanford, CA 94305, USA
[b] Stanford Sleep Medicine, 450 Broadway Street, M/C 5704, Pavilion C, 2nd Floor, Redwood City, CA 94063, USA
* Stanford Sleep Medicine, 450 Broadway Street, M/C 5704, Pavilion C, 2nd Floor, Redwood City, CA 94063.
E-mail address: mhtcao1@stanford.edu

Med Clin N Am 94 (2010) 541–555
doi:10.1016/j.mcna.2010.02.008
0025-7125/10/$ – see front matter © 2010 Elsevier Inc. All rights reserved.

medical.theclinics.com

Unwanted episodes of sleep attacks can occur several times a day. The duration of these sleep attacks may vary from a few seconds to several minutes and may happen in unusual circumstances, such as in the middle of a meal. Narcoleptic patients wake up feeling refreshed and there is a refractory period of 1 to several hours before the next episode occurs. Therefore, short (15–20 minute) naps are usually helpful and refreshing and help differentiate patients with narcolepsy from those with idiopathic hypersomnia, who take long and unrefreshing naps. Sleepiness is usually the first symptom to appear followed by cataplexy, sleep paralysis, and hypnagogic hallucinations. In approximately two-thirds of cases, cataplexy onset occurs within 5 years after the occurrence of EDS.[3,4]

Cataplexy occurs in 60% to 70% of narcoleptic patients.[5,6] It is an abrupt and reversible decrease or loss of muscle tone, most frequently elicited by emotional responses, with laughter and anger the 2 most common triggers. It may involve certain muscles or the entire voluntary musculature. Most typically the jaw sags, the head falls forward, the arms drop to the side, and the knees buckle. If it involves the upper limbs, patients may complain of clumsiness, such as dropping a cup when surprised. Awareness is preserved throughout the attack. The duration of each cataplectic attack is variable, in most cases lasting 30 seconds to 2 minutes. These short cataplectic attacks are the most common presentation of cataplexy. Status cataplecticus is a rare manifestation of cataplexy characterized by prolonged cataplexy lasting hours. Rarely in a cataplectic attack there is complete loss of muscle tone leading to total body collapse and serious injuries, such as bone fractures.

Sleep paralysis is often associated with hypnagogic hallucinations. It is best described as a terrifying experience occurring on falling asleep or awakening when individuals find themselves paralyzed, suddenly unable to move the limbs, speak, or even breathe deeply. During the event, individuals are fully aware of what is happening and afterwards are able to recall the event vividly. With time, individuals learn that episodes are brief and benign, rarely lasting longer than a few minutes and always ending spontaneously. Sleep paralysis may occur as an independent and isolated phenomenon, especially after sleep deprivation, and 3% to 5% of the general population may be affected by it. Abnormal vivid auditory or visual hallucinations that occur while falling asleep are known as hypnagogic hallucinations. Similarly, hypnopompic hallucinations occur on awakening. These hallucinations are unpleasant and associated with feelings of fear or major threat and sometimes associated with a feeling of dying. Hypnagogic hallucinations are often associated with sleep attacks.

Narcoleptic patients commonly experience disturbed nocturnal sleep and may complain of insomnia. Ironically, patients complain of difficulty falling asleep and staying asleep at night, but they fall asleep repeatedly during the daytime. The sleep disruption may be enhanced by the presence of periodic limb movements, which seem common in narcoleptics. Other associated sleep-related problems include REM sleep behavior disorder, obstructive sleep apnea, and non-REM parasomnias.

HYPOTHESES INTO THE PATHOPHYSIOLOGY OF NARCOLEPSY

The first major discovery came in 1980s when the tissue-type HLA-DR2 was found closely associated with narcolepsy.[7–9] Specifically, the HLA-DQB1*0602 is found in 95% of narcoleptic patients with cataplexy, 41% of patients with narcolepsy without cataplexy, and 18% to 35% of the general population.[9,10] This discovery led to the hypothesis that narcolepsy may be autoimmune mediated because many autoimmune diseases are associated with class II HLA haplotypes. In 1998, de Lecea and colleagues[11] discovered a hypothalamic peptide neurotransmitter, called hypocretin.

In the same year, this same peptide was discovered independently by Sakurai and colleagues,[12] who named it orexin. Hypocretin-1 and -2 are produced exclusively in the hypothalamus and project widely to the cerebral cortex, thalamus, hypothalamus, and brainstem and more densely to the locus coeruleus, tuberomamillary nucleus, raphe nucleus, and bulbar reticular formation, all of which are involved in wake-promoting mechanisms.[13]

Discovery of the hypocretin gene/ligand and its association with narcolepsy in canines and mice followed. In 1999, using a familial Doberman narcolepsy model, Stanford researchers identified an autosomal recessive mutation in the hypocretin receptor 2 gene (hcrtr-2) responsible for narcolepsy in canines.[14] Simultaneously, another group of researchers reported narcolepsy symptoms in hypocretin receptor (hcrtr) knockout mouse model.[15] The Hcrt receptor knockout mice exhibited short waking periods, frequent sleep-onset REM periods (SOREMs), and cataplexy. Hara and colleagues[16] produced the ataxin-3 (a gene product involved in cell apoptosis) transgenic mouse model in which mice are born with a normal number of hypocretin cells but with aging hypocretin neurons degenerate, leading to a deficiency in hypocretin, similar to human narcolepsy. The work of these researchers identified hypocretin as the major sleep-modulating neurotransmitter.

Narcolepsy in humans is not due to gene mutations; rather, narcoleptic humans were found to have very low levels of cerebrospinal fluid (CSF) hypocretin-1. There has been only 1 patient with a mutation in the hypocretin gene with very atypical early disease onset (6 months old).[17] Hypocretin neurons and functions are selectively damaged in patients with narcolepsy; however, the cause is still unknown.[18] Postmortem brain tissue of narcoleptic patients have undetectable levels of prehypocretin RNA and loss of hypocretin peptides. The melatonin-concentrating hormone neurons, however, located in the same region as the hypocretin neurons, were intact, suggesting that the loss of hypocretin was not a result of generalized neuronal degeneration in this region.[17,19]

After the discovery of hypocretin deficiency in humans, investigators discovered several substances that normally colocalize in hypocretin-containing neurons: dynorphin, neuronal activity-regulated pentraxin, and insulin-like growth factor-binding protein 3 (IGFBP3).[20] In postmortem human brain of narcoleptics, these substances were also found deficient.[20–22] This suggests that selective postnatal hypocretin neuronal cell death is the major pathophysiological process in human narcolepsy with cataplexy. Autoimmune mediated postnatal hypocretin neuronal cell death is an ongoing hypothesis under investigation. Multiple inflammatory markers have been tested (eg, erythrocyte sedimentation rate, serum immunoglobulin levels, C-reactive protein, and complement levels) in narcoleptic patients without any leads. Black and colleagues[23] tested neuron specific autoantibodies but did not find any association with narcoleptics. The same investigators also tested IgG reactivity to pre-prohypocretin and its major cleavage products (hypocretin-1 and -2) in serum and CSF but found no linkage.[24] It is possible that an autoimmune reaction may have occurred at the time of disease onset but then disappeared, as suggested by Dauvilliers and colleagues.[18]

Most recently, Honda and colleagues[20] discovered that the substance colocalizing with hypocretin neurons, IGFBP3, is a modulator of hypocretin cell function and is also involved in the regulation of sleep in normal individuals. Studies of transgenic mice overexpressing the human IGFBP3 protein reported decreased hypocretin messenger RNA and peptide contents and increased sleep. Overexpression of IGFBP3 resulting in increased serum IGFBP3 levels was associated with lower CSF hypocretin-1 levels in normal individuals.[20] No IGFBP3 autoantibodies or genetically associated IGFBP3 polymorphisms, however, were found in human narcolepsy.[20] Whether or not overexpression of IGFBP3 has something to do with hypocretin cell death and narcolepsy is undergoing further research.

Familial and twin studies have suggested that other genes as well as HLA are involved in human narcolepsy.[25] Specifically, the tumor necrosis factor (TNF)-α gene on chromosome 6, 3 narcolepsy predictive genes on chromosome 21, and 4 narcolepsy susceptible genes (CPT1B and CHKB) on chromosome 22 have been under investigation.[26–29] CPT1B is involved in regulating theta frequency of REM sleep, and CHKB is involved in choline metabolism, a precursor of REM and wake-regulating neurotransmitter acetylcholine. TNF polymorphisms are associated with increased risk of HLA-linked diseases. Researchers have found a positive association between polymorphisms of TNF-α gene in Japanese and Korean populations with narcolepsy and cataplexy.[27,30]

Most recently, Mignot and colleagues undertook a genome-wide association study in white populations in North America and Europe with replication in 3 ethnic groups.[31] Their work led to the discovery that narcolepsy is strongly associated with polymorphisms in the T-cell receptor α (TCRα) locus, with the highest significance at rs1154155.[31] This is the first documented genetic involvement of the TCRα locus, encoding a major receptor for the HLA-peptide presentation in any disease. Narcolepsy may then serve as a model on how HLA-TCR interactions can contribute to organ specific autoimmune targeting, which will lend insight into HLA-associated disorders. This finding also points to the direction that postnatal cell death of hypocretin neurons of human narcolepsy occurs by organ-specific autoimmune targeting with HLA-TCR interactions.

The Role of Hypocretins

If there is one neurotransmitter that influences almost every organ system in the human body, it is hypocretin. It is well established that hypocretin neurons project densely within the hypothalamus and widely to different regions of the cortex and brainstem as well as the periphery (spinal cord). In addition to its known involvement in the pathology of narcolepsy with wake and sleep, hypocretin seems to exert its influence on body homeostasis, feeding and appetite, endocrine functions, reward-seeking behaviors, cardiovascular states, and possibly ventilatory drive.[32–39] The Greek term, *orexin*, meaning appetite, used by Sakurai and colleagues,[12] came from the discovery that administration of supraphysiologic doses of this peptide caused an increase in food comsumption. Rodgers and colleagues[40,41] reported that intracerebroventricular (ICV) administration of hypocretin-1 indirectly results in increased feeding. Haynes and colleagues[42] administered SB-334867, a hypocretin-1 antagonist, resulting in suppression of food intake in rats despite fasting conditions. Other investigators, however, reported opposing results, that administration of hypocretin-1 in rats increased food intake only transiently, and continuous administration did not alter daily food intake, body weight, blood glucose, cholesterol, or free fatty acid levels.[43–45] The effects of hypocretin-1 on appetite and feeding remains controversial.

The role of hypocretin in mediating the state of arousal is evident.[32,33,46] There is a suggestion that the hypocretin system is involved in maintaining the body's homeostatic need for food intake, and it accomplishes this by increasing the state of arousal.[32,33] Low levels of glucose, triglycerides, and leptin have been shown to activate hypocretin activity.[47] Hypocretin is also involved in regulating obesity by acting on the arcuate nucleus of the hypothalamus. The arcuate nucleus of the hypothalamus functions in controlling leptin and insulin sensitivity, regulates metabolism and energy expenditure, and suppresses consumption of fatty foods.[48]

Hypocretin is also involved in the reward circuitry of the brain, which includes the nucleus accumbens and the ventral tegmental area (VTA).[32,33] Activation of the mesolimbic dopaminergic pathway of the VTA and the nucleus accumbens results from stimulation by drugs of abuse and natural rewards. Researchers found that direct ICV administration of hypocretin in the VTA induced drug/food-seeking behavior that was previously abolished in rodents.[39] Alternatively, administration of an investigational hypocretin antagonist SB-334867 prevents morphine-seeking behavior.[49] Preprohypocretin knockout mice had reduced susceptibility to morphine dependence.[50] These studies point to the influence of the hypocretin system on the brain's reward circuitry and may explain the importance of hypocretin in promoting "addictive" behaviors such as drug dependence.

Studies have shown hypocretin involvement in endocrine hormone secretion and cardiovascular responses.[32,33] The periventricular hypothalamic nucleus (PVN) is responsible for pituitary gland and neuroendocrine secretion and projections to the brainstem and spinal cord participate in regulation of cardiovascular responses.[51,52] ICV administration of hypocretin-1 activates corticotropin-releasing factor expressing neurons from the PVN, stimulates the hypothalamic pituitary adrenal axis, and decreases prolactin secretion[53,54]—all of which are involved in the stress response. Shirasaka and colleagues[55] reported that hypocretin ICV administration elevates blood pressure, heart rate, and plasma catacholamines in rats. Furthermore, hypocretin may have influences in thermoregulation. Mochizuki and colleagues[56] reported that hypocretin (orexin) knockout mice had blunted fall in core body temperature during sleep compared with wild-type mice.

Recently, Han and colleagues[57] tested the hypothesis that hypocretin plays a role in ventilatory chemosensitivity in 130 patients with narcolepsy and cataplexy by evaluating hyperoxia-hypercapnic and hypoxic responsiveness. All patients with narcolepsy and cataplexy (defined by low hypocretin-1 or positive HLA-DQB1*0602 status) had a higher apnea-hypopnea index ($P = .03$), a lower minimal oxygen saturation ($P = .0002$), and depressed hypoxic responsiveness ($P<.0001$) during sleep compared with controls. Controls with positive HLA status also had a lower hypoxic responsiveness compared with control with negative HLA status ($P<.0001$) but no significant differences in the hypercapnic responsiveness, indicating that a lower hypoxic responsiveness is a result of DQB1*0602 status. Further research needs to be performed to elucidate the significance of these findings.

Clinical Implications

These findings are likely to explain symptoms frequently observed in narcoleptics who are followed over several years. For example, weight gain is commonly seen in narcoleptics, and many of these patients have to cope with comorbidities of being overweight. Sleep-disordered breathing and obstructive sleep apnea are commonly associated with middle-aged narcoleptic patients. Increased autonomic nervous system instability has also been reported in narcoleptics, which may be related to animal findings (described previously).

DIAGNOSIS OF NARCOLEPSY

The diagnosis of narcolepsy requires a clinical history of EDS and a positive multiple sleep latency test (MSLT) with a mean sleep latency of less than or equal to 8 minutes and 2 or more SOREMs.[2] Ideally a polysomnogram of at least 6 hours of sleep and no other sleep-related disorders present is documented the night before the MSLT is performed. There is ongoing controversy regarding the diagnostic value of the MSLT in documenting narcolepsy in patients with EDS. Approximately 15% of narcoleptic patients with cataplexy do not have the MSLT criteria for narcolepsy.[58] Also, patients with sleep-disordered breathing may have MSLT findings similar to narcoleptics.[59] There is a progressive decrease in the number of SOREMs and an increase in the mean sleep latency on the MSLT as a function of age.[60] Furthermore, investigations have shown that normal subjects can present with 2 or more SOREMs.[61] Japanese researchers thought that the current diagnostic criteria for narcolepsy relies too much on polysomnographic and MSLT findings.[62] In Japan, a positive history of cataplexy associated with EDS is required for the diagnosis of narcolepsy.[62] Undoubtedly, the presence of cataplexy is pathognomonic for narcolepsy, but it can be difficult to rely on this criterion alone as cataplexy is not always present.

The discovery of CSF hypocretin (orexin) has led to a new diagnostic approach and brings clarification to the definition of narcolepsy. By performing a lumbar puncture, a low or absent level of hypocretin can confirm the diagnosis of narcolepsy with cataplexy.[13–15,63] Honda and colleagues[4] emphasized that narcolepsy with cataplexy as represented by a low or undetectable CSF hypocretin-1 level should be differentiated from narcolepsy without cataplexy or idiopathic hypersomnia, in which both diseases have normal CSF hypocretin-1 levels. CSF hypocretin-1 levels less than 110 ng/L have a high positive predictive value (94%) for narcolepsy with cataplexy.[18,64] HLA sensitivity is close to hypocretin deficiency sensitivity; however, the specificity of HLA is very low and about 30% of individuals without narcolepsy have the HLA haplotype. Currently, CSF hypocretin-1 measurement is the most accurate diagnostic technique.

SECONDARY NARCOLEPSY

Secondary narcolepsy, defined by ICSD-2 criteria for narcolepsy and an associated underlying neurologic condition, can be associated with low CSF hypocretin-1 levels and EDS. In a meta-analysis, Nishino and Kanbayashi[65] analyzed 116 symptomatic cases of secondary narcolepsy with EDS. The meta-analysis included patients with neurologic disorders, including inherited disorders, brain tumors, head trauma, multiple sclerosis, encephalomyelitis, vascular disorders, and degeneration. Reduced CSF hypocretin-1 was seen in most of these cases, and EDS was reversible when there is a corresponding improvement in the primary neurologic disorder and increase in CSF hypocretin levels. Kanbayashi and colleagues[66] reported 7 multiple sclerosis patients with hypothalamic lesions, low CSF hypocretin-1 levels, and EDS. CSF hypocretin-1 levels returned to normal with corresponding improvements in hypothalamic lesions and symptoms of EDS. Unlike secondary narcolepsy, hypocretin-1 levels never return to normal in the idiopathic form of narcolepsy. Based on these observations, the relationship between EDS and low hypocretin-1 levels is evident.

TREATMENT

Patient education and familiarity with the disease remain important parts of treatment. Career counseling regarding jobs that narcoleptics should avoid including shift-work, driving and transportation-related jobs, or any job necessitating continuous attention for long hours without breaks should be offered. Short 15- to 20-minute naps every 4 hours during the daytime are recommended. In addition to scheduled naps, other important behavioral treatment targets include maintaining a regular sleep-wake schedule, avoidance of frequent time zone changes, and good sleep hygiene.

Treatment of EDS, Major Symptoms of Narcolepsy (EDS, Cataplexy, Disturbed Nocturnal Sleep)

Sodium oxybate

Sodium oxybate is the treatment of choice for narcolepsy with cataplexy. γ-Hydroxybutyrate (GBH) is a naturally occurring central nervous system (CNS) metabolite found in highest concentrations in the hypothalamus and basal ganglia and acts as a sedative to consolidate REM sleep. In its endogenous form, it is a neurotransmitter and neuromodulator that affects dopamine, serotonin, γ-aminobutyric acid (GABA), and endogenous opioids. GHB is considered to be a GABA-β receptor agonist. GHB treats cataplexy through an unknown mechanism that is thought to be related to its consolidation of REM sleep or to a secondary interaction with dopamine secretion.[67–69]

The improvement in cataplexy is much more rapid than the effect on daytime sleepiness, which takes up to 6 to 8 weeks. The delayed improvement on daytime sleepiness suggests different modes of action of GHB on cataplexy and EDS. Huang and Guilleminault[70] conducted a study evaluating the actions of GHB (6 mg) and baclofen (10–20 mg) on cataplexy and EDS in 26 drug-naive teenagers (mean age 15 years) with narcolepsy and cataplexy. Baclofen is also a GABA-β agonist. It increases slow wave sleep and shortens sleep latencies as measured by polysomnography in patients with neurologic disorders.[71] Baclofen and sodium oxybate increased total sleep time and slow wave sleep, but only sodium oxybate had a positive effect on EDS and cataplexy at 3 months.[70] The effects on slow wave sleep are likely due to direct GABA-β agonist properties of both drugs; however, the effects of GHB on cataplexy and EDS are clearly distinguished from baclofen, which had no effect on these symptoms. This suggests that the effects of GHB on cataplexy and EDS may not be due to the immediate effect of GABA-β properties.

In an earlier double-blind placebo-controlled study evaluating the effect of sodium oxybate on EDS in 228 narcoleptic patients, compared with placebo, GHB produced statistically significant improvement in Epworth Sleepiness Scale scores and frequency of sleep attacks at doses of 6 and 9 g.[72] A more recent double-blind placebo-controlled study evaluated sleep-related parameters in 278 narcoleptic patients taking sodium oxybate as monotherapy or in combination with modafinil.[73] At 8 weeks, patients receiving sodium oxybate and the combination had a median increase in stage 3 and 4 sleep (43.5 and 24.5 minutes, respectively), delta power, and median decrease in nocturnal awakenings (6.0 and 9.5, respectively), compared with placebo or modafinil alone.

GHB is taken at bedtime and a second dose 2.5 to 4 hours later while patients are in bed. It has a short half-life of 90 to 120 minutes. The drug is progressively increased over 6 to 8 weeks to goal of 6 to 9 g, which is the effective dose. Due to the gradual improvement on daytime sleepiness, other alerting drugs must temporarily be given to control daytime sleepiness. It may take 2 to 3 months to see the full effects of the medication on EDS. Side effects include disorientation when awakened in the middle of the night, nighttime enuresis, nausea, and early morning grogginess, particularly at 9 g and during drug initiation. Patients generally prefer this drug to other anticataplectic drugs because of fewer side effects. The advantage of sodium oxybate is its slow but significant impact on daytime sleepiness and the possibility that after 2 to 3 months patients need to take only 1 medication for both cataplexy and daytime sleepiness.

Treatment of EDS

Modafinil

Modafinil is the first-line pharmacologic treatment for EDS and irresistible episodes of sleep in narcoleptic patients. It has a low abuse potential and is not associated with rebound hypersomnolence. Modafinil has no known anticataplectic effects or other REM-related sleep phenomenon. Its mechanism is hypothesized to selectively activate wake-generating sites in the hypothalamus. The data are controversial on the role of dopamine in mediating the wake-promoting effects of modafinil.[74,75] In narcoleptic dogs, the drug increases extracellular dopamine in a hypocretin receptor 2 independent manner.[74] In dopamine transporter knockout mice, the lack of response to the wake-promoting action of modafinil suggests that dopamine transporters do play a role and are necessary for wake-promoting actions of this drug.[74] Results from several multicenter studies indicated that modafinil has a significant impact on the objective measures of sleepiness and improves wakefulness in narcoleptic patients. Black and Houghton[76] performed a double-blind placebo-controlled comparison between modafinil, GHB, and a combination of both drugs for the treatment of EDS in 270 adult narcoleptic patients. The authors found that both drugs are effective in treating EDS and are additive when used together. Modafinil has no adverse effects on objective or subjective nocturnal sleep parameters in healthy volunteers and narcoleptics.

There is no reported evidence that tolerance develops to the effects of modafinil on EDS. Common side effects include headache, nervousness, nausea, and dry mouth. These symptoms can be reduced by a slow and progressive increase in dosage. Blood pressure should be monitored as the drug may cause elevated pressures. It is administered once, in the morning, or twice, in the morning and at lunchtime. Its elimination half-life is 10 to 12 hours. Modafinil produces best results in stimulant-naive individuals. It can reduce the efficacy of oral contraceptives and, therefore, patients need to be advised on additional forms of contraception.

Armodafinil
Armodafinil is the R-enantiomer of modafinil with a longer half-life of 10 to 14 hours. In 2007, armodafinil was approved for the treatment of EDS in narcoleptics. In a multicenter, randomized, double-blind, placebo-controlled trial of 196 subjects with narcolepsy, armodafinil significantly improved EDS throughout the day.[77-79] Compared with placebo, mean sleep latency was significantly improved with armodafinil (150 to 250 mg once daily) in patients with narcolepsy as measured by the MSLT or the MWT.[80] Side-effect profile is similar to modafinil.

Amphetamines and amphetamine-like CNS stimulants
These CNS stimulants include methylphenidate, dextroamphetamine, and methamphetamine. These stimulants have a significant side-effect profile, high abuse potential, and development of tolerance and, therefore, are generally not recommended any longer for use in EDS.

Treatment of Cataplexy

Selective norepinephrine/serotoninergic uptake inhibitors
Newer antidepressants have been effective for cataplexy, sleep paralysis, and hypnagogic/hypnopompic hallucinations and are the recommended drugs due to improved side-effect profile and greater efficacy. The most commonly used drug of this class is venlafaxine, a potent inhibitor of serotonin and norepinephrine. It is prescribed at a dosage of 75 to 150 mg twice a day for adults and children. The advantage of venlafaxin is that it is easily obtainable and can be taken during wakefulness.

Atomoxetine
Atomoxetine, a highly specific noradrenergic reuptake inhibitor, has been effective in improving cataplexy and EDS in children and in cases of resistant cataplexy after

failure of venlafaxine, fluoxetine, and the older serotonin reuptake inhibitors. The dosage is 18 to 100 mg once a day or in 2 divided doses. Its advantage is the use of 1 medication to deal with both symptoms, but it is less effective than modafinil and sodium oxybate in older teenagers and adults.[77]

Tricyclic antidepressants

The older tricyclic antidepressants (TCAs), imipramine, clomipramine, and protriptyline, are thought to increase muscle tone and suppress REM sleep. An unusual property of TCAs is the rebound cataplexy that occurs on abrupt discontinuation of the medication. TCAs are now used as a last resort due to significant side-effect profile and are not discussed further.

Selective serotonin reuptake inhibitors

Selective serotonin reuptake inhibitors (SSRIs), like TCAs, block presynaptic reuptake of catecholamines; however, they are more selective for serotonin, the prototype being fluoxetine and its active metabolite norfluoxetine. Similar to TCAs, SSRIs inhibit REM sleep. Fluvoxamine (25 to 200 mg/d) was mildly effective on cataplexy. Because of the availability and efficacy of newer agents, SSRIs are not recommended as first-line agents for cataplexy.

Investigative Agents for Narcolepsy

Emerging treatments undergoing investigation include hypocretin replacement therapies and hypocretin analogs, hypocretin gene therapy, stem cell transplant, immunotherapy, thyrotropin (TRH) analogs and promoters, and histamine (H_3) antagonists.[77,81] Replacement of hypocretin-1 seems promising; however, a major limitation is that hypocretin-1 does not cross the blood-brain barrier and, therefore, cannot reach the CNS. Potential possibilities of hypocretin replacement therapies include intranasal and ICV administration. In experiments on narcoleptic mouse models, ICV injection of hypocretin-1 compensated for hypocretin cell loss and reverse narcolepsy, including cataplexy.[82] ICV administration, however, is not the most feasible form of delivery. Nishino[83] administered high doses of hypocretin-1 (96–386 μg/kg) intravenously in ligand-deficient sporadic narcoleptic dogs and found that only a small portion of hypocretin-1 penetrated the CNS, producing only short-lasting anticataplectic effect. Administration of hypocretin-1 intranasally holds promise as this route delivers the compound directly into the brain and does not rely on bypassing the blood-brain barrier.[84,85] Development of centrally penetrable hypocretin agonists is needed.

There has been much interest in stem cell therapy to replace lost hypocretin-1 cells. Overexpression of the hypocretin gene has been effective in improving cataplexy in mouse models.[82] Mieda and colleagues[82] conducted a study on genetic rescue in mice with ablated hypocretin neurons, highlighting viral vectors as a potential future treatment for hypocretin-deficient narcoleptics. Autoimmune destruction of hypocretin neurons resulting in low or undetectable CSF hypocretin levels has been discussed. Because autoimmune mechanisms may be responsible for the development of narcolepsy, treatments have been undertaken focusing on the immune response soon after onset of narcolepsy. Steroids, plasmapheresis, and intravenous immunoglobulin (IVIG) therapy have had limited success, however. Several case series did show improvement in cataplexy or improved sleepiness with early IVIG administration soon after onset of symptoms.[86–88]

There is some evidence that TRH and TRH agonists have alerting properties, thus making it a possible treatment modality for narcolepsy.[89] TRH has increased wakefulness and decreased cataplexy in cataplectic canines.[90] Furthermore, there is ongoing research on the histaminergic system and its action on hypocretin signaling for promoting wakefulness.[91,92] Histamine H_3 receptors are abundant in the CNS and are inhibitory autoreceptors. Stimulation of H_3 receptors causes sedation, whereas antagonism causes wakefulness.[93] Thioperamide, a potent H_3 antagonist, significantly enhances wakefulness in hypocretin/orexin-deficient narcoleptic mice.[94] Leurs and colleagues[95] reported that H_3 receptor antagonists reduce the number and duration of narcoleptic attacks in a canine model of narcolepsy. Lin and colleagues[96] reported that an investigative drug, the H_3 receptor inverse agonist BF2.649, improved EDS compared with placebo. This gives promise that H_3 antagonists may be useful in treating EDS in human narcoleptics.

Other Investigational Treatments

Alteration of core body and peripheral skin temperature is documented in narcoleptic patients, which may contribute to increased sleepiness and impaired vigilance.[97] In normal subjects, higher distal skin temperature and lower proximal skin temperature are associated with falling asleep.[98] Fronczek and colleagues[99] conducted a study investigating the contribution of skin temperature changes to impairments in the ability to stay awake and maintain vigilance in 8 narcoleptic patients, as measured by the maintenance of wakefulness test (MWT) and the psychomotor vigilance task (PVT). Core body temperature was manipulated by hot or cold beverages or snacks whereas skin temperature was manipulated by use of a computer-controlled full-body thermosuit. Core body warming improved PVT response speed with increasing time on task by 25% ($P = .02$), and distal skin cooling increased the maintenance of wakefulness time by 24% ($P<.01$) in narcoleptics.[99] Although a small study, it gives hope in future directions for symptomatic treatment of narcolepsy.

SUMMARY

Narcolepsy with cataplexy is a rare but life-long and challenging disorder. Current insight into the pathophysiology of this condition seems to be autoimmune-mediated postnatal cell death of hypocretin neurons occurrence by organ-specific autoimmune targeting with HLA-TCR interactions. The hypocretin system seems to have an influence on multiple organ systems beyond its wake-promoting mechanisms, including body homeostasis, feeding-appetite, endocrine functioning, CNS reward system, cardiovascular regulation, and possibly ventilatory drive. The recent availability of CSF hypocretin-1 analysis has led to definitive diagnostic criteria for narcolepsy with cataplexy compared with the current MSLT criteria. First-line treatment for EDS and cataplexy is sodium oxybate, with modafinil for daytime sleepiness, in adults and children. Other investigative agents and treatment modalities hold promise in future directions for narcolepsy.

REFERENCES

1. Mignot E, Wang C, Rattazzi C, et al. Genetic linkage of autosomal recessive canine narcolepsy with a mu immunoglobulin heavy-chain switch-like segment. Proc Natl Acad Sci U S A 1991;88:3475–8.
2. American Academy of Sleep Medicine. International classification of sleep disorders: diagnostic and coding manual. 2nd edition. Westchester (IL): American Academy of Sleep Medicine; 2005.
3. Roth B. Narcolepsy and hypersomnia. Basel (Switzerland): Karger; 1980.

4. Honda Y. Clinical features of narcolepsy. In: Honda Y, Juji T, editors. HLA in narco-lepsy. Berlin: Springer-Verlag; 1988. p. 24–57.

5. Brooks S, Mignot E. Narcolepsy and idiopathic hypersomnia. In: Lee-Chiong T, Sateia M, Carskadon M, editors. Sleep medicine. Philadelphia: Hanley & Belfus, Inc; 2002. p. 193–202.

6. Bassetti C, Aldrich MS. Narcolepsy. Neurol Clin 1996;14(3):545–71.

7. Nishino S, Okuro M, Kotorii N, et al. Hypocretin/orexin and narcolepsy: new basic and clinical insights. Acta Physiol (Oxf) 2010;198:209–22.

8. Juji T, Satake M, Honda Y, et al. HLA antigens in Japanese patients with narco-lepsy. All the patients were DR2 positive. Tissue Antigens 1984;24:316–9.

9. Nishino S, Mignot E. Pharmacological aspects of human and canine narcolepsy. Prog Neurobiol 1997;52:27–78.

10. Mignot E, Hayduk R, Grumet FC, et al. HLA DQB1*0602 is associated with cataplexy in 509 narcoleptic patients. Sleep 1997;20:1012–20.

11. de Lecea L, Kilduff TS, Peyron C, et al. The hypocretins: hypothalamic-specific peptides with neuroexcitatory activity. Proc Natl Acad Sci U S A 1998;95:322–7.

12. Sakurai T, Amemiya A, Ishii M, et al. Orexins and orexin receptors: a family of hypothalamic neuropeptides and G protein-coupled receptors that regulate feeding behavior. Cell 1998;92:573–85.

13. Peyron C, Tighe DK, van den Pol AN, et al. Neurons containing hypocretin (orex-in) project to multiple neuronal systems. J Neurosci 1998;18:9996–10015.

14. Lin L, Faraco R, Li R, et al. The sleep disorder canine narcolepsy is caused by a mutation in the hypocretin (orexin) receptor 2 gene. Cell 1999;98:365–76.

15. Chemelli RM, Willie JT, Sinton CM, et al. Narcolepsy in orexin knockout mice: molecular genetics of sleep regulation. Cell 1999;98:437–51.

16. Hara J, Beuckmann CT, Nambu T, et al. Genetic ablation of orexin neurons in mice results in narcolepsy, hypophagia, and obesity. Neuron 2001;30:345–54.

17. Peyron C, Faraco J, Rogers W, et al. A mutation in a case of early onset narco-lepsy and a generalized absence of hypocretin peptides in human narcoleptic brains. Nat Med 2000;6:991–7.

18. Dauvilliers Y, Arnulf I, Mignot E. Narcolepsy with cataplexy. Lancet 2007;369: 499–511.

19. Thannickal T, Moore R, Nienhuis R, et al. Reduced number of hypocretin neurons in human narcolepsy. Neuron 2000;27:469–74.

20. Honda M, Erikson KS, Zhang S, et al. IGFBP3 colocalizes with and regulates hypocretin (orexin). PLoS One 2009;4:e4254.

21. Blouin AM, Thannickal TC, Worley PF, et al. Narp immunostaining of human hypo-cretin (orexin) neurons: loss in narcolepsy. Neurology 2005;65:1189–92.

22. Crocker A, Espana RA, Papadopoulou M, et al. Concomitant loss of dynorphin, NARP, and orexin in narcolepsy. Neurology 2005;65:1184–8.

23. Black JL III, Krahn LE, Pankratz VS, et al. Search for neuron-specific and non-neuron specific antibodies in narcoleptic patients with an without HLA DQB1*0602. Sleep 2002;25:719–23.

24. Black JL III, Silber MH, Krahn LE, et al. Studies of humoral immunity to pre-pro-hypocretin in human leukocyte antigen DQB1*0602 positive narcoleptic subjects with cataplexy. Biol Psychiatry 2005;58:504–9.

25. Mignot E. Genetic and familial aspects of narcolepsy. Neurology 1998;50: S16–22.

26. Hohjoh H, Nakayama T, Ohashi J, et al. Significant association of a single nucle-otide polymorphism in the tumor necrosis factor-alpha (TNF-alpha) gene promoter with human narcolepsy. Tissue Antigens 1999;54:138–45.

27. Park MH, Roh EY, Park H, et al. Association of TNF-alpha gene promoter polymorphism with narcolepsy-cataplexy in Koreans. Hum Immunol 2004;65:S110.

28. Kawashima M, Tamiya G, Oka A, et al. Genome wide association analysis of human narcolepsy and a new resistance gene. Am J Hum Genet 2006;79: 252–63.

29. Miyagawa T, Kawashima M, Nishida N, et al. Variant between CPT1B and CHKB associated with susceptibility to narcolepsy. Nat Genet 2008;40:1324–8.

30. Hohjoh H, Terada N, Kawashima M, et al. Significant association of the tumor necrosis factor receptor 2 (TNFR2) gene with human narcolepsy. Tissue Antigens 2000;56:446–8.

31. Hallmayer J, Faraco J, Lin L, et al. Narcolepsy is strongly associated with the T-cell receptor alpha locus. Nat Genet 2009;41:708–11.

32. De Lecea L. A decade of hypocretins: past, present, and future of the neurobiology of arousal. Acta Physiol (Oxf) 2010;198:203–8.

33. Kroeger D, de Lecea L. The hypocretins and their role in narcolepsy. CNS Neurol Disord Drug Targets 2009;8:271–80.

34. Horvath TL, Diano S, van den Pol AN. Synaptic interaction between hypocretin (orexin) and neuropeptide Y cells in the rodent and primate hypothalamus: a novel circuit implicated in metabolic and endocrine regulations. J Neurosci 1999;19: 1072–87.

35. Guan JL, Wang QP, Shioda S. Immunoelectron microscopic examination of orexin-like immunoreactive fibers in the dorsal horn of the rat spinal cord. Brain Res 2003;987:86–92.

36. Van den Pol AN. Hypothalamic hypocretin (orexin): robust innervation of the spinal cord. J Neurosci 1999;19:3171–82.

37. Cutler DJ, Morris R, Sheridhar V, et al. Differential distribution of orexin-A and orexin-B immunoreactivity in the rat brain and spinal cord. Peptides 1999;20: 1455–70.

38. Aston-Jones G, Smith RJ, Moorman DE, et al. Role of lateral hypothalamic orexin neurons in reward processing and addiction. Neuropharmacology 2009;56: 112–21.

39. Harris GC, Wimmer M, Aston-Jones G. A role for lateral hypothalamic orexin neurons in reward seeking. Nature 2005;437:556–9.

40. Rodgers RJ, Halford JCG, Nunes de Souza RL, et al. SB-334867, a selective orexin-1 receptor antagonist, enhances behavioral satiety and blocks the hyperphagic effect of orexin-A in rats. Eur J Neurosci 2001;13:1444–52.

41. Rodgers RJ, Ishii Y, Halford JCG, et al. Orexins and appetite regulation. Neuropeptides 2002;36:303–25.

42. Haynes AC, Jackson B, Chapman H, et al. A selective orexin-1 receptor antagonist reduces food consumption in male and female rats. Regul Pept 2000;96: 45–51.

43. Lin Y, Matsumura K, Tsuchihashi T, et al. Chronic central infusion of orexin-A increases arterial pressure in rats. Brain Res Bull 2002;57:619–22.

44. Haynes AC, Jackson B, Overend P, et al. Effects of single and chronic intracerebroventricular administration of orexins on feeding in the rat. Peptides 1999;20: 1099–105.

45. Yamanaka A, Sakurai T, Katsumoto T, et al. Chronic intracerebroventricular administration of orexin-A to rats increases food intake in daytime, but has no effect on body weight. Brain Res 1999;849:248–52.

46. Nambu T, Sakurai T, Mizukami K, et al. Distribution of orexin neurons in the adult rat brain. Brain Res 1999;827:243–60.

47. Sakurai T. The neural circuit of orexin (hypocretin): maintaining sleep and wakefulness. Nat Rev Neurosci 2007;8:171–81.
48. Funato H, Tsai AL, Willie JT, et al. Enhanced orexin receptor-2 signaling prevents diet-induced obesity and improves leptin sensitivity. Cell Metab 2009;9:64–76.
49. Narita M, Nagumo Y, Hashimoto S, et al. Direct involvement of orexinergic systems in the activation of the mesolimbic dopamine pathway and related behaviors induced by morphine. J Neurosci 2006;26:398–405.
50. Georgescu D, Zachariou V, Barrot M, et al. Involvement of the lateral hypothalamic peptide orexin in morphine dependence and withdrawal. J Neurosci 2003;23:3106–11.
51. Bernardis LL, Awad A, Fink C, et al. Metabolic and neuroendocrine indices one month after lateral hypothalamic area lesions. Physiol Behav 1992;52: 133–9.
52. Stern JE. Electrophysiological and morphological properties of pre-autonomic neurons in the rat hypothalamic paraventricular nucleus. J Physiol 2001;537: 161–77.
53. Kuru M, Ueta Y, Serino R, et al. Centrally administered orexin/hypocretin activates HPA axis in rats. Neuroreport 2000;11:1977–80.
54. Sakamoto F, Yamada S, Ueta Y. Centrally administered orexin-A activates corticotropin-releasing factor-containing neurons in the hypothalamic paraventricular nucleus and central orexins on stress-activated central CRF neurons. Regul Pept 2004;118:183–91.
55. Shirasaka T, Nakazato M, Matsukura S, et al. Sympathetic and cardiovascular actions of orexins in conscious rats. Am J Physiol Regul Integr Comp Physiol 1999;277:R1780–5.
56. Mochizuki T, Klerman EB, Sakurai T, et al. Elevated body temperature during sleep in orexin knock out mice. Am J Physiol Regul Integr Comp Physiol 2006; 1(3):R533–40.
57. Han F, Mignot E, Wei YC, et al. Ventilatory chemoresponsiveness, narcolepsy-cataplexy, and HLA DQB1*0602 staus. Eur Respir J 2010, in press.
58. Moscovitch A, Partinen M, Guilleminault C. The positive diagnosis of narcolepsy and narcolepsy's borderland. Neurology 1993;43:55–60.
59. Aldrich MS. The neurobiology of narcolepsy-cataplexy. Prog Neurobiol 1993;41: 533–41.
60. Dauvilliers Y, Gosselin A, Paquet J, et al. Effect of age on MSLT results in patients with narcolepsy-cataplexy. Neurology 2004;62:46–50.
61. Singh M, Drake CL, Roth T. The prevalence of multiple sleep-onset REM periods in a population-based sample. Sleep 2006;29(7):890–5.
62. Honda Y, Juji T, editors. HLA in narcolepsy. Berlin: Springer-Verlag; 1988. p. 10–57.
63. Nishino S, Ripley B, Overeem S, et al. Hypocretin (orexin) deficiency in human narcolepsy. Lancet 2000;35(5):39–40.
64. Mignot E, Lammers GJ, Ripley B, et al. The role of cerebrospinal fluid hypocretin measurement in the diagnosis of narcolepsy and other hypersomnias. Arch Neurol 2002;59:1553–62.
65. Nishino S, Kanbayashi T. Symptomatic narcolepsy, cataplexy and hypersomnia, and their implications in the hypothalamic hypocretin/orexin system. Sleep Med Rev 2005;9:269–310.
66. Kanbayashi T, Shimohata T, Nakashima I, et al. Symptomatic narcolepsy in patients with neuromyelitis optica and multiple sclerosis: new neurochemical and immunological implications. Arch Neurol 2009;66:1563–6.

67. Lammers GJ, Arends J, Declerk AC, et al. Gammahydroxybutyrate and narcolepsy: a double-blind placebo-controlled study. Sleep 1993;16:216–20.
68. U.S. Xyrem Multicenter Study Group. A randomized, double blind, multicenter trial comparing the effect of 3 doses of orally administered sodium oxybate with placebo for the treatment of narcolepsy. Sleep 2002;25:42–9.
69. Borgen LA, Okerholm RA, Lai A, et al. The pharmacokinetics of sodium oxybate oral solution following acute and chronic administration to narcoleptic patients. J Clin Pharmacol 2004;44:253–7.
70. Huang YS, Guilleminault C. Narcolepsy: action of two γ-aminobutyric acid type B agonists, baclofen and sodium oxybate. Pediatr Neurol 2009;41:9–16.
71. Bensmail D, Quera Salva MA, Roche N, et al. Effect of intrathecal baclofen on sleep and respiratory function in patients with spasticity. Neurology 2006;67: 1432–6.
72. Scharf MB, Brown D, Woods M, et al. The effects and effectiveness of gamma-hydroxybutyrate in patients with narcolepsy. J Clin Psychol 1985;46: 222–5.
73. Black J, Pardi D, Hornfeldt CS, et al. The nightly administration of sodium oxybate results in significant reduction in the nocturnal sleep disruption of patients with narcolepsy. Sleep Med 2009;10(8):829–35.
74. Wisor J, Nishino S, Sora I, et al. Dopaminergic role in stimulant-induced wakefulness. J Neurosci 2001;21(5):1787–94.
75. Mignot E, Nishino S, Guilleminault C, et al. Modafinil binds to the dopamine uptake carrier site with low affinity. Sleep 1994;15(5):436–7.
76. Black J, Houghton WC. Sodium oxybate improves excessive daytime sleepiness in narcolepsy. Sleep 2006;29(7):939–46.
77. Billiard M. Narcolepsy: current treatment options and future approaches. Neuropsychiatr Dis Treat 2008;4(3):557–66.
78. Lankford DA. Armodafinil: a new treatment for excessive sleepiness. Expert Opin Investig Drugs 2008;17:565–73.
79. Harsh JR, Hayduk R, Rosenberg R, et al. The efficacy and safety of armodafinil as treatment for adults with excessive sleepiness associated with narcolepsy. Curr Med Res Opin 2006;22:761–74.
80. Garmock-Jones KP, Dhillon S, Scott LJ. Armodafinil. CNS Drugs 2009;23(9): 793–803.
81. Thorpy M. Therapeutic advances in narcolepsy. Sleep Med 2007;8:427–40.
82. Mieda M, Willie JT, Hara J, et al. Orexin peptides prevent cataplexy and improve wakefulness in an orexin neuron-ablated model of narcolepsy in mice. Proc Natl Acad Sci U S A 2004;101:4649–54.
83. Nishino S. Clinical and neurobiological aspects of narcolepsy. Sleep Med 2007;8: 373–99.
84. Hanson LR, Martinez PM, Taheri S, et al. Intranasal administration of hypocretin 1 (orexin A) bypasses the blood-brain barrier & targets the brain: a new strategy for the treatment of narcolepsy. Drug Delivery Technol 2004;4:66–71.
85. Deadwyler SA, Porrino L, Siegel JM, et al. Systemic and nasal delivery of orexin-A (Hypocretin-1) reduces the effects of sleep deprivation on cognitive performance in nonhuman primates. J Neurosci 2007;27:14239–47.
86. Lecendreux M, Maret S, Bassetti C, et al. Clinical efficacy of high-dose intravenous immunoglobins near the onset of narcolepsy in a 10-year old boy. J Sleep Res 2003;12(4):347–8.
87. Zuberi SM, Mignot E, Ling L, et al. Variable response to intravenous immunoglobulin therapy in childhood narcolepsy. J Sleep Res 2004;13(Suppl 1):828.

88. Dauvilliers Y, Carlander B, Rivier F, et al. Successful management of cataplexy with intravenous immunoglobulins at narcolepsy onset. Ann Neurol 2004;56(6): 905–8.

89. Gemkow MJ, Davenport AJ, Harich S, et al. The histamine H3 receptor as a therapeutic drug target for CNS disorders. Drug Discov Today 2009;14:509–15.

90. Nishino S, Arrigoni J, Shelton J, et al. Effects of thyrotropin-releasing hormone and its analogs on daytime sleepiness and cataplexy in canine narcolepsy. J Neurosci 1997;17:6401–8.

91. Le S, Gruner JA, Mathiasen JR, et al. Correlation between ex vivo receptor occupancy and wake-promoting activity of selective H3 receptor antagonists. J Pharmacol Exp Ther 2008;325:902–9.

92. Parmentier R, Anaclet C, Guhennec C, et al. The brain H3-receptor as a novel therapeutic target for vigilance and sleep-wake disorders. Biochem Pharmacol 2007;73:1157–71.

93. Barbier AJ, Berridge C, Dugovic C, et al. Acute wake-promoting actions of JNJ-5207852, a novel, diamine-based H3 antagonist. Br J Pharmacol 2004;143(5): 649–61.

94. Shiba T, Fujiki N, Wisor JP, et al. Wake promoting effects of thioperamide, a histamine H3 antagonist in orexin/ataxin-3 narcoleptic mice. Sleep 2004;27(Abstract Suppl):S241–2.

95. Leurs R, Bakker RA, Timmerman H, et al. The histamine H-3 receptor: from gene cloning to H-3 receptor drugs. Nat Rev Drug Discov 2005;4(2):107–20.

96. Lin JS, Dauvilliers Y, Arnulf I, et al. An inverse agonist of the histamine H-3 receptor improves wakefulness in narcolepsy: studies in orexin(-/-) mice and patients. Neurobiol Dis 2008;30(1):74–83.

97. Fronczek R, Overeem S, Lammers GJ, et al. Altered skin-temperature regulation in narcolepsy relates to sleep propensity. Sleep 2006;11:1444–9.

98. Krauchi K, Cajochen C, Werth E, et al. Warm feet promote the rapid onset of sleep. Nature 1999;6748:36–7.

99. Fronczek R, Raymann R, Romeijn N, et al. Manipulation of core body and skin temperature improves vigilance and maintenance of wakefulness in narcolepsy. Sleep 2008;31(2):233–40.

Kleine-Levin Syndrome: Current Status

Yu-Shu Huang, MD[a,b], Clair Lakkis, MD[c,*],
Christian Guilleminault, MD, DBiol[c]

KEYWORDS

- Kleine-Levin syndrome • Periodic hypersomnia
- Upper respiratory tract infections • Thalamic hypoperfusion

Kleine-Levin syndrome (KLS) is a periodic hypersomnia characterized by recurrent episodes of hypersomnia and at least one of the following symptoms: (1) cognitive or mood disturbances, (2) megaphagia with compulsive eating; (3) hypersexuality with inappropriate behaviors; and (4) abnormal behavior.[1,2]

The syndrome was essentially described by Critchley[1] who designated the name Kleine-Levin Syndrome based on historical reports made by these two specialists. Critchley originally linked the syndrome to boys, but later studies showed that girls could also be affected but at a much lower frequency.

Recently, mostly in Europe, Israel, and Far-East Asia, specific programs have been established aimed at collecting initial and follow-up clinical information and finding volunteers agreeable to participate in research protocols to resolve the enigma behind this syndrome that may be devastating to a teenage individual.

One of the most successful programs has been established in Taiwan at Chang-Gung University Memorial Hospital (Taoyuan, Taiwan) to which most, if not all, cases of periodic hypersomnia seen on the island are referred, and where a team of physicians is in continuous contact with families and affected individuals. Most of the recent advances have come from this group, which also has international collaborations. Despite the efforts made to include as many individuals with the disorder as possible, and to have the strictest follow-up program possible, the Taiwan group has only 33 subjects (out of a population of 23 million) who have been regularly followed. The fact that there is only one pediatric sleep clinic, which is staffed by very knowledgeable individuals and accessible by fast transportation throughout the territory, makes it a low probability that any new case is missed. In parallel to this single, specialized

[a] Sleep Center, Chang Gung Memorial Hospital and University, Taoyuan, Taiwan
[b] Department of Child Psychiatry, Chang Gung Memorial Hospital and University, Taoyuan, Taiwan
[c] Division of Sleep Medicine, Stanford University School of Medicine, Stanford Medical Outpatient Center, 450 Broadway Street, Pavillon C, Redwood City, CA 94063-5074, USA
* Corresponding author.
E-mail address: cllakkis@yahoo.com

Med Clin N Am 94 (2010) 557–562
doi:10.1016/j.mcna.2010.02.011
0025-7125/10/$ – see front matter © 2010 Elsevier Inc. All rights reserved.

referral center, receiving all cases from a geographically well-delineated area, others have tried to obtain information from many different sources such as clinical reports, biologic samples, and other pieces of information. Such efforts have brought in information, but limitations in the collected data due to the "noise" are important to note and cannot be resolved. "Noise" includes cases where individuals were seen by nonspecialists, the lack of systematic data collection on all aspects of the problem, the lack of long term follow-up data, and, at times, questions on the validity of the diagnosis. Such collaboration, however, has lead to the collection of 106 cases, the largest compilation of possible KLS cases ever collected and reported.[3]

The clinical symptoms have been reviewed in *The International Classification Of Sleep Disorders*, 2nd edition.[2] This compilation shows that patients present with many psychiatric symptoms and the most common diagnostic difficulty is to differentiate KLS from the onset of a psychiatric syndrome in a teenage individual. This is even more evident when looking at the data obtained in Taiwan and presented in **Table 1**.

Most commonly, the syndrome involves teenagers and significantly disturbs the daily life of families, affecting schooling and any planned activities, but it can persist through adulthood and some adult onset cases have been reported.

EVOLUTION

Each episode lasts between 7 and 21 days and reoccurrences vary in frequency but often are seen several times during a year, at least at the beginning of the clinical

Table 1
Symptoms reported by 33 Taiwanese KLS patients

Clinical Symptoms	%	Clinical Symptoms	%
Hypersomnia	100	*Autonomic dysfunction*	60
Disinhibition	54	*Personality changes*	98
Eating behavior disorder	80	Irritability	60
Megaphagia	58	Decreased motivation	35
Apathy	85	Negative thoughts	13
Decreased appetite	37	Depressive symptoms	23
Increased drinking	0	Impulsive thoughts	23
Craving for sweets	25	Fearful	40
Hyperphagia after episode	16	Anxiety	23
Large increase in BW	10	*Compulsions*	10
Large decrease in BW	3	Aggressive tendencies	25
Cognitive disorder	100	Impatient	30
Confusion	32	Childish	53
Dreamy feeling	61	*Psychotic signs or symptoms*	60
Abnormal speech	17	Auditory hallucinations	30
Derealization	95	Visual hallucinations	27
Impaired concentration	27	*Sleep disturbances*	49
Amnesia	27	Dreamy sleep	20
Slow response	10	Dream talking	3
Mutism	65	Sleep terrors	13
Delusions	13		

Abbreviation: BW, body weight.

manifestations of the syndrome. If the acute, symptomatic phase is of variable dura-tion the recurrent episodes most commonly oscillates between 5 and 10 days. As a group the Taiwan data show a tendency toward a reduction of the number of symp-tomatic days over time during recurrent episodes, despite the fact that there is a variability not only in the number of episodes per year within subjects and between subjects.

TESTS

No specific marker for KLS is yet available. Although numerous blood biologic tests have been performed in patients, there is still no clue as to the origin of the disease.

Cerebral fluid analysis is within normal limits, including level measurements of hypo-cretin-1, a hypothalamic peptide that has been shown to be deficient in the narcolepsy syndrome.[4] Many neurologic tests have been normal such as electro-encephalogram, eliminating seizure disorder as a possibility.

Sleep laboratory findings have been of greater interest. Decreased sleep efficiency and increased wake time have been reported in nocturnal polysomnograms. However, a study performed on 19 patients during symptomatic and asymptomatic periods, with subjects acting as their own controls, did not show a significant difference for any sleep stage or sleep efficiency, and there was a nonsignificant tendency for reduc-tion in slow wave sleep (SWS).[5] The study showed that the timing of the sleep study during the symptomatic period is an important variable. If data from all subjects is taken together without taking into account the timing of the test in relationship to the onset of clinical symptoms, the common outcome is the absence of significant results. If an analysis is performed taking into consideration the relationship between clinical onset and timing of test, the results are different. There is a clear reduction of SWS during the first few days. In contrast, rapid eye movement (REM) sleep remains normal during that period. During the second phase of the symptomatic period, a decrease in REM sleep is seen while SWS comes back to normal. When comparing the changes in the two sleep states, the decrease in SWS during the first half of the symptomatic period, is always more important than any REM sleep decrease seen during the second half of the same period.[5]

It is difficult to perform recordings and obtain collaboration of patients during the symptomatic period, particularly at the beginning of the period. Therefore, the perfor-mance of multiple sleep latency tests has been infrequent and, most commonly, they were obtained later during the symptomatic period when aggressive behavior is not as prominent. In the majority of the cases, the mean sleep latencies were longer than 10 minutes. However, some patients, particularly when monitored early in the symptom-atic period, presented with shorter sleep latencies. In some cases, but not in the majority, two sleep onset REM periods were recorded. The more recent investigations show thus that the beginning of the symptomatic period is much more disturbed and the sleep tests indicate these disturbances. Subjectively, however, subjects still report sleepiness during the second phase of the total period.[5]

BRAIN IMAGING

The results of brain imaging using CT scan and simple MRI were normal in all the well-documented cases of KLS. There have been cases associated with clear lesions, but these cases were associated with additional neurologic signs and symptoms related to the noted lesions. They have to be considered as "secondary" cases, and the question is often raised concerning their relationship to KLS.

The most interesting findings have come from at single-photon emission computed tomography (SPECT) analysis.[6] Recently, several authors reported similar findings. The initial and largest study included seven patients studied during an asymptomatic period, five of whom also were also studied during a symptomatic period. In that study, each subject underwent brain CT scanning, brain magnetic resonance imaging, and Tc-99mECD SPECT. The results showed that hypoperfusion was seen during the symptomatic period at different localizations, in the basal ganglia in four out of five of the cases, and in occipital and frontal cortex in a fewer number of subjects. The thalamus was the only region where hypoperfusion was systematically seen. During follow-up testing, while in the asymptomatic period, a complete resolution of the perfusion problem was noted in the five cases and no defect was noted in the thalamus in the two additional cases. Also, during the asymptomatic period, the other areas of hypoperfusion noted in cortex were diminished or completely disappeared in most, but not all, cases.[6] Subsequently, it has been confirmed that the consistent finding during the symptomatic period is that of thalamic hypoperfusion, which is not seen during the asymptomatic period.[7,8] It was suggested that the hypoperfusion was more marked on the left hypothalamus, but such observations will have to be confirmed.

COGNITIVE DEFICITS

Patients with long evolutions appear to present with persistent hypoperfusion in different locations in the cerebral cortex. Swedish researchers[9,10] have shown that in association with these areas of persistent cortical hypoperfusion and abnormal functional magnetic resonance imaging (fMRI) findings, particularly in the frontotemporal regions, persistent specific cognitive deficits could be demonstrated during the asymptomatic period in cognitive testing—specifically a reduced working memory capacity. The Swedish team found that the deficit correlates with lower activation of the cingular cortex and adjacent dorsomedial prefrontal cortex. Persistent changes in the frontotemporal regions were noted also in the subject with the longest evolution in the Taiwan SECT study.[6] All studied patients with cognitive deficits were adult subjects that had the evolution of the syndrome over years.

WHAT TRIGGERS THE NEW SYMPTOMATIC PERIOD?

The cause of KLS remains unknown, although some have hypothesized involvement of an autoimmune disorder.[11] In the hypothesis of an immune mediation of KLS, the HLA phenotypes or genotypes were determined. In a controlled study of 30 European patients, the DQB1-0201 genotype allele was twice more frequent in the KLS patients than in controls matched for ethnicity.[12] However, none of the 10 Taiwanese KLS-tested patients presented this haplotype. Recently, the relationship between the occurrence of mild, upper respiratory tract infections (URIs) in the general population and the occurrence and seasonality of episodes of URIs and hypersomnia in KLS patients was investigated. The timing of hypersomnolent episodes in 30 KLS patients was compared with calendar reports of URI events obtained from 2004 to 2007 from the Taiwan National Health Insurance Research Database, National Health Research Institutes, on age-matched subjects from the Taiwanese general population.[13] Results showed a significant bivariate correlation between KLS episodes and URI in the general population. The causative agent behind, or the consequences of, the URI were associated with a significant increased incidence of KLS episodes. The repetitive presentation of a brain syndrome suggests the presence of an immune disorder; but, to date, the cause of KLS remains unknown. Several hypotheses can be generated from this successive information. An immune-related dysfunction may be a cause in the symptomatic recurrence of symptoms of KLS patients. In addition, the by-product of a mild infection, such as fever, or the sleep fragmentation or deprivation, may modify the permeability of the blood-brain barrier. In association with a certain genetic background, this may lead to recurrence of symptoms for a short period, but there is no definitive proof to date.

TREATMENT

There is suspicion that several case reports indicating successful response to treatments have been erroneous because there is no established objective test to affirm presence of the syndrome. One of the goals of the long-term follow-up of the Taiwanese KLS patients is the evaluation of treatment trials that involve at least eight KLS patients initiated on a medication reported in the literature to have helped KLS cases, for a duration sufficient to see reoccurrence of at least four symptomatic episodes. To date, not a single treatment trial has been successful. Medications such as psychotropic (including Lithium[14,15]), antidepressants, and stimulants have been systematically tried. Drugs possibly having an effect on brain edema (including acetazolamide) have been also looked at, particularly during the symptomatic period, without any significant changes in the reoccurrence of the periodic hypersomnia.[16] Only stimulants have had an effect, not on the reoccurrence, but on the duration of the symptomatic period. The best-tolerated stimulant has been modafinil, a non-amphetaminic alerting agent. Compared with placebo, the medication has significantly decreased the duration of the symptomatic period, but it has never reduced the overall frequency of relapses and has not changed symptoms during the initial days of the symptomatic phase. It is probably best administered at the very beginning of the symptomatic phase during the first 24 hours with symptoms. The usual dose of modafinil has been 200 mg/day. However, to date, there is no effective consistent treatment of recurrences.

REFERENCES

1. Critchley M. Periodic hypersomnia and megaphagia in adolescent males. Brain 1962;85:627–56.
2. American Academy of Sleep Medicine. The international classification of sleep disorders: diagnostic and coding manual. 2nd edition. Westchester (NY): Illinois American Academy of Sleep Medicine; 2005.
3. Arnulf I, Lin L, Gadoth N, et al. Kleine-Levin syndrome: a systematic study of 106 patients. Ann Neurol 2008;63:482–92.
4. Mignot E, Lammers GJ, Ripley B, et al. The role of cerebro-spinal hypocretin measurement in the diagnostic of narcolepsy and other hypersomnias. Arch Neurol 2002;59:1255–62.
5. Huang YS, Lin YH, Guilleminault C. Polysomnography in Kleine-Levin syndrome. Neurology 2009;70:795–801.
6. Huang YS, Guilleminault C, Kao PF, et al. SPECT findings in the Kleine-Levin syndrome. Sleep 2005;28:955–60.
7. Hong SB, Joo EY, Tae WS, et al. Episodic diencephalic hypoperfusion in Kleine-Levin syndrome. Sleep 2006;29:1091–3.
8. Poryazova R, Schnepf B, Boesiger P, et al. Magnetic resonance spectroscopy in a patient with Kleine-Levin syndrome. J Neurol 2007;254:1445–6.

9. Landtblom AM, Dige N, Schwerdt K, et al. A case of Kleine-Levin syndrome examined with SPECT and neuropsychological testing. Acta Neurol Scand 2002;105:318–21.

10. Landtblom AM, Dige N, Schwerdt K, et al. Short-term memory dysfunction in Kleine-Levin syndrome. Acta Neurol Scand 2003;108:363–7.

11. Manni R, Martinetti M, Ratti MT, et al. Electrophysiological and immunogenetic findings in recurrent monosymptomatic-type hypersomnia: a study of two unrelated Italian cases. Acta Neurol Scand 1993;88:293–5.

12. Dauvillies Y, Mayer G, Lecendreux M, et al. Kleine-Levine syndrome: an autoimmune hypothesis based on clinical and genetic analyses. Neurology 2002;59: 1739–45.

13. Huang YS, Lin KL, Guilleminault C. Relationship between Kleine-Levin syndrome and upper respiratory infection in Taiwan [abstract]. Sleep 2010, in press.

14. Kellett J. Lithium prophilaxis of periodic hypersomnia. Br J Psychiatry 1977;130: 312–6.

15. Muratori F, Bertini N, Masi G. Efficacy of lithium treatment in Kleine-Levin syndrome. Eur Psychiatry 2002;17:232–3.

16. Huang YS, Tafti M, Chen NH, et al. Characteristics and long term outcomes of treatment trials of Kleine-Levin syndrome [abstract]. Sleep 2005;33:831.

Insomnia Pharmacology

Shannon S. Sullivan, MD[a,b]

KEYWORDS

• Hypnotics • Insomnia • Sleep-wake

With an astounding 10% to 15% of the United States population meeting criteria for an insomnia disorder,[1,2] insomnia is not only the most common sleep disorder in the population, it is a frequent complaint heard overall by primary care physicians and specialists alike: in data from 127 general practitioners caring for 11,810 patients (55% women), 26% of all patients complained of insomnia and 10% used sleep-promoting medication.[3] Treatment is recommended when chronic insomnia has a significant impact on sleep quality, health, daytime function, or comorbid conditions.[4] The National Sleep Foundation estimates that one of every four adult Americans takes sleep medication at some time point during the year, and it is estimated that the United States market for sleep drugs will be $5 billion by 2010.[2,5] Given the high prevalence of this disorder, its tendency to persist, and the frequency with which patients complain of symptoms in practice, it is imperative to have an understanding of basic sleep-wake mechanisms and the evolving field of pharmacologic approaches to enhance sleep.

Currently, pharmacologic approaches are among the most widely used therapies for insomnia. Several neurotransmitter and peptide systems are targeted, including γ-aminobutyric acid (GABA), serotonin, and histamine. Classically, the underpinnings of sleep-wake have been described as the balance between two predominant modes of transmission: excitation (mediated largely by glutamate) and inhibition (mediated largely by GABA).[6] This article reviews sleep-wake mechanisms, the neuroanatomic targets for sleep and wake-promoting agents, and discusses currently used agents to promote sleep and investigational hypnotics.

SLEEP-WAKE MECHANISMS
Neural Circuitry

As the understanding of the key central nervous system pathways that govern wake and sleep continue to grow, so does the ability to design and evaluate targeted therapies for insomnia, and indeed excessive sleepiness. The so-called "sleep circuit" of the brain[7] is comprised of a number of key nuclei in the brainstem and hypothalamus

[a] Stanford Sleep Medicine Center, Redwood City, CA, USA
[b] Center for Sleep Sciences, Stanford University, Palo Alto, CA, USA
E-mail address: shannon.s.sullivan@stanford.edu

Med Clin N Am 94 (2010) 563–580
doi:10.1016/j.mcna.2010.02.012
0025-7125/10/$ – see front matter © 2010 Elsevier Inc. All rights reserved.

(**Fig. 1**). An ascending arousal pathway starting in the rostral pons and running through the midbrain reticular system, known as the "ascending reticular activating system,"[8] is comprised of a loose network of well-defined cell groups dominated by certain neurotransmitters. First described by Moruzzi and Magoun,[9] the ascending brainstem reticular receives inputs from a large number of somatic and visceral sensory systems and extends excitatory projects to subcortical targets, such as the thalamus, hypothalamus, and basal forebrain.[10] Some centers within the activating network, including the locus ceruleus (dominated by neurotransmitter norepinephrine), dorsal and median raphe nuclei (dopamine), ventral periaqueductal gray matter (dopamine), and tuberomammillary nuclei (histamine), project by way of the hypothalamus and basal forebrain to the cortex, forming what has been termed the "ventral pathway." These signals are augmented by neurons of the lateral hypothalamus (orexin-hypocretin or melanin-concentrating hormone) and neurons of the basal forebrain (containing acetylcholine or GABA). A second branch of this activating system involves the pedunculopontine nucleus (dominated by acetylcholine) and laterodorsal tegmental nuclei (acetylcholine) in the upper brainstem, which project to the thalamus (see **Fig. 1**). Their firing facilitates thalamic relay neurons, which project to the cerebral cortex, which is important for wakefulness.[11]

Inhibition of these arousal centers occurs with sleep. Such inhibition is generated by hypothalamic nuclei, such as the ventrolateral preoptic nucleus ([VLPO] dominated by GABA and galanin) and the median preoptic nucleus (**Fig. 2**). GABA is the most common inhibitory neurotransmitter in the brain, and a major target for hypnotic agents. The VLPO sends outputs to all of the major arousal nuclei of the hypothalamus and brainstem and is most active during sleep.[12] The VLPO also receives inhibitory afferents from each of the major monoaminergic nuclei. These nuclei (summarized

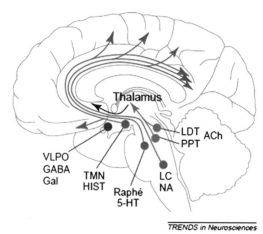

TRENDS in Neurosciences

Fig. 1. The ascending arousal system. Projections from the brainstem and posterior hypothalamus travel throughout the forebrain. Neurons of the laterodorsal tegmental (LDT) and pedunculopontine tegmental (PPT) nuclei send cholinergic (Ach) fibers to many targets including the thalamus, which regulates cortical activity. Aminergic wake centers also project diffusely throughout the forebrain, including the tuberomammillary nucleus (TMN) containing histamine (HIST), raphe nuclei neurons containing serotonin (5-HT), and locus ceruleus (LC) neurons containing norepinephrine (NA). The sleep-promoting neurons of the ventrolateral preoptic nucleus contain GABA and galanin. (*From* Saper CB, Chou TC, Scammell TE. The sleep switch: hypothalamic control of sleep and wakefulness. Trends Neurosci 2001;24:726–31; with permission.)

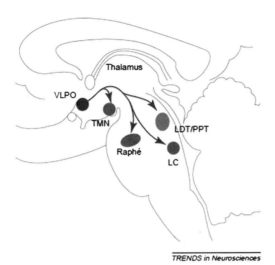

Fig. 2. The sleep-promoting ventrolateral preoptic nucleus (VLPO) projects to the main components of the ascending arousal system. The VLPO containing GABA and galanin has projections to the main centers of the ascending arousal system. LC, locus ceruleus; LDT, laterodorsal tegmental nucleus; PPT, pedunculopontine tegmental nucleus; TMN, tuberomammillary nucleus. (*From* Saper CB, Chou TC, Scammell TE. The sleep switch: hypothalamic control of sleep and wakefulness. Trends Neurosci 2001;24:726–31; with permission.)

in **Table 1**) form a circuit with mutually inhibitory elements in a self-reinforcing loop, with arousal centers active and inhibiting the sleep-promoting centers during wake, and sleep-promoting centers inhibiting arousal centers during sleep. This circuit has been described as a "flip-flop switch," such that one is in either one state or the other, with a rapid transition state between the two.[13] Saper and colleagues[13] have pointed to mathematical models showing that when either side of a flip-flop neural circuit is weakened, homeostatic forces cause the switch to ride closer to its transition point during both states,[14] resulting in more frequent transitions during both wake and sleep periods. Interestingly, these complex multicentered arousal and sleep circuits are in part overlapping and redundant, and manipulation of a single system may not strongly influence sleep or wakefulness.

It is understood that reducing wake-promoting systems to merely groups of neurons producing acetylcholine, hypocretin-orexin, and monoamines, such as dopamine, norepinephrine, and histamine, oversimplifies the dynamic, coordinated expression of behaviors and mechanisms that are constantly responding to internal and external cues.[10] Equally, sleep is not merely the result of absent or reduced activity of ascending arousal systems; rather, specific brain regions actively control non–rapid eye movement (NREM) and rapid eye movement (REM) sleep in concert with permissive physiologic and environmental cues. Somnogens, such as inflammatory factors, may promote sleep during infection. Cytokines interleukin-1β and tumor necrosis factor-α are produced within the brain and may promote sleep. Cytokines also induce production of certain prostaglandins that promote sleep. Other putative somnogens, such as the peptides somatostatin, cortistatin, growth hormone–releasing hormone, α-melanocyte-stimulating hormone, and others, have been proposed.[10,15]

Table 1
Major nuclei and neurotramitters involved in sleep and wake

Activating/Arousal Promoting	Location
Acetylcholine	Basal forebrain/basalocortical system
	Pedunculopontine tegmentum/laterodorsal tegmentum
Dopamine	Ventral periaquaductal gray matter
	Substantia nigra
	(D1/D2 receptors facilitate arousal; D2/D3 receptors facilitate sedation)
Glutamate	Ascending reticular activating system
	Thalamocortical system
Histamine	Tuberomammillary nucleus/posterior hypothalamus
Hypocretin/orexin	Lateral hypothalamus, periformical region
Norepinephrine	Locus ceruleus
Serotonin	Raphe nuclei, thalamus
Sleep promoting	Location
Adenosine	Basal forebrain
Melatonin	Pineal gland
GABA	VLPO
Galanin	VLPO

Abbreviations: GABA, γ-aminobutyric acid; VLPO, ventrolateral preoptic area.

Models of Sleep-Wake

There are two major concepts that largely describe propensity for sleep and wake when considered from a macroscopic perspective. The first is the concept of homeostatic sleep drive (termed "process S"), the idea that one accumulates increasing sleep need the longer one is awake; somnogens, such as extracellular adenosine, which accumulates during wake, may be the biologic correlate of homeostatic sleep drive. The second is circadian sleep drive (process C), the brain's intrinsic, approximately 24-hour sleep rhythm that helps time wakefulness and REM sleep, and may be environmentally influenced.[16] Models of the interaction of these two processes predict sleep propensity at any given time during an individual's subjective day, and these influences are important to consider when evaluating the impact of hypnotics or other sleep aides. Insomnia is modeled as a disorder of hyperarousal; targeting the brain's arousal pathways by pharmaceuticals and targeting cognitive and behavioral components of arousal by cognitive behavioral therapy are considered the mainstays of insomnia therapy.

PRACTICAL ISSUES IN PHARMOCOLOGIC INSOMNIA TREATMENT
Clinically Meaningful End Points and Goals of Treatment

Practically speaking, the goals of treatment include improvements in nighttime and daytime symptoms. Typical measures in insomnia intervention trials include sleep latency; number of awakenings; wake after sleep onset (WASO); total sleep time (TST); and frequency and nature of complaints, distress, and daytime symptoms.[17] Although sleep-promoting agents have been shown to improve sleep latency and maintenance, the daytime benefits of these changes are not fully understood.

The definition of insomnia is largely based on subjective elements, including symptoms of poor sleep and reports of daytime dysfunction. Hypnotic drug efficacy is judged generally by objective, and sometimes subjective, measures of sleep. Although trials to determine efficacy of agents to promote sleep tend to focus on polysomnographic improvements, other dimensions receive less attention, such as daytime function and quality of life. Furthermore, most studies of hypnotic medications select patients with primary insomnia, without association with comorbidities, such as depression, anxiety spectrum disorders, and circadian rhythm disorders, such as shift work disorder. Yet, in both clinic and population data, it is estimated that primary insomnia accounts for only 25% to 30% of the chronic insomnia population.[18] Finally, study populations are generally limited to otherwise healthy, nonelderly adults. Although pharmacologic trials in the elderly exist, meaningful end points such as fall risk, balance, memory, and unintentional naps, are usually neglected. Prospective pediatric studies are few, and there is little consensus on indication for hypnotics; benefit-risk assessment; and hypnotic selection, dose, and duration.

Coexisting Medication Use

Because the processes of sleep are known to be actively influenced by multiple neuronal loci in the brain with a variety of neurotransmitters, hormones, peptides, and others, it follows that changes in these signals may influence sleep. Many medications may influence sleep. One often overlooked aspect of pharmacologic insomnia treatment is a clear assessment of potential insomnia-producing drugs included in an individual's medication routine. A host of common medications have insomnia side effects. At times, changing dose or timing or swapping to a different drug for the same indication can assist with insomnia treatment. This practical approach to insomnia management may be daunting for practitioners when patients are on multiple medications, but Web-based and digital resources can be helpful in detecting possible medication triggers of insomnia. History may also be helpful, if symptoms of poor sleep started around the time of introduction of the offending medication. **Table 2** summarizes some common offenders. Finally, the symptom of unrefreshing sleep may be indirectly produced by medication; for example, a patient with chronic pain may be taking significant doses of methadone, a long-acting opiate with known association with sleep-disordered breathing and complex sleep apnea, which may be influencing arousals from sleep and sleep quality.

Characteristics of Hypnotics

Insomnia may be broadly categorized into sleep onset–type, sleep maintenance–type, or a combination of the two. Hypnotic choice should be based on when symptoms occur. Onset of action of a drug is affected by both the rate of drug absorption (Tmax) and rate of distribution in the central nervous system. Tmax is a useful indicator of onset of action. Duration of action, however, is affected by the dose administered, the elimination half-life, and the rate of metabolism. The parameter most predictive of sleep maintenance (and residual effects) is half-life. **Table 3** lists elimination half-lives of commonly used medications for sleep. These features influence sleep maintenance. Generally speaking, short-acting medications may be used for sleep initiation insomnia, whereas a drug half-life of greater than 4 hours is needed for sleep maintenance insomnia. Especially with such longer half-life medications, it is important to counsel patients that they may have morning-after symptoms of sleepiness, cognitive changes, and so forth. When using such agents, adequate sleep time opportunity must exist. Finally, potency of action is determined by both dose and receptor affinity.

Table 2
Drugs commonly associated with insomnia

Drug	Comments
Antidepressants	
Tricyclic antidepressants	Mechanism may be worsening of periodic limb movements of sleep
	More alerting: protriptyline, nortriptyline
	Sedating: tertiary amines
	Associated with nightmares
Monoamine oxidase inhibitors	Insomnia is frequent
	Segeline has partial metabolism to amphetamine
Selective serotonin reuptake inhibitors	Citalopram and fluoxetine are most alerting
	Fluvoxamine and paroxetine are most sedating
	Can worsen periodic limb movements of sleep; associated with nightmares and RBD-type presentation
Venlafaxine	Insomnia in 4%–18% of patients
	May produce PSG features of RBD
Bupropion	DA and NE reuptake inhibitor, insomnia 11%–20%
Antipsychotics	
Aripiprazole	Insomnia 8%–18%, may also cause sedation or sleepiness
Antiparkinsonian drugs	
Levodopa	Dopamine precursor, insomnia at higher doses
Anticonvulsants	
Felbamate	Insomnia is common
Cardiovascular drugs	

β-Blockers	Most common with metoprolol and propranolol Decrease rapid eye movement sleep; more lipophilic drugs cause sleep disruption Commonly associated with nightmares or night terrors
Decongestants	Pseudoephedrine, phenylpropanolamine
Antibiotics Levofloxacin Ciprofloxacin Amphotericin B Antivirals	Especially amantidine, DA reuptake inhibitor
Asthma medications Albuterol Theophylline Systemic corticosteroids	
Stimulants Caffeine Dextroamphetamine Methamphetamine Methylphenidate Modafinil	Attention to total 24-hour dose and time of dosing is important

Abbreviations: DA, dopamine; NE, norepinephrine; PSG, polysomnogram; RBD, rapid eye movement sleep behavior disorder.

Table 3
Common prescription drugs used for insomnia

Drug Class	Medication	Typical Dose Range (mg)	Half-Life (h)	Comments
Antidepressant	Trazodone	25–100	8	Falls, orthostatic hypotension, priapism
Antidepressant	Doxepin	Older 10–50; newer 3–6	Active metabolite: 28+	Anticholinergic side effects
Antidepressant	Mirtazapine	7.5–15	26–40	Weight gain
Antipsychotic	Quetiapine	12.5–50	6	Weight gain, metabolic syndrome
Benzodiazepine	Triazolam	0.25–0.5	2–5	
Benzodiazepine	Estazolam	1–2	10–24	
Benzodiazepine	Temazepam	7.5–30	8 (range, 4–18)	Incoordination, falls, cognitive impairment
Benzodiazepine	Clonazepam	0.5–2	30–40	
Benzodiazepine	Flurazepam	15–30	40+	Infrequently used
Benzodiazepine	Quazepam	7.5–30	40+	Infrequently used
Benzodiazepine receptor agonist	Zaleplon	5–20	1	
Benzodiazepine receptor agonist	Zolpidem	5–10	2.5 (1.4–4.5)	
Benzodiazepine receptor agonist	Eszopiclone	1–3	4–6	
Benzodiazepine receptor agonist	Zolpidem extended release	6.25–12.5	2.8 (1.6–4)	Biphasic release
Melatonin receptor agonist	Melatonin	1–3	0.5	
Melatonin receptor agonist	Ramelteon	8	<1	

Term of Use

Before 2005, Food and Drug Administration (FDA) class labeling for hypnotics implied short-term treatment durations. Since 2005, there have been no durations indicated in hypnotic labeling, and neither eszopiclone nor ramelteon have usage term restrictions.[4] Recent evidence suggests that efficacy and safety of eszopiclone, zaleplon, and zolpidem is sustained over periods of 6 to 12 months.[19–22] Consensus recommendations do support the possibility of long-term hypnotic use in those with severe or refractory insomnia, or with chronic comorbid illnesses, although emphasis is placed on providing interventions, such as cognitive behavioral therapy, and on-going follow-up, reassessment of efficacy, and monitoring for adverse events related to medication usage.[4]

Although hypnotic drug treatment is well-described over shorter, well-defined time horizons, psychological and behavioral interventions have shown short- and long-term efficacy. Cognitive behavioral therapy for insomnia in the setting of comorbid depression has been recently shown to improve depression outcomes and insomnia, and this therapy also has been shown in a randomized trial to be equally effective for primary insomnia and comorbid insomnia.[23,24] Studies have also demonstrated the cognitive behavioral therapy for insomnia is arguably superior to benzodiazepine and benzodiazepine receptor agonists (BzRA) in terms of rates of relapse after cessation of therapy.[25] There are also fewer concerns regarding tolerance effects, and efficacy is equivalent or better.[26] Barriers to this form of treatment exist, however, because it involves multiple visits to a practitioner, of whom there are not nearly enough to meet demand.

CURRENT THERAPY

Most drugs used to promote sleep have not been approved for this indication by the FDA. In a recent Physician Drug and Diagnosis audit, three of the top four prescription medications (ranked according to frequency of mention) were antidepressants (trazodone, amitryptyline, and mirtazepine).[18] Of all of the drugs used to treat insomnia, only a handful have been approved by the FDA for this indication. Broadly categorized, sleep aids fall into several categories: hypnotic agents FDA-approved for the indication of insomnia (benzodiazepines, nonbenzodiazepine BzRAs, and ramelteon); antidepressants (eg, trazodone); antipsychotics (eg, quetiapine); anticonvulsants (eg, gabapentin); and over-the-counter medications (eg, diphenyhydramine) and agents considered to be supplements (eg, melatonin). Off-label use of medications for sleep is common. What follow is a summary of features of currently used agents for sleep induction.

Benzodiazepines and Nonbenzodiazepine BzRAs

The prototypical class of hypnotics, benzodiazepines, modulate $GABA_A$ receptors, which are gated ion channels that mediate effects of GABA. These agents decrease the time to sleep onset and enhance stage 2 sleep. The oldest of the benzodiazepine sedatives, chlordiazepoxide, was introduced in 1960. This class of compounds is more potent than previously used sedatives, such as barbiturates, and had an improved profile in toxicity and overdose. These drugs bind to the GABA-benzodiazepine receptor complex, rather than directly on GABA. Benzodiazepines bind to the benzodiazepine receptor so that the inhibitory action of GABA is allosterically enhanced. There are a number of subtypes of the benzodiazepine receptor that mediate different actions. Traditional benzodiazepines bind nonselectively to GABA-benzodiazepine receptor subtypes BZ1, BZ2, and BZ3, which mediate sedation and amnesia, anxiolysis, and myorelaxation and anticonvulsants effects, respectively. Benzodiazepines vary widely in their biologic half-life, which along with dose determines the duration of action of the drug. The time needed to reach Tmax shows less variability between the various benzodiazepines and BzRA, however, with virtually all of them reaching peak plasma concentrations within 1 to 2 hours, which has been shown to shorten sleep latency. Like the barbiturates before them, benzodiazepines may be associated with tolerance, abuse potential, morning-after sedation, and cognitive impairment.[27,28] They are also associated with rebound insomnia (especially with short- and intermediate-acting agents). With discontinuation, withdrawal symptoms (anxiety, irritability, restlessness) may occur. Additionally, there may be worsening of obstructive sleep apnea and an increase in falls in older adults. Contraindications to use include pregnancy or lactation; significant renal or hepatic impairment (dose adjustment); untreated obstructive sleep apnea; or severe ventilatory impairment.

More recently, nonbenzodiazepine BzRAs have been developed with varying degrees of increased selectivity hypnotic action compared with benzodiazepine predecessors. This class includes zolpidem, zaleplon, zopiclone, and eszopiclone, the so-called "z drugs" or BzRAs. Despite evidence suggesting that BzRAs are preferred over traditional benzodiazepines,[29] evidence pointing to improvements in efficacy or safety is limited.[30,31] In contrast to traditional benzodiazepines, these agents selectively bind to the BZ1 (α_1-subunit–containing) receptor subtype, explaining their more targeted action as sleeping agents with far fewer anxiolytic or myorelaxant properties. There are three distinct drugs in this class: zaleplon, zolpidem, and eszopiclone. Zolpidem, one of the leading hypnotic medications, is currently the only agent of this class to be available as a generic medication. Compared with conventional benzodiazepines, these agents have similar hypnotic action, but an improved profile for rebound insomnia, withdrawal, tolerance, and abuse or dependence potential. There is less sleep architectural change and no muscle relaxation, anticonvulsant, or anxiolytic activity associated with these agents. FDA-approved for use in insomnia, these are Drug Enforcement Agency Schedule IV controlled substances, just as conventional benzodiazepines. Concerns regarding potential adverse effects of BzRAs include behaviors during sleep, such as sleepwalking; drug interactions; residual sedation; memory and daytime performance alterations; and concern for increased risk of motor vehicle accidents and falls.[32] There is also the possibility of tolerance and lack of effectiveness over time, and dependence in some patients.[33]

Melatonin Receptor Agonists

The high-affinity melatonin receptor (MT1-MT2) agonist ramelteon has been on the market in the United States since 2005 for the treatment for insomnia and is not scheduled like its $GABA_A$ agonist counterparts. It has an advantageous safety profile, and dependence and abuse potential is considered to be minimal; however, the overall effectiveness of this medication has been called into question.[7] Subjective measures of sleep quality have not been improved,[34] and lack of head-to-head reports published between ramelteon and other agents and clinical data suggests that its efficacy may be relatively modest compared with other insomnia therapeutics.[34]

Sedating Antidepressants and Antipsychotic Medications

Despite the widespread use of these medications for insomnia, there are limited published data on the appropriate use of such agents in insomnia. Nonetheless, use of antidepressants and, increasingly, antipsychotics, is commonplace in insomnia therapy. This may be in part because these agents are not Drug Enforcement Agency–scheduled and a wide variety of practitioners are familiar with them. Typically, the doses used to treat insomnia are below the antidepressant dose. Nonetheless, the safety profile of sedating antidepressants is not impressive compared with the BzRAs; however, most safety data is for antidepressant doses, not hypnotic doses.

The sedating tricyclic antidepressants, which include amitriptyline, doxepin, nortryptiline, trimipramine, and others, act by inhibiting the uptake of norepinephrine and serotonin, and by blocking histamine and acetylcholine. They can increase TST and stage 2 sleep, but suppress REM sleep. The tricyclics are known to impair cognition and psychomotor performance, a finding more pronounced in the elderly.[35] Other first-generation antidepressants, the monoamine oxidase inhibitors, inhibit the enzymes involved in metabolism of norepinephrine, serotonin, and dopamine either irreversibly or reversibly depending on the agent. These are not considered sedating but can disturb nighttime sleep with shorter TST and REM suppression, thereby increasing daytime symptoms.

Several serotonin-modulating antidepressants, such as trazodone and nefazodone, are used for insomnia, especially depression-associated insomnia.[36,37] Trazodone, a sedating antidepressant with inhibition of serotonin, α_1, and histamine receptors, causes daytime hypersomnolence and increases TST. It has no significant potential for abuse or dependence, but may affect daytime performance.[38] It is associated with cardiac arrhythmias, orthostatic hypotension, and, notably, priapism, which may limit its use. It can also give rise to serotonin syndrome when administered in conjunction with other serotonergic agents. Although this agent may have use in those with comorbid depression, data in nondepressed patients with insomnia are limited and side effects including weight gain, dizziness, and psychomotor impairment have led to relatively high rates of discontinuance.[36] Nefazodone is similar to trazodone in its serotonin receptor blockade, but is less active at α_1-receptors and has no activity at histamine receptors. Drowsiness is a dose-dependent side effect.[39]

The selective serotonin reuptake inhibitors selectively block reuptake of serotonin and are commonly used as first-line agents in the treatment of depression. As a whole, this class of drugs is considered less sedating, and may decrease TST, but drugs in this class are associated with both somnolence and insomnia. Selective serotonin reuptake inhibitors also are associated with suppression of REM sleep. Mirtazepine, a selective α_2, serotonin, and histamine receptor blocker,[40] is another antidepressant associated with daytime sedation and an increase in TST. Weight gain may be a deal-breaking side effect, however, in some patients. Sedating newer antipyschotics have also been increasingly used in the treatment of insomnia, especially comorbid insomnia, but have not been studied extensively for this purpose. Quetiapine, a dopamine, serotonin, and norepinephrine antagonist, and olanzapine, a cholinergic, histaminergic, and dopaminergic antagonist, have been used for the purpose of sleep promotion.

Nonprescription Medications Used for Insomnia

Although over-the-counter agents are not recommended for the treatment of insomnia, they are the most commonly used sleep agents.[41] They are inexpensive and easily available to insomnia sufferers, who invariably have tried them before considering prescription agents. There are little published data on the efficacy of over-the-counter medications in insomnia, and side effects may be considerable in some populations.

Diphenhydramine and other first-generation histamine antagonists (with activity at H_1 receptors) are the usual sleep-promoting agent in over-the-counter sleep promoting agents. They are sedating because they cross the blood-brain barrier to work at central nervous system histamine receptors. Diphenhydramine has been shown to extend sleep duration.[18] These agents, however, are associated with rapid tolerance to hypnotic effect (within two to three administrations for diphenyhydramine); residual daytime sedation associated with long half-life; and anticholinergic side effects, such as confusion, dizziness, delirium, blurred vision, urinary retention, constipation, and increased intraocular pressure. They should be used with great caution in the elderly and in those with narrow-angle glaucoma.

Melatonin and Other Nutritional Supplements

The hormone melatonin is released from the pineal gland during the night, starting at dim light onset in the early evening, and is important for maintaining circadian rhythms. Low levels of melatonin have been linked to insomnia and depression, and administration of melatonin has mild sleep-promoting properties[42]; however, there are limited clinical trial data to support efficacy. Clinically, melatonin is used both for sleep initiation insomnia and in lower doses for managing circadian rhythm disorders. Considered a nutritional supplement, it is not FDA-approved for the indication of insomnia, nor is it regulated by the FDA. High levels of discrepancy of melatonin content in over-the-counter preparations have been reported.

There is inconsistent evidence for kava, valerian, skullcap, passionflower, and other botanic compounds in the treatment of insomnia. Additionally, hepatotoxicty has been described for some of these agents.[43,44] Although several placebo-controlled trials of valerian root formulations have demonstrated short-term, mainly subjective improvements in insomnia, objective data are largely lacking. Studies of the impact of supplements and herbals on sleep in insomnia have been summarized as "absent, uncontrolled, negative, or indicative of safety concerns."[41]

New Agents

Despite decades of GABAergic therapies for insomnia, GABA continues to be a target for development of new insomnia drugs. The more recent addition of ramelteon exemplifies heightened interest in new targets and pathways, however, namely serotonin antagonists and inverse agonists, histamine antagonists, melatonin agonists, and hypocretin-rexin agonists. As thinking about pharmacologic targets for insomnia therapy moves beyond the traditional GABA realm, the field is opened to the possibility of targeted therapy for certain comorbid conditions or demographics; in addition, synergistic combinations of agents targeting different pathways may become possible. What follows is an introduction to newer or proposed agents for insomnia and currently used agents with other indications that have a proposed expanded indication for insomnia.

Several $GABA_A$ receptor agonists have been recently investigated. EVT-201 is a partial positive allosteric modulator of the $GABA_A$ receptor complex that has shown positive results in two Phase II proof of concept trials in both elderly and adult insomnia patients.[45] In a randomized, placebo-controlled Phase II trial of EVT-201 at doses of 1.5 and 2.5 mg for two consecutive nights (with a 5–12 day washout period) in 75 patients with primary insomnia (mean age, 45 ± 11 years), WASO and TST improved.[46] Improvements in secondary end points including sleep latency and number of awakenings were also shown. There was no subjective residual sedation; it was safe and well-tolerated. A second Phase II double-blind study of 149 elderly patients with chronic insomnia and daytime sleepiness showed that after 7 days of use, the 1.5-mg dose also demonstrated increased TST compared with placebo,[47] and there were improvements in objective measurements of daytime sleepiness and significant overall improvement in multiple sleep latency test compared with placebo. There was no significant difference in daytime function or in the benzodiazepine withdrawal questionnaire. Common adverse events were dizziness, headache, and somnolence. Regarding Phase III trials, no data are available.

Other $GABA_A$ receptor agonists have also reached later stages of development, but are not currently being pursued. These include indiplon, adipiplon, and a selective extrasynaptic $GABA_A$ receptor agonist gaboxadol. Gaboxadol was extensively studied for treatment of insomnia, but Phase III trials suggested that the overall clinical profile did not support further development.[48] Of interest, gaboxadol garnered interest as an agent that demonstrated enhanced slow wave sleep in models of insomnia[49]; and during experimentally induced sleep restriction, gaboxadol enhanced slow wave sleep without changes in TST, and was associated with less physiologic and subjective sleepiness on multiple sleep latency testing and other measures, respectively.[50]

Finally, although by no means a new drug, a sublingual form of zolpidem tartrate (OX22) is being developed, representing a new delivery platform for a well-described medication. This is anticipated to be targeted for middle-of-the-night awakenings associated with insomnia.

Some agents already on the market with non-GABA$_A$ activity are being proposed for the indication of insomnia. Low-dose doxepin is now being considered for an indication of insomnia because of its antihistaminergic activity. Doxepin is a tricyclic antidepressant that has been used for more than 35 years to treat depression at typical doses of 75 to 300 mg; at low dose (1–6 mg) its activity is selective for mainly histamine (H$_1$) receptor blockade. Unlike the antihistamine diphenyhydramine, which has antagonism at muscarinic cholinergic receptors at doses that are clinically useful for histamine blockade (leading to increased anticholinergic side effects), doxepin has a wide separation of binding potency at H$_1$ receptors compared with other receptors.[51] Doxepin doses of less than or equal to 6 mg have been shown to exhibit highly selective H$_1$ antagonism. The low-dose formulation has completed four Phase III trials,[52] in which, for example, doses of 3 and 6 mg improved WASO and TST in 229 patients with chronic insomnia. In a 4-week, randomized, double-blind, parallel group, placebo-controlled trial of 255 elderly chronic insomniacs, sustained improvement of TST (primary end point) and significant improvements in WASO and sleep quality were shown compared with placebo at the 6-mg dose. Elderly patients with chronic insomnia (N = 240) in a 3-month, double-blind, parallel-group study had significant improvements in WASO (primary end point) and multiple secondary end points at both 1- and 3-mg doses.[17] The drug has been well-tolerated and in all Phase III trials somnolence was the only dose-related adverse event. Unlike BzRAs, low-dose doxepin is not expected to be restricted as a scheduled medication by the FDA.

Another drug approved for another indication with recent increased interest for use in chronic insomnia, especially that associated with fibromyalgia, is sodium oxybate. This drug was launched in 2002 in the United States for the treatment of cataplexy associated with narcolepsy. The active metabolite of this agent, γ-hydroxybutyrate, inhibits presynaptic dopamine release and is known to increase slow wave sleep; however, its mechanisms of action are incompletely understood. Subsequently approved for use in the European Union for narcolepsy with cataplexy and released in multiple countries around the world, this drug is classified as a psychostimulant, but it has dose-dependent hypnotic properties when administered. In a Canadian and United States 8-week randomized, double-blind trial of 147 patients (of 188 enrolled), doses of 4.5 or 6 g per day produced significant benefit for symptoms of fibromyalgia, including sleep disturbance.[53] In a 12-week trial of 49 patients (32 female) with chronic insomnia (mean age, 53.2 years; range, 20–76 years) with a double-dummy, randomized, blinded design with sodium oxybate plus placebo, zolpidem plus placebo, or placebo nightly, and blinded flexible-dose titration for 1 month and fixed doses for 2 months, all groups had improvement in overall insomnia, daytime sleepiness, and sleep quality indices. There was no treatment effect seen, however, for TST, WASO, sleep efficiency, or sleep latency. Furthermore, dizziness (67%) and nausea (60%) were reported with sodium oxybate.[54] Further studies are needed in larger populations to explore the potential and efficacy of sodium oxybate in the treatment of chronic insomnia.

Regarding agents in the development pipeline with novel targets, serotonin antagonists and inverse agonists have also been the focus of recent attention. Eplivanserin is principally a 5HT-2A antagonist, although the compound also has some affinity for the 5HT-2C receptor. Developed originally to treat psychiatric disorders, this agent had completed three Phase III clinical trials for the treatment of insomnia but its application for approval was recently withdrawn in both the United States and the European Union.[55] Pimavanserin tartrate (ACP-103) is also a neuroleptic with antagonist and inverse agonist activity at 5HT-2A receptors, which is being investigated as a treatment for Parkinson disease psychosis; this agent too has been proposed to have hypnotic-sedative activity and has reached phase II trials for insomnia.[56,57] Administration of ACP-103 to healthy volunteers was found to be well tolerated at a dose of 10 mg,[58] and in a Phase I, randomized, proof-of-concept double-blind, placebo-controlled study of 45 healthy volunteers, pimavanserin tartrate, 1 to 20 mg, included increased slow wave sleep in a dose-dependent manner, decreasing both WASO and number of awakenings after sleep onset. Finally, nelotanserin, a 5HT-2A receptor inverse agonist, has shown some early signs of promise in human and murine studies.[59]

New agents with melatonin receptor agonism are also showing promise. Agomelatine is a melatonin MT1 and MT2 receptor agonist and a 5HT-2C antagonist. It was recently approved for clinical use in the European Union for depression. FDA application in the United States is expected in the coming years. This novel melatonergic agent has strong affinity for hypothalamic melatonin-binding sites in the superchiasmatic nucleus and garnered early interest in resynchronization of circadian rhythms. Its unique 5HT-2C properties have been hypothesized to have an impact on sleep. This agent has been shown to improve sleep in depressed patients and to have an antidepressant efficacy that is partially attributable to its effects on sleep. The agent has been shown to decrease the severity of anxiety associated with depression, and may be especially useful for improving disrupted sleep patterns in patients with depression without affecting daytime vigilance.[60] It should be noted, however, that agomelatine is not marketed for insomnia, and that this indication is currently unapproved.

Tasimelteon is a MT1-MT2 melatonin receptor agonist in Phase III trials for the treatment of insomnia. With tested doses of 20, 50, and 100 mg, tasimelteon demonstrated statistically significant improvements in sleep onset, sleep maintenance, and TST using subjective and objective measures.[61] On its Web site, the manufacturer emphasizes the indication of treatment for circadian rhythm disorders, such as transient insomnia caused by jet lag. Study results have demonstrated decreased sleep latency and WASO and increased sleep efficiency, and a dose-dependent shift in plasma melatonin rhythm to an earlier hour.

Hypocretin-orexin is yet another emerging target showing promise in the insomnia field. Almorexant is a potent orexin 1 and 2 receptor antagonist currently in Phase III clinical trials in Israel, Australia, and Switzerland. Evidence was presented in 2007 that this dual receptor antagonist could facilitate sleep induction and maintenance in preclinical and clinical models.[62] When administered in healthy human subjects, almorexant decreased wakefulness in a dose-dependent manner without evidence of cataplexy.[63] The RESTORA 1 trial, which involved 670 adults with chronic primary insomnia in Asia, Australia, Europe, Israel, and Latin America, assessed almorexant compared with zolpidem in primary insomnia, and increases in sleep efficiency, reductions in latency to sleep onset, and reductions in WASO were demonstrated.[64] Thus far, no significant safety concerns have been identified and the agent has been well-tolerated, supporting further development; results from Phase III trials are not yet available.[65] Another orexin receptor antagonist, MK-4305, is under development for indications of schizophrenia and insomnia.

SUMMARY

Traditional therapeutic targets of GABA$_A$ agonism are far from being overlooked, but the field is expanding rapidly, as understanding of the multiple pathways influencing sleep-wake states grows and as agents become available to target these pathways. Although the mainstay of insomnia therapy currently resides with GABA$_A$ agonism, emerging drugs feature much more than just new formulations of existing insomnia treatments. Several GABA$_A$ agonists have recently been in Phase II and Phase III development, but further development has recently been suspended or discontinued. The melatonin MT1-MT2 receptor agonist and serotonin 2C receptor antagonist agomelatine has demonstrated efficacy in treating depression and insomnia, and another melatonergic agent, tasimelteon, is also in Phase III trials for transient insomnia, such as jet lag. Multiple serotonin 2A receptor antagonists have also progressed to mid to late stages of development. Orexin 1 and 2 receptors represent a novel target for insomnia therapy, and at least two companies are pursuing this target in Phase II and anticipated Phase III trials. Finally, agents already on the market for other indications, such as low-dose doxepin, an H$_1$ receptor blocker, are at later stages of investigation for hypnotic use. As novel targets are explored, synergistic combinations may become possible to customize insomnia pharmacotherapy for comorbid conditions and special populations. In this era of pharmacologic exploration for improved insomnia therapy, a more complete view of meaningful outcomes should also be sought when evaluating therapies. Finally, the success of cognitive behavioral therapy for insomnia demonstrates that nonpharmacologic approaches hold a great deal of promise; awareness about and access to such therapy should be expanded.

REFERENCES

1. Ohayon M. Epidemiology of insomnia: what we know and what we still need to learn. Sleep Med Rev 2002;6:97–111.
2. National Sleep Foundation. 2005 sleep in America poll. Washington, DC: National Sleep Foundation; 2005.
3. Ohayon M, Caulet M, Arbus L, et al. Are prescribed medications effective in the treatment of insomnia complaints? J Psychosom Res 1999;47(4):359–68.
4. Schutte-Rodin S, Broch L, Buysse D, et al. Clinical guideline for the evaluation and management of chronic insomnia in adults. J Clin Sleep Med 2008;4(5): 487–504.
5. Available at: www.hypnion.com/programs/seepfacts.htm. Accessed May 25, 2009.
6. Winsky Sommerer R. Role of GABA$_A$ receptors in the physiology and pharmacology of sleep. Eur J Neurosci 2009;29:1779–94.
7. Wafford KA, Ebert B. Emerging anti-insomnia drugs: tackling sleeplessness and the quality of wake time. Nat Rev Drug Discov 2008;7:530–40.
8. Starzi TE, Taylor CW, Magoun HW. Ascending conduction in reticular activating system with special reference to the diencephalon. J Neurophysiol 1951;14: 461–77.
9. Moruzzi G, Magoun HW. Brain stem reticular formation and activation of the EEG. Electroencephalogr Clin Neurophsyiol 1949;1:455–73.

10. Espana RA, Scammell TE. Sleep neurobiology for the clinician. Sleep 2004;27(4): 811–20.
11. MCormick DA. Cholinergic and noradrenergic modulation of thalamocortical processing. Trends Neurosci 1989;12:215–20.
12. Sherin JE, Shiromani PJ, McCarley RW, et al. Activation of ventrolateral preoptic neurons during sleep. Science 1996;271:216–9.
13. Saper CB, Scammell TE, Lu J. Hypothalamic regulation of sleep and circadian rhythms. Nature 2005;437:1257–63.
14. Chou TC. Regulation of sleep-wake timing: circadian rhythms and bistability of sleep-wake states [thesis]. Cambridge (MA): Harvard University; 2003. p. 82–99.
15. Qureshi A, Lee-Chiong T. Medications and their effects on sleep. Med Clin North Am 2004;88:751–66.
16. Borbely AA, Achermann P. Concepts and models of sleep regulation: an overview. J Sleep Res 1992;1:62–79.
17. Sullivan SS, Guilleminault C. Emerging drugs for insomnia: new frontiers for old and novel targets. Expert Opin Emerg Drugs 2009;14(3):411–22.
18. Roth T. Sedative hypnotics. In: Opp MR, editor. Sleep Research Society basics of sleep guide. 1st edition. Westchester (IL): Sleep Research Society; 2005. p. 147–9.
19. Walsh JK, Krystal AD, Amato DA, et al. Nightly treatment of primary insomnia with eszopiclone for six months: effect on sleep, quality of life, and work limitations. Sleep 2007;30(8):959–68.
20. Roth T, Walsh JK, Krystal A, et al. An evaluation of the efficacy and safety of eszopiclone over 12 months in patients with chronic primary insomnia. Sleep Med 2005;6(6):487–95.
21. Ancoli-Israel S, Richardson GS, Mangano RM, et al. Long-term use of sedative hypnotics in older patients with insomnia. Sleep Med 2005;6(2):107–13.
22. Krystal AD, Erman M, Zammit GK, et al. Long term efficacy and safety of zolpidem extended-release 12.5 mg, administered 3 to 7 nights per week for 24 weeks, in patients with chronic primary insomnia: a 6-month, randomized, double-blind, placebo-controlled, parallel-group, multicenter study. Sleep 2008; 31(1):79–90.
23. Edinger JD, Olsen MK, Stechuchak KM, et al. Cognitive behavioral therapy for patients with primary insomnia or insomnia associated predominantly with mixed psychiatric disorders: a randomized clinical trial. Sleep 2009;32(4): 499–510.
24. Manber R, Edinger JD, Gress JL, et al. Cognitive behavioral therapy for insomnia enhances depression outcome in patients with comorbid major depressive disorder and insomnia. Sleep 2008;31(4):489–95.
25. Morin CM, Bootzin RR, Buysse DJ, et al. Psychological and behavioral treatment of insomnia: update of the recent evidence (1998–2004). Sleep 2006;29(11): 1398–414.
26. Sivertsen B, Omvik S, Pallesen S, et al. Cognitive behavioral therapy vs zopiclone for treatment of chronic primary insomnia in older adults: a randomized controlled trial. JAMA 2006;295(24):2851–8.
27. O'brien CP. Benzodiazepine use, abuse, and dependence. J Clin Psychiatry 2005;66(Suppl 2):28–33.
28. Barker MJ, Greenwood KM, Jackson M, et al. Cognitive effects of long-term benzodiazepine use: a meta-analysis. CNS Drugs 2004;18(1):37–48.
29. Ozminkowski RJ, Wang S, Walsh JK. The direct and indirect costs of untreated insomnia in adults in the United States. Sleep 2007;30(3):263–73.

30. Buscemi N, Vandermeer B, Friesen C, et al. The efficacy and safety of drug treatments for chronic insomnia in adults: a meta-analysis of RCTs. J Gen Intern Med 2007;22(9):1335–50.
31. Montplaisir J, Hawa R, Moller H, et al. Zopiclone and zaleplon vs benzodiazepines in the treatment of insomnia: Canadian consensus statement. Hum Psychopharmacol 2003;18(1):29–38.
32. Vermeeren A. Residual effects of hypnotics. CNS Drugs 2004;18:297–328.
33. Hajak G, Müller WE, Wittchen HU, et al. Abuse and dependence potential for the non-benzodiazepine hypnotics zolpidem and zopiclone: a review of case reports and epidemiological data. Addiction 2003;98:1371–8.
34. Borja NL, Daniel KL. Ramelteon for the treatment of insomnia. Clin Ther 2006;28: 1540–55.
35. van Laar MW, vanWillingenburg AP, Volkerts ER. Acute and subacute effects of nefazodone and imipramine on highway driving, cognitive functions, and daytime sleepiness in healthy adults and elderly subjects. J Clin Psychopharmacol 1995;15:30–40.
36. Mendelson WB. A review of the evidence for the efficacy and safety of trazodone in insomnia. J Clin Psychiatry 2005;66(4):469–76.
37. James SP, Mendelson WB. The use of trazodone as a hypnotic: a critical review. J Clin Psychiatry 2004;65:752–5.
38. Haria M, Fitton A, McTavish D. Trazodone: a review of its pharmacology, therapeutic use, in depression and therapeutic potential in other disorders. Drugs Aging 1994;4:331–55.
39. Robinson DS, Roberts DL, Smith JM, et al. The safety profile of nefazodone. J Clin Psychiatry 1996;57:31–8.
40. Nutt D. Mirtazepine: pharmacology in relation to adverse effects. Acta Psychiatr Scand Suppl 1997;391:31–7.
41. Sateia MJ, Pigeon WR. Identification and management of insomnia. Med Clin North Am 2004;88:567–96.
42. Cajochen C, Krauchi K, Wirz-Justice A. Role of melatonin in the regulation of human circadian rhythms and sleep. J Neuroendocrinol 2003;15:432–7.
43. Wheatley D. Medicinal plants for insomnia: a review of their pharmacology, efficacy and tolerability. J Psychopharmacol 2005;19(4):414–21.
44. Vassiliadis T, Anagnostis P, Patsiaoura K, et al. Valeriana hepatotoxicity. Sleep Med 2009;10(8):935.
45. Available at: http://www.evotec.com/display/articleCategorizedDetail/cms_article_id/63/website_part_id/4/selected_category_id/6. Accessed February 5, 2010.
46. Walsh JK, Thacker S, Knowles LJ, et al. The partial positive allosteric GABA$_A$ receptor modulator EVT201 is efficacious and safe in the treatment of adult primary insomnia patients. Sleep Med 2009;10(8):859–64.
47. Evotec. Available at: http://www.evotec.com/display/archiveDetail/website_part_id/1/selected_year/2007/cms_article_id/1553. Accessed March 21, 2010.
48. Saul S. Merck cancels work on a new insomnia medication, in NYT 3/29/2007. Available at: http://www.nytimes.com/2007/03/29/business/29sleep.html. Accessed February 16, 2010.
49. Walsh JK, Deacon S, Dijk DJ, et al. The selective extrasynaptic GABAA agonist, gaboxadol, improves traditional hypnotic efficacy measures and enhances slow wave activity in a model of transient insomnia. Sleep 2007;30(5):593–602.
50. Walsh JK, Mayleben D, Guico-Pabia C, et al. Efficacy of the selective extrasynaptic GABA A agonist, gaboxadol, in a model of transient insomnia: a randomized, controlled clinical trial. Sleep Med 2008;9(4):393–402.

51. Stahl S. Selective histamine H1 antagonism: novel hypnotic and pharmacologic actions challenge classical notions of antihistamines. CNS Spectr 2008;13(12): 1–12.

52. Available at: http://www.somaxon.com/pages/pc_silenor.htm. Accessed May 25, 2009.

53. Russell IJ, Perkins AT, Michalek JE. Sodium oxybate relieves pain and improves function in fibromyalgia syndrome: a randomized, double-blind, placebo-controlled, multicenter clinical trial. Arthritis Rheum 2009;60(1):299–309.

54. Kuo TF, Stowers P, Tortora L, et al. Sodium oxybate and zolpidem in the treatment of chronic insomnia: a randomized, doule-blind, double dummy, placebo controlled 3-arm, parallel group study [abstract]. Sleep 2009;32(A Suppl): A273.

55. Mimosa S, Berton E. Sanofi-Aventis discontinues eplivanserin for insomnia. Dow Jones & Co. Available at: http://english.capital.gr/news.asp?id=876133. Accessed February 5, 2010.

56. Abbas A, Roth B. Pimavanserin tartrate: a 5-HT2A inverse agonist with potential for treating various neuropsychiatric disorders. Expert Opin Pharmacother 2008; 9(18):3251–9.

57. Teegarden BR, Al Shamma H, Xiong Y. 5HT-2A inverse-agonists for the treatment of insomnia. Curr Top Med Chem 2008;8:969–76.

58. Nordstrom AL, Mansson M, Jovanovic H, et al. PET analysis of the 5-HT2A receptor inverse agonist ACP-103 in human brain. Int J Neuropsychopharmacol 2008;11(2):163–71.

59. Al-Shamma HA, Anderson C, Chuang E, et al. Nelotanserin, a novel selective human 5-Hydroxytryptamine2A inverse agonist for the treatment of insomnia. J Pharmacol Exp Ther 2010;332:281–90.

60. Rivara S, Mor M, Bedini A, et al. Melatonin receptor agonists: SAR and applications to the treatment of sleep-wake disorders. Curr Top Med Chem 2008;8: 954–68.

61. Birznieks G, Scott C, Baroldi P, et al. Melatonin agonist VEC-162 improves sleep onset and maintenance in a model of transient insomnia [abstract]. Sleep 2007; 30(A Suppl):A264.

62. Brisbare-Roch C, Dingemanse J, Koberstein R, et al. Promotion of sleep by targeting the orexin system in rats, dogs and humans. Nat Med 2007;13(2):150–5.

63. Roecker A, Coleman P. Orexin receptor antagonists: medicinal chemistry and therapeutic potential. Curr Top Med Chem 2008;8(11):977–87.

64. Actelion presentations, World Sleep Congress, Cairns, Australia, September 3–6, 2007.

65. Neubauer DN. Almorexant, a dual orexin receptor antagonist for the treatment of insomnia. Curr Opin Investig Drugs 2010;11(1):101–10.

Insomnia and Its Effective Non-pharmacologic Treatment

Allison T. Siebern, PhD*, Rachel Manber, PhD

KEYWORDS

• Insomnia • CBTI • Non-pharmacologic treatment

Insomnia is the most common sleep disorder characterized by nocturnal symptoms; difficulties initiating or maintaining sleep; and daytime symptoms, such as difficulty with concentration, memory, fatigue, decrease in pleasurable activities, and impairment in function and mood. Insomnia symptoms and insomnia disorder have been often used interchangeably in the literature. In 2004, sleep researchers proposed the term "insomnia disorder" defined as sleep difficulties associated with daytime impairment or distress about the difficulty sleeping.[1] Insomnia disorder also requires the presence of symptoms for at least 1 month and it is often classified by its duration: transient (<1 month); short term (between 1 to 6 months); and chronic insomnia (more than 6 months). Estimates of prevalence of insomnia disorders vary based on methodologies, with best estimates arising from epidemiologic studies. Such studies suggest that chronic insomnia is present in approximately 6% to 10% of persons in the United States[2,3] and between 5% and 12% in other countries.[4–6]

There are two classification systems for the diagnosis of insomnia: the *Diagnostic and Statistical Manual for Mental Disorders* (DSM), which is published by the American Psychiatric Association[7] and used by mental health professionals, such as psychologists and psychiatrists; and the *International Classification of Sleep Disorders* (ICSD), which is most commonly used by sleep specialists.[8] The two diagnostic classifications identify subtypes of insomnia. The current version of the DSM includes primary insomnia, insomnia related to another mental disorder, insomnia caused by a general medical condition, and substance-induced insomnia. The current ICSD system includes insomnia that has 10 subcategories: adjustment insomnia, psychophysiologic insomnia, paradoxical insomnia, idiopathic insomnia, inadequate sleep hygiene, insomnia caused by mental disorder, insomnia caused by drug or substance, insomnia caused by medical

Sleep Medicine Center, Stanford University School of Medicine, 450 Broadway Street, M/C 5704, Redwood City, CA 94063, USA
* Corresponding author.
E-mail address: Asiebern@stanford.edu

Med Clin N Am 94 (2010) 581–591
doi:10.1016/j.mcna.2010.02.005
0025-7125/10/$ – see front matter © 2010 Elsevier Inc. All rights reserved.

medical.theclinics.com

condition, insomnia unspecified, and physiological (organic) insomnia. The DSM-V (diagnostic and statistical manual of mental disorders, 5th edition) advisory committee on sleep nosology has proposed a single diagnosis of insomnia disorder with the use of qualifiers to specify presence of medical and psychiatric comorbidities. This proposed diagnosis will replace the existing DSM diagnoses of primary insomnia and insomnia related to other medical or psychiatric conditions, thus eliminating causal implications inherent with the use of terms, such as "sleep disorder due to a general medical condition" and "sleep disorder related to another mental disorder".[9]

INSOMNIA IS A PUBLIC HEALTH PROBLEM

In 1995 the direct cost of substances used and health care costs related to insomnia in the United States were estimated to be $13.9 billion per year.[10] A broader insomnia-related estimate includes direct costs (inpatient, outpatient, emergency room health care utilization, over-the-counter supplements and pharmaceuticals); indirect costs (workplace absenteeism, loss of work productivity); and related costs (those that do not fall into direct/indirect, such as damages caused by on the job accidents). With this broader definition, a 1994 study estimated that the cost of insomnia is $30 billion to $35 billion per year.[11] More recent estimates for direct and indirect costs in the United States are even higher, more than $100 billion.[12] The relative direct and indirect costs for adults (under 64 years of age) with and without insomnia is $1253 per 6 calendar months, with slightly lower differential cost among people aged 65 years or older ($1143).[13] Emerging data underscore the public health and economic burden of insomnia. These data can be divided into the following three categories: health risks, health utilization, and work domain deficits (absenteeism and reduced productivity).

HEALTH RISKS

Prolonged insomnia is associated with significant health problems. In a study of 3445 primary care subjects, in which 50% had chronic insomnia, individuals who experienced insomnia symptoms defined as most or all nights a week for the previous 4 weeks were more likely to also have physician-diagnosed myocardial infarction (odds ratio [OR]: 0.9); congestive heart failure (OR: 2.5); and diabetes mellitus (OR: 1.0); and patient-reported comorbidities, such as osteoarthritis (OR: 1.6); rheumatoid arthritis (OR: 1.3); peptic ulcer (OR: 1.8); and bowel problems (OR: 0.9).[14] A new study of 1440 women suggests that the well-documented association between anxiety and cardiovascular diseases is mediated by insomnia as evidenced by a threefold reduction in the association between anxiety and cardiovascular symptoms when insomnia was added as a predictor.[15] Poor sleep quality is also associated with next morning worsening of irritable bowel syndrome symptoms [16] and pain associated with rheumatologic disorders.[17,18] Recent data also suggests an association between poor sleep and obesity.[19] The direction of the link between poor sleep and health indices has not been fully explored. For pain conditions, this relationship appears to be a bidirectional relationship[20] but less is known about other conditions.

HEALTH UTILIZATION

Insomnia is associated with increased health care utilization, such as medical visits and hospitalizations.[21] In a sample of 350 subjects with insomnia in a sleep clinic, who were receiving behavioral management of insomnia, 82% reported having a medical office visit in the past 2 months and 44% had reported having a mental health visit in the past 2 months.[22] Simon and VonKorff found a relationship between insomnia and greater general medical service utilization. Specifically, those with insomnia had significantly higher total health services costs than those without.[23] Insomnia is more strongly associated with health problems thus it is not surprising that there is an increase in use of health care services and subsequently increased cost. Data is lacking on the cost savings and reduction in health care utilization that result from treating insomnia.

Impact on Work Domain

Insomnia is associated with lost work days and reduced productivity. It is estimated that employees who meet ICD diagnosis of insomnia miss on average 3.1 more days per year than those who do not.[24] In addition to absences, insomnia is associated with an average of 27.6 days in lost productivity on the job, likely related to poor concentration and fatigue.[25] Absenteeism and lost productivity related to insomnia have a significant economic toll. A recent study of 948 participants estimated that $970 million Canadian dollars are lost annually because of absences related to insomnia and an additional $5 billion Canadian dollars annually are lost because of lost productivity on the job.[25] Leger and colleagues[21] suggest that greater absenteeism in people with insomnia might be attributable to the health issues that are comorbid with insomnia but this possibility has not been directly tested.

INSOMNIA IS UNDERTREATED

Only one in five individuals with difficulty sleeping in the United States makes an appointment to see a physician with a chief complaint of difficulty sleeping.[26] Of the 30% that have discussed sleep with their doctor four out of five mentioned concern about sleep within the context of a visit about a different chief complaint.[26] Predictors of whether patients would discuss insomnia with a physician include perceived daytime fatigue, symptoms of depression and anxiety,[27] poor physical well being, longer insomnia duration, older age, and higher income level.[28] Less is known about the reasons patients are hesitant to bring up insomnia symptoms with their doctor. Some possibilities may include uncertainty whether insomnia will be taken seriously, concern that only medication treatment is available, ambivalence about taking medication, and being unaware of alternative non-pharmacologic treatments for insomnia; however, these possibilities have not been examined systematically in representative samples. There is also a lack of systematic investigations of how patients who do not seek treatment cope with insomnia. One study found that two thirds of people with insomnia reported lacking knowledge of available treatments for insomnia and 4 out of 10 reported self medicating with over-the-counter medication or alcohol.[29]

Physician-specific reasons for under treating insomnia include insufficient time[30] and a belief that insomnia is secondary to another medical or mental disorder and will resolve when the parent disorder is treated. Indeed, in primary and tertiary settings insomnia is often comorbid with other medical or psychiatric conditions.[31] However, the belief that insomnia will resolve with the treatment of the parent disorder has been challenged by new evidence to the contrary. For example, 44% of patients with a depressive disorder continue to experience poor sleep even after their depression improves. It is now believed that when insomnia is experienced in the context of another disorder, the two conditions impact each other. Insomnia may hinder treatment of the coexisting condition. For example, a person with insomnia and depression may not respond as favorably to treatment of the depression as would those with only depression and no insomnia. Conversely, coexisting medical and psychiatric conditions may impact response to insomnia treatment. Terminology, such as secondary insomnia, is not helpful for patient care in that it does not change how the provider would approach treatment. The challenge for the clinician is in determining when the insomnia is significant enough to warrant clinical attention.

WHO IS AT RISK FOR THE DEVELOPMENT OF INSOMNIA

Some groups have been identified as being more at risk for the development of insomnia. One such group is women who are two times more likely than men to have insomnia.[31] Sleep disruptions increase during certain junctures in a woman's life, such as pregnancy, postpartum,[32] and menopause.[33] However, the prevalence of insomnia disorder during these junctures has not been fully assessed. Another risk factor for insomnia is aging. Older adults are more likely to have insomnia, which may be related to poor health, chronic illnesses, and multiple medication use.[34] Those that have irregular sleep-wake schedules, such as workers with rotating shifts; frequent travel across time zones (such as airline personnel); or those that frequently sleep irregular schedules, are at significant risk for developing insomnia. This risk is because irregular sleep-wake schedules can dampen the circadian clock signals that help regulate sleep and wakefulness, as described later in this article. Self described night owls tend to have more irregular sleep-wake schedules than those who are not.[35] People with some medical or psychiatric conditions and those who describe themselves as worriers are at an increased risk for the development of insomnia. People who have experienced insomnia disorder in the past have a lower threshold for the reemergence of insomnia.[36]

NON-PHARMACOLOGIC TREATMENT OF INSOMNIA

Cognitive behavioral therapy for insomnia (CBTi) is a brief and effective non-pharmacologic treatment for insomnia that is grounded in the science of sleep medicine, the science of behavior change and psychological theories. There is strong empirical evidence that CBTi is effective.[37,38] Direct comparisons of CBTi with sleep medication in randomized control trials demonstrate that CBTi has comparable efficacy with more durable long-term maintenance of gains after treatment discontinuation.[39-41] These studies carefully selected subjects with insomnia with no comorbid medical, sleep, or psychiatric disorders. Evidence is mounting that CBTi is also effective when insomnia is experienced in the context of medical disorders (eg, cancer, HIV, fibromyalgia, and pain) and psychiatric disorders, such as depression and anxiety.[42] National Institutes of Health consensus and the American Academy of Sleep Medicine Practice Parameters recommend that CBTi be considered standard treatment for insomnia.[43,44] Despite the high level of empirical support, health care providers and consumers are largely unaware of this treatment option. The remainder of this article is dedicated to describing CBTi, beginning with a conceptual model of insomnia that underlies the therapy, continuing with descriptions of the components of CBTi, and concluding with practical issues related to its implementation in primary care.

A MODEL OF INSOMNIA

A behavioral model of insomnia, put forth by Spielman and colleagues[45] in 1987, identifies predisposing characteristics, precipitating events, and perpetuating attitudes and practices – three factors that together explain the development and course of insomnia. Predisposing characteristics are individual attributes that lower the threshold for the development of insomnia during unsettling or stressful periods and hence increase the likelihood of the development of insomnia.[45] These characteristics include biological and psychological factors. For example, people who tend to be restless or anxious and those who worry excessively are at increased risk for insomnia during periods of increased stress and distress.

Precipitating events are life events, such as significant loss, that lead to increased stress and trigger sleep disruptions. Approximately 75% of people with insomnia can identify a clear trigger.[46] Sleep disruptions that emerge during periods of acute stress often resolve when the stress subsides, but in some cases poor sleep persists and insomnia develops.

An individual's response to the experience of poor sleep may perpetuate the problem. Exaggerated distress about poor sleep leads to increased sleep effort, characterized by worrying about not getting enough sleep, apprehension about sleep at bedtime, and frustration when sleep onset is delayed. It is as if the person develops performance anxiety about sleep, which of course interferes with the process of sleep. Trying to get to sleep, stay asleep, or get more sleep may take different forms, such as extending time in bed by going to bed earlier than before, avoiding previously enjoyable activities in the evening for fear that they will interfere with sleep, cancelling engagements or obligations during the day, and using alcohol to induce sleep.

In addition, continued frustration and distress when unable to sleep leads to conditioned arousal, which means that the bed or the bedroom become a trigger for increased arousal, rather than sleep. Some patients with insomnia report that as they get into the bed at night their minds become active and their heart rate increases even though they were dozing on the couch just before going to bed. CBTi targets perpetuating attitudes and practices. It is a set of interventions aimed at modifying cognitions and behaviors that interfere with sleep and breaking the cycle of conditioned arousal. The interventions that constitute CBTi are time-in-bed restriction, stimulus control, relaxation therapy, cognitive therapy, and sleep hygiene.

TIME-IN-BED RESTRICTION (SLEEP RESTRICTION)

Time-in-bed restriction (also known as sleep restriction) is a procedure designed to increase the homeostatic sleep drive, one of two components involved in the regulation of sleep. The homeostatic drive to sleep, known as process S, increases in a linear fashion from rise time to bedtime. The longer we are awake the stronger the sleep drive. The second component involved in the regulation of sleep is the circadian clock, known as process C. Process C, generated in the suprachiasmatic nucleus, opposes process S by sending alerting signals that initially increase in magnitude as the homeostatic drive to sleep increases and later wanes in magnitude, thus permitting sleep. The alerting signals increase again approximately 2 hours before rise time. The optimal time to sleep is when the homeostatic drive (process S) to sleep is high and the alerting signals (process C) begin to dampen.

Time-in-bed restriction (sleep restriction) was initially developed by Spielman to address middle-of-the-night awakenings, but it has since been used even for initial sleep onset difficulties.[47] It is an iterative process that starts with limiting the allowed time in bed to the patients' current average reported actual sleep time and subsequently slowly increasing the allowed time in bed as sleep improves by small increments. Typically, improvement in sleep quality is seen within the first week of implementing this procedure. Individuals with insomnia tend to underestimate their total sleep time.[48,49] Therefore limiting time in bed to the reported sleep time is likely to result in mild sleep deprivation and increased homeostatic sleep drive, thus reducing sleep latency or time awake in the middle of the night. Increased sleep drive may lead to sleepiness during the day. Patients should therefore be cautioned against driving while sleepy when undergoing this procedure. The decision to increase the allowed time in bed is based on the percent of actual sleep time relative to the time spent in bed (sleep efficiency). When the average sleep efficiency for more than 1 week is at least 0.85, the time in bed is extended by 15 minutes. The initial time in bed is never less than 5.5 hours, even if the initial reported sleep time is less than that. Each new time-in-bed prescription is followed for at least 1 week before the next extension is proposed. The process stops when the patients' sleep need is met as reflected by optimal daytime alertness and functioning. Sleep logs that are completed each morning are very helpful during this process as they aid in providing more accurate estimates of total sleep time than retrospective recollection.

Ideally the placement of the sleep window (the times in and out of bed) should maximize the likelihood that sleep will occur and therefore needs to be informed by the patients' circadian tendency (chronotype). For example, the prescribed bedtime is not at a time during which the circadian clock still generates strong alerting signals. To maximize the likelihood of adherence with the prescribed time in bed, the decision of the times in and out of bed should be done in collaboration with patients. Consideration of the patients' current sleep-wake schedule and life constraints that might impact bed time and rise time, such as work schedule, child care, and so forth, impact the chosen sleep window.

A caveat to time-in-bed restriction and CBTi is that unresolved medical conditions may continue to cause sleep disruption, such as those associated with pain, abnormal thyroid function, acid reflux disorder, increased nighttime urinary frequency, dementia, depression, and anxiety. Trouble breathing during sleep can also lead to fragmented sleep, such as with sleep apnea, asthma, and congestive heart failure.

STIMULUS CONTROL

Stimulus control, developed by Bootzin, is a set of instructions aimed at breaking conditioned arousal and strengthening the bed and bedroom as stimuli for sleep.[50] Stimulus control is used for sleep onset and sleep maintenance insomnia. The four instructions and their rationale are

- Go to sleep only when sleepy. This instruction will likely increase the probability of sleeping by aligning the bedtime to coincide with low arousal and strong homeostatic drive to sleep. It is important that patients learn to distinguish sleepiness from fatigue and tiredness. Sleepiness is a state requiring effort to stay awake. It is more closely associated with low arousal and high homeostatic drive and is therefore more conducive for sleep. Fatigue and tiredness are states of low energy but may also be accompanied by an active mind and high arousal, which are not conducive to sleep. Patients with insomnia often report feeling "tired but wired" at bedtime, wishing to sleep but not feeling sleepy, most likely because of conditioned arousal and high activation of the arousal system.
- If unable to sleep at the beginning or middle of the night get out of bed and return only when sleepy. When out of bed engage in quiet non-arousing activities and use the minimum amount of lighting necessary for the activity. This instruction removes the frustration and other negative emotions experienced by individuals with insomnia when they are unable to sleep, which helps break the conditioned arousal.
- Set a regular morning wake time. This instruction applies irrespective of how much total sleep was acquired the night before. This important instruction aims at strengthening the circadian clock, as rise time is important for the

entrainment of the clock. This instruction also reduces sleep effort by eliminating the end of the night tossing and turning.
- Avoid napping during the day. For people with insomnia who also experience daytime sleepiness, this original stimulus control instruction can be modified to allow short (15–20 minutes) naps. Naps are kept short to avoid reducing the homeostatic drive. It is recommended that when naps are taken they are initiated 7 to 9 hours after the morning wake time.

RELAXATION THERAPY

There are a variety of factors, such as cognitions and emotions, that influence the activation of the arousal system that can interfere with or supersede the sleep promoting system. A person should attempt to sleep when they feel calm because wakefulness and sleep are two distinct systems and do not operate like an on-off switch but rather on a continuum of continual communication. Research has shown that those with insomnia compared with good sleepers have higher heart rates, stress hormones, and metabolic levels.[51,52] Techniques to help in reducing this hyperarousal activation are relaxation therapy, such as progressive muscle relaxation, diaphragmatic breathing, visual imagery, and stress management skills. They are designed to reduce somatic and psychic anxiety related to sleep.

A common reaction to difficulties with sleeping is to try harder to sleep or to force sleep to happen, which may actually lead to an increase in arousal activation. This process has been likened to the Chinese finger trap; you put your fingers into the trap and the harder you try to pull them out the more stuck you become. The key to getting your fingers out is letting go and easing them out.[53] Relaxation therapy can be an adaptive replacement to trying and forcing sleep to occur, but with the goal of using the techniques to calm the mind and relax the body thus decreasing the hyperarousal. However, the caveat to relaxation therapy is to not use the relaxation techniques for the purpose of trying to get to sleep.

COGNITIVE THERAPY

The cognitive therapy component of the CBTi targets thoughts and beliefs that interfere with sleep directly by increasing arousal in bed or indirectly by interfering with adherence to sleep restriction and stimulus control. A common reaction to difficulties with sleeping is to worry about sleep or lack thereof. As times goes on and poor sleep continues, an anticipation of not sleeping well each night begins to emerge. The daytime consequences of not sleeping well also become worries, such as "how will I function at work tomorrow"; "I will be unable to get through my day"; or "I may lose my job because I am not functioning optimally." These worries about getting to sleep and daytime consequences of not getting enough sleep serve to increase the arousal response. Cognitive therapy is employed to address these sleep-related cognitions and worries. In some patients, the behavioral components of treatment (time-in-bed restriction and stimulus control) may increase patients' anxiety about getting enough sleep leading to a paradoxical reaction. In these instances treatment may focus more on components that reduce the anxiety and arousal activation.

SLEEP HYGIENE

Standard sleep hygiene therapy includes "limiting caffeine intake, avoiding alcohol before bed, incorporating daily exercise, having a bedtime snack, and keeping the bedroom quiet, dark, and at a comfortable temperature." There is insufficient evidence to support sleep hygiene as a lone intervention[44] but it is often included along with other more potent interventions. A comparison of standard sleep hygiene with CBTi in a sample of 81 subjects revealed that CBTi produced greater decrease in wakefulness after sleep onset than standard sleep hygiene education.[54] Sleep hygiene recommendations, like dental hygiene, might be best conceptualized as a set of preventative rather than therapeutic strategies.

MULTIMODAL APPROACH

CBTi is a multimodal approach that combines behavioral and cognitive strategies. The most commonly used behavioral components are time-in-bed restriction and stimulus control, which can be combined into a single set of instructions. The cognitive component is added as a means for reducing cognitive and emotional hyperarousal and for increasing adherence with the behavioral components. Sleep restriction and stimulus control are counter-intuitive. Some patients may respond to a reduction in the time they are allowed to spend in bed with a significant increase in anxiety about sleep, which may interfere with sleep. The task of the CBTi provider is to tailor its components to each individual based on the unique presentation. A brochure with instruction is often not sufficient. Research has shown that for individuals with insomnia and no comorbid conditions, four individual sessions, each approximately 1 hour, are optimal length of therapy.[55] When the presentation is more complex, additional sessions are needed. CBTi can also be provided effectively in a group format. In fact, one of the seminal randomized control trials compared group CBTi to the benzodiazepine temazepam and pill placebo.[39] The study found that the two active interventions were statistically equivalent in reducing time awake after sleep onset after 8 weeks of treatment and both were more effective than pill placebo. The study also found that group CBTi had more durable effects 2 years later.[39]

COGNITIVE BEHAVIORAL THERAPY FOR INSOMNIA PROVIDERS AND WHERE TO FIND THEM

CBTi is a form of cognitive behavioral therapy, an approach to therapy that was developed by psychologists to deal with many psychiatric conditions and aims to modify cognitions and behaviors relevant to each disorder. Historically, CBTi was developed and provided by psychologists whose training included the science of behavior change, cognitive and behavioral interventions, psychological assessment, and additional specialized training in sleep medicine. Specialized training in sleep medicine is important for an effective delivery of CBTi. General psychotherapy is not effective for improving sleep.[56] At the same time, knowledge of sleep medicine alone, without training in the science of behavioral change and principles of cognitive behavioral therapy, is not likely to produce optimal results. Currently, the American Academy of Sleep Medicine offers certification for providers of behavioral sleep medicine, including CBTi. A list of certified providers can be found at http://www.aasmnet.org/BSMSpecialists.aspx.

SUMMARY

Cognitive behavioral therapy for insomnia is an effective non-pharmacologic treatment for insomnia. In direct comparisons with sleep medication in randomized control trials, CBTi demonstrates that it has comparable efficacy with more durable long-term maintenance of gains after treatment discontinuation. Because of the strong empirical support of CBTi, the National Institutes of Health Consensus and the American

Academy of Sleep Medicine Practice Parameters recommend that CBTi be considered standard treatment for insomnia. The importance of identifying and treating insomnia is underscored by the public health and economic burden of insomnia currently estimated at $100 billion annually. Increased awareness is needed in the primary and tertiary settings for health care providers and patients regarding the availability and the short- and long-term efficacy of CBTi.

REFERENCES

1. Edinger JD, Bonnet MH, Bootzin RR, et al. Derivation of research diagnostic criteria for insomnia: report of an American Academy of Sleep Medicine Work Group. Sleep 2004;27(8):1567–96.
2. Ohayon MM. Epidemiology of insomnia: what we know and what we still need to learn. Sleep Med Rev 2002;6(2):97–111.
3. Ford DE, Kamerow DB. Epidemiologic study of sleep disturbances and psychiatric disorders. An opportunity for prevention? JAMA 1989;262(11):1479–84.
4. Ohayon MM, Hong SC. Prevalence of insomnia and associated factors in South Korea. J Psychosom Res 2002;53(1):593–600.
5. Ohayon MM, Partinen M. Insomnia and global sleep dissatisfaction in Finland. J Sleep Res 2002;11(4):339–46.
6. Leger D, Guilleminault C, Dreyfus JP, et al. Prevalence of insomnia in a survey of 12,778 adults in France. J Sleep Res 2000;9(1):35–42.
7. Association AP. Diagnostic and statistical manual of mental disorders-IV-TR (text revision). 4th edition. Washington, DC: American Psychiatric Publishing, Inc; 2000.
8. American Academy of Sleep Medicine. International classification of sleep disorders: diagnostic & coding manual. 2nd edition. Westchester (IL): American Academy of Sleep Medicine; 2005.
9. Reynolds CF, Redline S, DSM-V Sleep-Wake Disorders Workgroup and Advisors. The DSM-V sleep-wake disorders nosology: an update and an invitation to the sleep community. Sleep 2010;33(01):10–1.
10. Walsh JK, Engelhardt CL. The direct economic costs of insomnia in the United States for 1995. Sleep 1999;22(Suppl 2):S386–93.
11. Chilcott LA, Shapiro CM. The socioeconomic impact of insomnia. An overview. Pharmacoeconomics 1996;10(Suppl 1):1–14.
12. Fullerton DS. The economic impact of insomnia in managed care: a clearer picture emerges. Am J Manag Care 2006;12(Suppl 8):S246–52.
13. Ozminkowski RJ, Wang S, Walsh JK. The direct and indirect costs of untreated insomnia in adults in the United States. Sleep 2007;30(3):263–73.
14. Katz DA, McHorney CA. Clinical correlates of insomnia in patients with chronic illness. Arch Intern Med 1998;158(10):1099–107.
15. Olafiranye O, Jean-Louis G, Magai C, et al. Anxiety and cardiovascular symptoms: the modulating role of insomnia. Cardiology 2009;115(2):114–9.
16. Goldsmith G, Levin JS. Effect of sleep quality on symptoms of irritable bowel syndrome. Dig Dis Sci 1993;38(10):1809–14.
17. Affleck G, Arrows S, Tennen H, et al. Sequential daily relations of sleep, pain intensity, and attention to pain among women with fibromyalgia. Pain 1996; 68(2–3):363–8.
18. Smith MT, Quartana PJ, Okonkwo RM, et al. Mechanisms by which sleep disturbance contributes to osteoarthritis pain: a conceptual model. Curr Pain Headache Rep 2009;13(6):447–54.

19. Patel SR. Reduced sleep as an obesity risk factor. Obes Rev 2009;10(Suppl 2): 61–8.
20. McCracken LM, Iverson GL. Disrupted sleep patterns and daily functioning in patients with chronic pain. Pain Res Manag 2002;7(2):75–9.
21. Leger D, Guilleminault C, Bader G, et al. Medical and socio-professional impact of insomnia. Sleep 2002;25(6):625–9.
22. Lee C, Kuo T, Manber R. Chronic insomnia and health care utilization [abstract supplement]. Sleep 2005;28:A236.
23. Simon GE, VonKorff M. Prevalence, burden, and treatment of insomnia in primary care. Am J Psychiatry 1997;154(10):1417–23.
24. Kleinman NL, Brook RA, Doan JF, et al. Health benefit costs and absenteeism due to insomnia from the employer's perspective: a retrospective, case-control, database study. J Clin Psychiatry 2009;70(8):1098–104.
25. Daley M, Morin CM, LeBlanc M, et al. The economic burden of insomnia: direct and indirect costs for individuals with insomnia syndrome, insomnia symptoms, and good sleepers. Sleep 2009;32(1):55–64.
26. Dement W. Sleep in America: 1995 Gallup Poll, 1999. Available at: http://www. stanford.edu/~dement/95poll.html. Accessed March 11, 2010.
27. Morin CM, LeBlanc M, Daley M, et al. Epidemiology of insomnia: prevalence, self-help treatments, consultations, and determinants of help-seeking behaviors. Sleep Med 2006;7(2):123–30.
28. Shochat T, Umphress J, Israel AG, et al. Insomnia in primary care patients. Sleep 1999;22(Suppl 2):S359–65.
29. Ancoli-Israel S, Roth T. Characteristics of insomnia in the United States: results of the 1991 National Sleep Foundation Survey. I. Sleep 1999;22(Suppl 2):S347–53.
30. National Sleep Foundation. The National Online Healthcare Professional Insomnia Poll, 2008. Available at: http://www.sleepfoundation.org/sleep-facts-information/sleep-report-card. Accessed March 11, 2010.
31. Mellinger GD, Balter MB, Uhlenhuth EH. Insomnia and its treatment. Prevalence and correlates. Arch Gen Psychiatry 1985;42(3):225–32.
32. Soares CN, Murray BJ. Sleep disorders in women: clinical evidence and treatment strategies [abstract xi]. Psychiatr Clin North Am 2006;29(4):1095–113.
33. Eichling PS, Sahni J. Menopause related sleep disorders. J Clin Sleep Med 2005; 1(3):291–300.
34. Bloom HG, Ahmed I, Alessi CA, et al. Evidence-based recommendations for the assessment and management of sleep disorders in older persons. J Am Geriatr Soc 2009;57(5):761–89.
35. Ong JC, Huang JS, Kuo TF, et al. Characteristics of insomniacs with self-reported morning and evening chronotypes. J Clin Sleep Med 2007;3(3):289–94.
36. LeBlanc M, Mérette C, Savard J, et al. Incidence and risk factors of insomnia in a population-based sample. Sleep 2009;32(8):1027–37.
37. Morin CM, Culbert JP, Schwartz SM. Nonpharmacological interventions for insomnia: a meta-analysis of treatment efficacy. Am J Psychiatry 1994;151(8):1172–80.
38. Smith MT, Perlis ML, Park A, et al. Comparative meta-analysis of pharmacotherapy and behavior therapy for persistent insomnia. Am J Psychiatry 2002; 159(1):5–11.
39. Morin CM, Colecchi C, Stone J, et al. Behavioral and pharmacological therapies for late-life insomnia: a randomized controlled trial. JAMA 1999;281(11):991–9.
40. Sivertsen B, Omvik S, Pallesen S, et al. Cognitive behavioral therapy vs zopiclone for treatment of chronic primary insomnia in older adults: a randomized controlled trial. JAMA 2006;295(24):2851–8.

41. Jacobs GD, Pace-Schott EF, Stickgold R, et al. Cognitive behavior therapy and pharmacotherapy for insomnia: a randomized controlled trial and direct comparison. Arch Intern Med 2004;164(17):1888–96.
42. Smith MT, Huang MI, Manber R. Cognitive behavior therapy for chronic insomnia occurring within the context of medical and psychiatric disorders. Clin Psychol Rev 2005;25(5):559–92.
43. NIH state-of-the-science conference statement on manifestations and management of chronic insomnia in adults. NIH Consens State Sci Statements 2005; 22(2):1–30.
44. Morgenthaler T, Kramer M, Alessi C, et al. Practice parameters for the psychological and behavioral treatment of insomnia: an update. An American academy of sleep medicine report. Sleep 2006;29(11):1415–9.
45. Spielman AJ, Caruso LS, Glovinsky PB. A behavioral perspective on insomnia treatment. Psychiatr Clin North Am 1987;10(4):541–53.
46. Bastien CH, Vallieres A, Morin CM. Precipitating factors of insomnia. Behav Sleep Med 2004;2(1):50–62.
47. Spielman AJ, Saskin P, Thorpy MJ. Treatment of chronic insomnia by restriction of time in bed. Sleep 1987;10(1):45–56.
48. Harvey AG. A cognitive model of insomnia. Behav Res Ther 2002;40(8):869–93.
49. Frankel BL, Coursey RD, Buchbinder R, et al. Recorded and reported sleep in chronic primary insomnia. Arch Gen Psychiatry 1976;33(5):615–23.
50. Bootzin RR, Nicassio PM. Behavioral treatment for insomnia. In: Eisler R, Hersen M, Miller P, editors. Progress in behavior modification. New York: Academic Press; 1978.
51. Bonnet MH, Arand DL. 24-Hour metabolic rate in insomniacs and matched normal sleepers. Sleep 1995;18(7):581–8.
52. Vgontzas AN, Chrousos GP. Sleep, the hypothalamic-pituitary-adrenal axis, and cytokines: multiple interactions and disturbances in sleep disorders. Endocrinol Metab Clin North Am 2002;31(1):15–36.
53. Manber R. Insomnia: risk factors, diagnosis, & treatment, 2009. Available at: http://www.knol.google.com/k/insomnia#. Accessed March 11, 2010.
54. Edinger JD, Olsen MK, Stechuchak KM, et al. Cognitive behavioral therapy for patients with primary insomnia or insomnia associated predominantly with mixed psychiatric disorders: a randomized clinical trial. Sleep 2009;32(4):499–510.
55. Edinger JD, Wohlgemuth WK, Radtke RA, et al. Dose-response effects of cognitive-behavioral insomnia therapy: a randomized clinical trial. Sleep 2007;30(2): 203–12.
56. Kopta SM, Howard KI, Lowry JL, et al. Patterns of symptomatic recovery in psychotherapy. J Consult Clin Psychol 1994;62(5):1009–16.

REM Sleep Behavior Disorder

Eric Frenette, MD, FRCP(C)

KEYWORDS

- REM sleep behavior disorder • α-Synucleinopathy
- Parkinson disease • Dementia of the Lewy body
- Multiple system atrophy • REM sleep without atonia

HISTORICAL PERSPECTIVE

Jouvet and Delorme,[1] in the 1960s, described persistent motor behavior during rapid eye movement (REM) sleep in cats with bilateral mediodorsal pontine tegmental lesions. Tachibana and colleagues,[2] in the 1970s, described a condition similar to REM sleep behavior disorder (RBD) in patients abusing alcohol and meprobamate. Quera-Salva and Guilleminault,[3] in 1986, reported on 2 patients with olivopontocerebellar degeneration who had abnormal motor activity during REM sleep. However, it was Schenck and colleagues,[4] in a seminal paper published in the June 1986 issue of the journal *Sleep*, that established RBD as a bona fide sleep disorder and brought attention to this disorder.

DEFINITION

Normal REM sleep is characterized by phasic REMs; decreased or absent muscle tone; desynchronization of the electroencephalogram, with presence of sawtooth waves; and autonomic instability.[5] It alternates with non-REM sleep (NREM) in an ultradian pattern, with cycles lasting about 90 minutes until waking up. REM sleep becomes more prominent with each subsequent cycle and overall makes up about 20% of the adult total sleep time; it is also the sleep stage in which dreams occur.[5] RBD, as its name suggests, is a parasomnia arising from REM sleep. It is characterized by an active behavior causing sleep disruption and occasional bodily harm to oneself or to a bed partner, in response to dream content.[6] This is rendered possible by a lack of muscle atonia otherwise present in normal REM sleep.

EPIDEMIOLOGY

Using telephone interviews with the validated Sleep-EVAL questionnaire, Ohayon and colleagues[7] screened 2078 men and 2894 women and found a prevalence of 0.5% in this general population (**Table 1**). Chiu and colleagues,[8] collecting data from a sample

Department of Neurology, University of Sherbrooke, 3001 12e Avenue Nord, Sherbrooke, QC, J1H 5N4, Canada
E-mail address: eric.frenette@usherbrooke.ca

Med Clin N Am 94 (2010) 593–614
doi:10.1016/j.mcna.2010.02.010
0025-7125/10/$ – see front matter © 2010 Elsevier Inc. All rights reserved.

Table 1	
Prevalence of RBD in the general population	
A complaint of violence or injurious behavior during sleep and	2.1%
Limb or body movement associated with dream mentation and	0.8%
Harmful or potentially harmful sleep behavior or Dreams appear to be acted out or Sleep behaviors disrupt sleep continuity	0.5%

Data from Ohayon MM, Caulet M, Priest RG. Violent behavior during sleep. J Clin Psychiatry 1997;58(8):369–7.

of more than 1000 elderly people living in Hong Kong, estimated a prevalence of 0.38%. Data from a group of 703 consecutive patients referred to a sleep laboratory yielded a prevalence of 4.8% in this selected population. If not for a comprehensive sleep questionnaire and a video polysomnogram (PSG) recording,[9] more than 80% of patients with RBD would have been ignored. In all studies, men are more likely to be affected than women, comprising 80% to 90% of all cases.[10–14] The age of onset for RBD is in the sixth or seventh decade, the disorder being commonly present for many years before the diagnosis.[10–14] The special features related to RBD in childhood and the form associated with narcolepsy are discussed separately.

CLINICAL FEATURES

The cardinal feature of RBD is physical motion in response to dream content.[6] Dreams are action filled or violent, patients frequently reporting having to defend themselves or responding to attacks from foes. Complex and spectacular behaviors can be witnessed, but conversely, more subtle manifestations are probably missed, as the overt dream enactment can give way to simple limb movements, somniloquy, and other gestures (**Box 1**).[6,10,11,15,16] Walking and leaving the room are rare occurrences.[6,10,11,15,16] Chewing, feeding, drinking, sexual behaviors, urination, or defecation should not be considered part of the RBD spectrum and lead the clinician to other diagnostic possibilities.[6,10,11,15,16] Episodes are also said to be isomorphic, that is, the actions are congruent with the dream content.[10] If awakened shortly after the event, the individual should be able to recollect what he was dreaming about and what he was trying to do.[10,11] The eyes usually remain closed.[10] Episode frequency is somewhat variable, ranging from once a week to sometimes multiple times during the same night.[11] In a population with Parkinson disease (PD), patients with RBD had a higher percentage of violent dreams compared with non-RBD patients.[15] Although dream content seems to be more aggressive in patients with PD and clinical RBD, the presence of violent dreams or clinical RBD is associated neither with daytime aggressiveness in a mixed RBD subset[16] nor with increased testosterone levels in men with RBD and PD.[17] Medical attention is habitually sought because of recurrent aggressive or violent behavior, sometimes in the wake of self or bed partner injury.[10,11]

CLASSIFICATION

RBD has been classified as idiopathic or symptomatic. The latter encompasses all cases associated with an underlying disorder.[18] Numerous conditions associated with RBD have been described (**Box 2**), but by far the most studied and prevalent

Box 1
RBD common symptoms
Talking
Laughing
Shouting
Swearing
Gesturing
Reaching
Grabbing
Flailing
Slapping
Punching
Kicking
Sitting up
Leaping from bed
Crawling
Running
Data from Refs.[6,10,11,15,16]

have been the α-synucleinopathies, which consist primarily of PD, dementia with Lewy body (DLB), and multiple system atrophy (MSA).[18]

IDIOPATHIC RBD

The idiopathic form of the disorder has been questioned by numerous authors.[74,75] In well-characterized cohorts, 50% to 70% of idiopathic RBD (iRBD) subjects eventually evolve toward a clearly established α-synucleinopathy over a 10- to15-year period.[10,11,20,76–79] Investigators have tried to find clues to be able to predict the occurrence of full-blown neurodegenerative diseases.[80] Early features present in patients with α-synucleinopathies have been sought in patients with iRBD. Olfaction, color vision, neurocognitive function, and autonomic function have been studied in iRBD. Correlations with baseline REM electromyographic (EMG) tonic and phasic activity, electroencephalographic (EEG) spectral analysis, and midbrain sonography imaging have also been looked at.

Olfaction

Olfactory impairment is observed in more than 60% of subjects.[81] Inability to identify paint thinner is the most specific anomaly found.[81] Odor identification in a Japanese population yielded the same results in iRBD when compared with PD, confirming the general involvement of the olfactory tract even in the absence of other neurologic signs.[82]

Color Vision

Using the Farnsworth-Munsell 100 Hue test, significant color identification impairment was seen in all 4 color groups (red-yellow, yellow-green, green-blue, blue-red) compared with controls, mimicking results already found in PD.[83]

Box 2
Causes of symptomatic RBD

1. α-Synucleinopathies
   a. Parkinson disease[10,11,19,20]
   b. Dementia with Lewy bodies[11,21–23]
   c. Multiple system atrophy[11,24,25]
2. Tauopathies
   a. Progressive supranuclear palsy[26–29]
   b. Alzheimer disease[30]
   c. Corticobasal degeneration[27,31]
   d. Guadalupean atypical parkinsonism[32]
3. Genetically determined
   a. Machado-Joseph disease (SCA-3)[33–36]
   b. Parkin gene mutation[37,38]
   c. Huntington disease[39]
   d. DJ-1 mutations and parkinsonism-dementia-amyotrophic lateral sclerosis complex[40]
   e. Möbius syndrome[41]
   f. Type A xeroderma pigmentosum[42]
4. Focal anatomic brainstem lesion
   a. Tumor[43]
   b. Multiple sclerosis[44,45]
   c. Stroke[46,47]
   d. Hemorrhage[48]
5. Nonfocal lesion
   a. Limbic encephalitis[49,50]
   b. Epilepsy[51–54]
   c. Autism[55]
   d. Gilles de la Tourette syndrome[56]
   e. Amyotrophic lateral sclerosis[57]
   f. Guillain-Barré syndrome[1]
   g. Subarachnoid hemorrhage[1]
6. Sleep disorder
   a. Narcolepsy[58–60]
   b. Periodic leg movements[61,62]
   c. Restless legs syndrome[38]
   d. Bruxism[63]
7. Medication induced
   a. Tricyclic antidepressants[64,65]
   b. Selective seronin recapture inhibitors (SSRIs)[66,67]
   c. Serotonin noradrenalin recapture inhibitors[68]

d. Mirtazapine[69]

e. Bisoprolol[70]

8. Substance induced

a. Alcohol[71]

b. Chocolate[72]

c. Caffeine[73]

Neurocognitive Function

Comprehensive neurocognitive testing has been performed in iRBD in the presence of a normal mini-mental status examination. Visuospatial constructional dysfunction and altered visuospatial learning, memory impairment and executive dysfunctions in association with visuoconstructional learning impairment, attention, executive functions, and verbal memory alterations have all been found by different groups of investigators[75,80,84–86] (**Box 3**). Recent data found a prevalence of mild cognitive impairment (MCI) in 50% of patients with iRBD. However, compared with a population with PD and RBD, they did not have visuoconstructional and visuoperceptual abilities impairment.[87]

Autonomic Function

Autonomic nervous system dysfunction is seen early in iRBD. Small controlled series of patients with RBD (both idiopathic and symptomatic) have shown a 74% rate of abnormalities on at least 1 autonomic test (R-R interval variation during deep breathing, Valsalva ratio, blood pressure and heart rate changes on standing) during wakefulness.[88] During sleep, tonic and phasic R-R variability assessment has shown a significantly reduced variability in NREM and REM sleep. There was no difference between the 2 subsets of RBD.[88] Spectral analysis of R-R interval and respiration in patients with iRBD has shown that normally observed NREM-to-REM-sleep variability in breathing rate, cardiac excitatory response, and parasympathetic withdrawal are absent compared with controls.[89] Myocardial iodine 123–labeled metaiodobenzylguanidine (^{123}I-MIBG) scintigraphy has also been used to assess the sympathetic nervous system in iRBD.[90–96] Decreased heart/mediastinum (H/M) ratio indicates weakened capacity of ^{123}I-MIBG uptake to the terminal of postganglionic sympathetic fibers,

---

Box 3
Neurocognitive dysfunction in RBD

Consistent impairment in iRBD

1. Executive functions

2. Verbal learning and memory

3. Visual learning and memory

Inconsistent impairment in iRBD

1. Visual-spatial constructional ability

2. Working memory/attention

3. Verbal fluency

4. Processing speed

Data from Refs.[75,80,84–86]

and increased washout rate (WR) suggests a ^{123}I-MIBG retention failure.[93] Patients with iRBD consistently show decreased HR and increased WR, even at the beginning of the disease, suggesting early autonomic involvement.[93] The magnitude of the changes parallels those encountered in DLB and PD.[93] Patients with MSA and patients with tauopathies did not experience significant changes compared with controls.[93] These disorders lack the presence of Lewy bodies at pathology, even if MSA has α-synuclein inclusions.[97] Follow-up data in 2 patients diagnosed initially with iRBD showed no differences in ^{123}I-MIBG uptake, even as one of them had progressed toward PD.[94] Clinical symptoms of erectile dysfunction, orthostatism, and constipation are also more common in iRBD.[83]

Motor Control

Unified Parkinson Disease Rating Scale (UPDRS) part 2 and 3 results revealed that subtle motor manifestations are common in patients with iRBD compared with controls, patients with possible PD were carefully excluded from that study.[83]

Electromyogram

Two recent studies looked at the progression of EMG activity with time in patients with iRBD. The first one confirmed that tonic and phasic EMG activities increase during a 5-year interval in a study of 11 patients, suggesting a progression of the disease even as the patients remain free of α-synucleinopathies.[98] Postuma and colleagues[99] looked at it from another angle, as they analyzed initial PSG data of patients with symptomatic RBD when they were diagnosed as iRBD and compared it with controls and patients who remained with iRBD. They found that the baseline tonic, but not the phasic, EMG activity in patients who developed symptomatic RBD was significantly higher than the ones who remained with iRBD. This was true only for iRBD patients who developed PD compared to the ones who acquired DLB.

Electroencephalogram

Initial work by the Montreal group has shown significant quantitative EEG slowing in different frequencies in wakefulness and in REM sleep in patients with iRBD compared with controls.[100] Moreover, another study by the same group confirmed an increase of slow wave sleep and of delta power during NREM sleep in patients with iRBD compared with control subjects.[101] Hypothesizing that this increase might represent an early sign of central nervous system dysfunction, further studies comparing spectral EEG analysis with cognitive testing have been pursued, showing a co-occurrence of impaired cognitive profile and waking EEG slowing in patients with iRBD, similar to that observed in early stages of some synucleinopathies.[84]

Midbrain Sonography

An increased prevalence of midbrain hyperechogenicity on transcranial sonography is found in patients with iRBD,[102] which is also present in PD, supporting the potential role of hyperechogenicity as a risk marker for PD in that population.[103] This is supported by the absence of substantia nigra (SN) hyperechogenicity in narcoleptic patients with RBD,[86] indicating that SN hyperechogenicity in patients with presumed iRBD is not an RBD-immanent finding.[102,103]

SYMPTOMATIC RBD

As a group and in relation to RBD, α-synucleinopathies comprise PD, DLB, and MSA.[104] This trio displays extrapyramidal symptoms and signs (PD), associated with prominent cognitive alterations (DLB) or autonomic and/or cerebellar manifesta-tions (MSA). Idiopathic RBD can be the presenting feature of any of these entities, and some of them are almost invariably associated with RBD.

Parkinson Disease

PD is the prototypical α-synucleinopathy. Its association with RBD has been recog-nized since Schenck and Mahowald's[76] report in 1996, which commented on the appearance of PD after the onset of RBD in 11 male patients. Point prevalence of RBD in PD is reported to be between 14.6% and 33%.[19,105] In one study, counting REM sleep without atonia (RSWA), this number increased to 58%.[19] The clinical mani-festations of PD differ depending on the presence or absence of RBD. Patients with PD who have RBD tend to have akinetic-rigid disease, an increased frequency of falls, and less clinical response to medication.[106] If tremor-dominant PD is present, RBD will occur after diagnosis of PD and not precede it.[107] RBD in PD is also associated with nonmotor symptoms, particularly orthostatic hypotension.[108] EEG slowing was found in patients with RBD-PD but not in PD patients without RBD, suggesting that RBD might be a marker of cognitive dysfunction in PD patients.[109] The same group later confirmed that hypothesis by demonstrating that patients with PD and concomitant RBD performed significantly worse on standardized tests measuring episodic verbal memory, executive functions, as well as visuospatial and visuoperceptual processing compared with patients with PD without RBD and control subjects.[110] Patients with PD alone had no detectable cognitive impairment compared with controls.[110] The presence of RBD in PD is associated with an increased risk of manifesting hallucina-tions and delusions.[111] Patients with PD presenting RBD but not hallucinations were found to show impairment of some logical abilities, suggesting frontal dysfunction. Patients with PD without RBD and hallucinations had normal cognitive function.[112] A longitudinal evaluation 2 years after the initial testing revealed that patients with hallucinations presented more severe cognitive impairment, involving not only execu-tive functions but also short- and long-term memory and nonverbal logical abilities.[113] The presence of RBD increased the probability of cognitive decline and presence of hallucinations, especially in older patients with greater impairment of motor and exec-utive functions.[112] Finally, recent data suggest that MCI is present in 73% of patients with PD with RBD compared with 11% in patients with PD without RBD, making RBD an important determinant of cognitive impairment in PD.[87]

Multiple System Atrophy

MSA, formerly known through its 3 subtypes[97] (olivopontocerebellar atrophy, Shy-Drager syndrome, striatonigral degeneration), was already associated with RBD in the original publication of Schenck and colleagues.[4] In an unselected series of 39 consecutive patients with MSA, RBD was a prominent feature in 69% of them. RBD preceded MSA in nearly half the subjects.[25] Counting RSWA, 90% of patients with MSA had abnormal muscle tone in REM sleep.[25] Sleep talk (somniloquy) seems to be an early feature of RBD associated with MSA.[114] Women are more affected in this condition than in other synucleinopathies, although male prevalence is still predominant.[25]

Dementia of the Lewy Body Type

The link between RBD and DLB was first recognized in 1995 by Uchiyama and colleagues.[21] In 1998, Boeve and colleagues[23] reported on a series of 37 patients with dementia presenting symptoms of RBD. In that series, more than 90% fulfilled the criteria for probable DLB, and RBD occurred first in all but 2 patients.[23] To date, all patients with dementia who have been autopsied have Lewy bodies, including those believed to have Alzheimer disease (AD).[115,116] Differences have been found between the RBD/dementia group and AD group.[117] The RBD/dementia group performed significantly worse on attention, perceptual organization, visual memory, and letter fluency than the AD group, who performed significantly worse on confrontation naming and verbal memory.[117] Because most of the patients in this RBD/dementia subset also met criteria for possible or probable DLB, dementia associated with RBD may represent DLB.[117]

RDB ASSOCIATED WITH OTHER SLEEP DISORDERS
Narcolepsy

RBD was initially reported in association with narcolepsy by Schenck and Mahowald[58] in 1992. Prevalence ranging from 7% to 36% has been reported, with a significant number having RSWA (50%) without the abnormal behavior.[58–60] RBD as a presenting feature of narcolepsy has been reported in children and in adults.[118,119] Narcolepsy is also associated with olfactory dysfunction, independently of the presence of RBD.[120] It is unlikely to be a predictor for developing a neurodegenerative disorder because narcolepsy is viewed as a dysregulation of REM sleep.[58] It is hypothesized that dysfunctions in the hypocretin/dopaminergic system are likely to be the most important mechanisms involved in the pathophysiology of RBD in narcolepsy, as the lack of hypocretinergic neurons in the lateral hypothalamus is the hallmark of narcolepsy.[60] Treatment of cataplexy with SSRIs can increase muscle tone in REM sleep; therefore, one has to be careful that RSWA induced by medication is not mistaken for a marker of RBD.[65–67]

Periodic Leg Movements of Sleep

Periodic leg movements of sleep (PLMSs) are common in RBD, occurring in up to 85% of patients.[61,62] They are more prevalent in REM sleep in patients with RBD than in patients without RBD.[61,62] They are associated with fewer arousals and lesser autonomic activation in patients with RBD compared with controls.[61]

Some data suggested that PLMSs were shorter in duration, less often bilateral, and with a higher intermovement interval in patients with RBD compared with patients with restless legs syndrome (RLS).[62]

RLS, Bruxism, and Rhythmic Movement Sleep Disorder

RLS and RBD have been reported in patients presenting a parkin mutation.[38] One case report mentions bruxism as a motor manifestation of RBD.[63] Childhood onset rhythmic movement disorder persisting into adulthood has also been associated with RBD.[121]

RBD IN CHILDREN AND ADOLESCENTS

Stores,[122] in 2008, authored a comprehensive review of this subject. RBD starting in childhood is never idiopathic.[122] It has been associated with brainstem tumors,[123] narcolepsy,[118,124] autism,[55] Tourette syndrome,[56] and juvenile PD.[125]

PATHOPHYSIOLOGY

Clues from case reports[126] and animal models suggest that a final common pathway exists in the generation of motor behavior in RBD.[127] It has been proposed that the sublaterodorsal (SLD) or analogous nucleus projects directly to spinal interneurons, causing active inhibition of muscle activity in REM sleep.[127] An indirect pathway is also hypothesized, which suggests that the SLD neurons project to the magnocellular reticular formation and from there to the spinal interneurons.[127] Lesions of the SLD region decrease activation of the spinal interneurons, through the direct or indirect pathway, the final effect being a lack of muscle tone inhibition.[127] The locomotor generators, which are presumed to project to the spinal motoneurons directly or indirectly via other brainstem nuclei, are yet to be identified and characterized.[117] Increased phasic locomotor drive and/or loss of REM sleep atonia has been suggested as the likely mechanism for the clinical expression of RBD.[127]

NEUROIMAGING

Neuroimaging studies have been numerous.[128] Dorsal mesopontine tegmentum lesions have been demonstrated by magnetic resonance imaging.[129] Decreased blood flow in the pons and superior frontal regions has been documented.[130] Decreased activity in frontal and temporoparietal cortices and increased activity in the pons, putamen, and right hippocampus were seen in single-photon emission computed tomographic (SPECT) study.[131] Increased choline/creatine ratio in the brainstem, suggesting local neural dysfunction, was shown by proton magnetic resonance spectroscopy in one study but not in another.[132,133] Using SPECT, the binding of ligands of striatal presynaptic dopamine transporters in patients with RBD during wakefulness was found to be lower than in normal controls but higher than in patients with PD.[134,135] This finding provides evidence for a continuum of striatal presynaptic dopaminergic dysfunction in patients with RSWA, clinical RBD, and PD, as the number of presynaptic dopamine transporters decreases in patients with PD and RBD.[135] No differences were found for a marker of postsynaptic D_2 receptor density in patients with RDB.[134] Significant reductions in striatal ^{11}C-dihydrotetrabenazine (^{11}C-DTBZ, a marker for dopamine nerve terminals) binding were found in all striatal nuclei, suggesting a loss of dopamine midbrain neurons in chronic RBD.[135] A recent SPECT study using a radiomarker of the presynaptic dopamine transporter showed that patients with iRBD had degeneration of presynaptic nigrostriatal neurons, as determined by reduced dopamine transporter binding. It was assumed that this finding is related to the long duration of RBD symptoms.[136] Neuroimaging studies have thus revealed that RDB can affect several levels of cerebral organization, from neurotransmission (presynaptic striatal dopamine) to neuroanatomic integrity (lesions in mesopontine tegmentum) and brain function (frontal, temporoparietal, and cingulate cortex dysfunctions). It is still unclear whether these cerebral anomalies play a causal role in the pathophysiology of RBD or mainly reflect pharmacologic consequences or adaptations to the pathologic condition.[128]

LABORATORY FINDINGS

Besides PSG data, which is discussed in detail later, and the findings associated with symptomatic RBD, no reliable blood test has emerged to help diagnose RBD. HLA typing has not yielded reproducible results,[137,138] and the search for serum antilocus ceruleus antibodies has been inconclusive.[139]

DIAGNOSIS

Diagnosis is essentially made with the history and examination and confirmed by PSG. Some have devised questionnaires to help sort the different symptoms,[140] but the key elements are the precise description of events by a reliable eyewitness and the corroboration of the dream content by the patient. The International Classification of Sleep

Disorders second edition has come forth with revised diagnostic criteria to ensure the proper identification of RBD, rendering video-PSG confirmation mandatory (**Box 4**).[6]

An abnormal PSG is thus necessary to fulfill criteria 1. The American Academy of Sleep Medicine (AASM) issued a set of scoring rules for PSG in 2007.[141] One of these rules was specifically introduced for RBD and EMG scoring (**Box 5, Fig. 1**).

These criteria stem directly from the pioneering work of Lapierre and Montplaisir[142] at the beginning of the 1990s. The investigators scored 20-second epochs for tonic chin EMG in REM sleep. Increased tone had to be present for more than 50% of the epoch to be considered abnormal. They also allowed for scoring 2-second mini-epochs within REM epochs for phasic EMG burst and REM phasic density. The bursts had to last for more than 0.1 seconds but less than 5 seconds, and their amplitude had to be at least 4 times that of the background EMG.[142] These criteria were later adapted to the 30-second epoch.[143] Although many investigators tried to refine the EMG analysis,[144-147] some of the more interesting work came from the Sleep Innsbruck Barcelona (SINBAR) group who studied activity in different muscles and devised that the best yield for EMG electrode placement would be a combination of submentalis, flexor digitorum superficialis, and extensor digitorum brevis,[148] differing from the usual PSG montage, which includes EMG recording of the submentalis and tibialis anterior muscles.[141] Most investigators agree on a 20% cutoff for RSWA, meaning that more than 20% of REM epochs have to be spent with elevated muscle tone and/or muscle phasic activity.[142-148] The AASM adopted the more conservative 50% criteria.[141] The search for a secondary cause is also important (see **Box 2**), especially looking for precipitating events (medication, alcohol), symptoms and signs of α-synucleinopathies (PD, DLB, MSA), and evidence for a concurrent sleep disorder (narcolepsy, PLMs). If acute onset of RBD occurs, search for a structural brainstem lesion is warranted.

DIFFERENTIAL DIAGNOSIS

Sometimes a clear account of the situation is not possible (**Box 6**). The patient might be living alone, the depiction of the behavior not satisfying, and so forth. Other conditions are to be considered. RBD-like symptoms have been reported in patients with severe obstructive sleep apnea, with relief occurring with positive pressure treatment.[149] Epileptic seizures, especially the one originating from the frontal lobe, can give rise to

---

Box 4
Diagnostic criteria

1. Presence of RSWA: the EMG finding of excessive elevation of submental EMG tone or excessive phasic submental or (upper or lower) limb EMG twitching.

2. At least one of the following is present:

   Sleep-related injurious, potentially injurious, or disruptive behaviors by history.

   Abnormal REM sleep behaviors documented during PSG monitoring.

3. Absence of EEG epileptiform activity during REM sleep unless RBD is clearly distinguished from any concurrent REM sleep–related seizure disorder.

4. The sleep disturbance is not better explained by another sleep disorder, medical or neurologic disorder, mental disorder, medication use, or substance use disorder.

Data from American Sleep Disorders Association, Diagnostic Classification Steering Committee. International Classification of Sleep Disorders: Diagnostic and Coding Manual, ICSD-R. Westchester (IL): American Academy of Sleep Medicine; 2005.

Box 5
Criteria for RSWA

PSG in RBD is characterized by either or both of the following features:

1. Sustained muscle activity in REM sleep in the chin EMG

   An epoch of REM sleep with at least 50% of the duration of the epoch having a chin EMG amplitude greater than the minimum amplitude than in NREM

2. Excessive transient muscle activity during REM in the chin of limb EMG

   In a 30-second epoch of REM sleep divided into 10 sequential 3-second miniepochs, at least 5 (50%) of the miniepochs contain bursts of transient muscle activity. In RBD, excessive transient muscle activity bursts are 0.1 to 5.0 seconds in duration and are at least 4 times higher in amplitude as the background EMG activity

Data from Consens FB, Chervin RD, Koeppe RA, et al. Validation of a polysomnographic score for REM sleep behavior disorder. Sleep 2005;28(8):993–7.

---

bizarre behavioral features.[150] The Frontal Lobe Epilepsy Parasomnia scale has been created as a tool to help distinguish parasomnias from epileptic manifestations.[151] NREM sleep parasomnias (sleepwalking) also need to be carefully excluded.[6] However, REM and NREM sleep parasomnias can coexist in the same individual in overlap syndrome.[152,153] RBD, sleep terrors, and sleepwalking are encountered. Onset is in the second decade, and treatment is usually achieved with clonazepam.[152]

TREATMENT
General

Before drug treatment, general measures need to be established to ensure the safety of patients with RBD and the patient's bed partner. In a well-documented series,

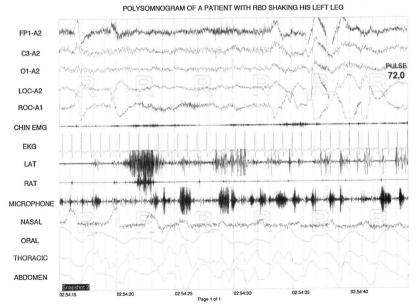

Fig. 1. Example of PSG in a patient with RBD.

Box 6
RBD differential diagnosis

Obstructive sleep apnea

NREM sleep parasomnia

Parasomnia overlap syndrome

Nocturnal frontal lobe epilepsy

Data from Refs.[149–153]

injuries related to an episode have been reported in 32% of RBD, including a subdural hematoma.[11] In the same series, 64% of bed partners have reported being assaulted, causing injuries to 16% of them.[11] Removing furniture from the bedroom, putting a mattress on the floor to prevent falls from bed, sleeping in separate bedrooms, have all been advocated to promote a safe sleeping environment.[11]

Medical

Since the first standardized description of RBD, clonazepam has consistently been the preferred treatment option.[4] In 2 large series, complete or partial benefit was achieved in nearly 90% of patients.[10,11] A dose of 0.5 to 2 mg is usually effective.[10,11] The mode of action seems to be related to its ability to suppress phasic REM activity.[65] One has to be aware that usage of clonazepam can exacerbate obstructive sleep apnea, warranting PSG evaluation before starting the medication.[154] A recent series has issued concerns about potentially limiting side effects, because more than 50% of their patient base had side effects related to clonazepam, including excessive daytime sedation, confusion, and cognitive changes.[155] In that study, zopiclone at a dosage of 3.75 to 7.5 mg nightly was effective as an alternative to clonazepam.[155] A few controlled studies of melatonin at doses ranging from 3 to 12 mg have revealed success rates ranging from 40% to 100%.[156–160] Melatonin is believed to act by decreasing tonic REM.[65] Levodopa preparations have also been used in patients

Box 7
Forensic considerations

1. There should be reason, by history and/or formal PSG evaluation, to suspect RBD.

2. The duration of the action is usually brief (seconds to minutes).

3. The behavior is usually confined to the bed or to the bedroom.

4. The behavior is usually abrupt, immediate, impulsive, and without apparent reason.

5. The victim is someone who merely happened to be present.

6. Immediately on awakening, there is perplexity or horror, without attempt to escape, conceal, cover-up, or rationalize the action.

7. There is amnesia for the event (but not the dream).

8. PSG evaluation reveals RSWA as a persistent abnormality.

Data from Schenck CH, Lee SA, Bornemann MA, et al. Potentially lethal behaviors associated with rapid eye movement sleep behavior disorder: review of the literature and forensic implications. J Forensic Sci 2009;54(6):1475–84.

with RBD preceding PD[161] and in association with DLB.[162] Pramipexole has been the subject of mixed reviews.[163–165] Donepezil at doses up to 15 mg provided partial relief.[166] Anecdotal evidence of benefit from carbamazepine[167]; yi-gan san, a Chinese herbal remedy that is believed to be a serotonin modulator[168]; sodium oxybate[169]; and even paroxetin[170] has also been reported.

SPECIAL CONSIDERATION

Because of the violent nature of the behavior encountered in the dream enactment of RBD, potentially lethal or severe injuries to the individual or others present can lead to misinterpretation on the nature of their occurrence by the medical team. One has to be aware of the forensic implications of such events when reporting them, thus avoiding to label them as homicidal or suicidal behavior.[171] A brief summary of elements to look for is put forward in **Box 7**.

SUMMARY

RBD is an REM sleep parasomnia occurring in older men. Its cardinal manifestation is dream enactment leading to active or aggressive behavior. Diagnosis is made through careful history and characteristic polysomnographic findings (lack of REM sleep atonia). It is commonly associated with neurodegenerative disorders, particularly α-synucleinopathies. Clonazepam is the treatment of choice and is effective in most patients.

REFERENCES

1. Jouvet M, Delorme F. Locus coeruleus et sommeil paradoxal. CR Soc Biol 1965; 159:895–9.
2. Tachibana M, Tanaka K, Hishikawa Y, et al. A sleep study of acute psychotic states due to alcohol and meprobamate addiction. Adv Sleep Res 1976; 2:177–205.
3. Salva MA, Guilleminault C. Olivopontocerebellar degeneration, abnormal sleep, and REM sleep without atonia. Neurology 1986;36(4):576–7.
4. Schenck CH, Bundlie SR, Ettinger MG, et al. Chronic behavioral disorders of human REM sleep: a new category of parasomnia. Sleep 1986;9(2):293–308.
5. Carskadon MA, Dement WC. Normal human sleep: an overview. In: Kryger MH, Roth T, Dement WC, editors. Principles and practice of sleep medicine. 4th edition. Philadelphia: Saunders; 2005. p. 13–23.
6. American Sleep Disorders Association. Diagnostic Classification Steering Committee. International Classification of Sleep Disorders: Diagnostic and Coding Manual, ICSD-R. Westchester (IL): American Academy of Sleep Medicine; 2005.
7. Ohayon MM, Caulet M, Priest RG. Violent behavior during sleep. J Clin Psychiatry 1997;58(8):369–76.
8. Chiu HF, Wing YK, Chung DW, et al. REM sleep behaviour disorder in the elderly. Int J Geriatr Psychiatry 1997;12(9):888–91.
9. Frauscher B, Gschliesser V, Brandauer E, et al. REM sleep behavior disorder in 703 sleep-disorder patients: the importance of eliciting a comprehensive sleep history. Sleep Med 2010;11(2):167–71.
10. Schenck CH, Hurwitz TD, Mahowald MW. Symposium: Normal and abnormal REM sleep regulation: REM sleep behaviour disorder: an update on a series

of 96 patients and a review of the world literature. J Sleep Res 1993;2(4): 224–31.

11. Olson EJ, Boeve BF, Silber MH. Rapid eye movement sleep behaviour disorder: demographic, clinical and laboratory findings in 93 cases. Brain 2000;123(Pt 2): 331–9.

12. Iranzo A, Santamaría J, Rye DB, et al. Characteristics of idiopathic REM sleep behavior disorder and that associated with MSA and PD. Neurology 2005; 65(2):247–52.

13. Wing YK, Lam SP, Li SX, et al. REM sleep behaviour disorder in Hong Kong Chinese: clinical outcome and gender comparison. J Neurol Neurosurg Psychiatr 2008;79(12):1415–6.

14. Postuma RB, Gagnon JF, Vendette M, et al. Quantifying the risk of neurodegenerative disease in idiopathic REM sleep behavior disorder. Neurology 2009; 72(15):1296–300.

15. Borek LL, Kohn R, Friedman JH. Phenomenology of dreams in Parkinson's disease. Mov Disord 2007;22(2):198–202.

16. Fantini ML, Corona A, Clerici S, et al. Aggressive dream content without daytime aggressiveness in REM sleep behaviour disorder. Neurology 2005;65(7):1010–5.

17. Chou KL, Moro-De-Casillas ML, Amick MM, et al. Testosterone not associated with violent dreams or REM sleep behavior disorder in men with Parkinson's. Mov Disord 2007;22(3):411–4.

18. Mahowald MW, Schenck CH. REM sleep parasomnias. In: Kryger MH, Roth T, Dement WC, editors. Principles and practice of sleep medicine. 4th edition. Philadelphia: Saunders; 2005. p. 897–916.

19. Gagnon JF, Bédard MA, Fantini ML, et al. REM sleep behavior disorder and REM sleep without atonia in Parkinson's disease. Neurology 2002;59(4):585–9.

20. Schenck CH, Bundlie SR, Mahowald MW. Delayed emergence of a parkinsonian disorder in 38% of 29 older men initially diagnosed with idiopathic rapid eye movement sleep behaviour disorder. Neurology 1996;46(2):388–93.

21. Uchiyama M, Isse K, Tanaka K, et al. Incidental Lewy body disease in a patient with REM sleep behavior disorder. Neurology 1995;45(4):709–12.

22. Turner RS, Chervin RD, Frey KA, et al. Probable diffuse Lewy body disease presenting as REM sleep behavior disorder. Neurology 1997;49(2):523–7.

23. Boeve BF, Silber MH, Ferman TJ, et al. REM sleep behavior disorder and degenerative dementia: an association likely reflecting Lewy body disease. Neurology 1998;51(2):363–70.

24. Tison F, Wenning GK, Quinn NP, et al. REM sleep behaviour disorder as the presenting symptom of multiple system atrophy. J Neurol Neurosurg Psychiatr 1995;58(3):379–80.

25. Plazzi G, Corsini R, Provini F, et al. REM sleep behavior disorders in multiple system atrophy. Neurology 1997;48(4):1094–7.

26. Arnulf I, Merino-Andreu M, Bloch F, et al. REM sleep behavior disorder and REM sleep without atonia in patients with progressive supranuclear palsy. Sleep 2005;28(3):349–54.

27. Cooper AD, Josephs KA. Photophobia, visual hallucinations, and REM sleep behavior disorder in progressive supranuclear palsy and corticobasal degeneration: a prospective study. Parkinsonism Relat Disord 2009;15(1): 59–61.

28. Sixel-Döring F, Schweitzer M, Mollenhauer B. et al. Polysomnographic findings, video-based sleep analysis and sleep perception in progressive supranuclear palsy. Sleep Med 2009;10(4):407–15.

29. Compta Y, Martí MJ, Rey MJ, et al. Parkinsonism, dysautonomia, REM behaviour disorder and visual hallucinations mimicking synucleinopathy in a patient with progressive supranuclear palsy. J Neurol Neurosurg Psychiatr 2009;80(5):578–9.

30. Gagnon JF, Petit D, Fantini ML, et al. REM sleep behavior disorder and REM sleep without atonia in probable Alzheimer disease. Sleep 2006;29(10):1321–5.

31. Kimura K, Tachibana N, Aso T, et al. Subclinical REM sleep behavior disorder in a patient with corticobasal degeneration. Sleep 1997;20(10):891–4.

32. De Cock VC, Lannuzel A, Verhaeghe S, et al. REM sleep behavior disorder in patients with guadeloupean parkinsonism, a tauopathy. Sleep 2007;30(8): 1026–32.

33. Fukutake T, Shinotoh H, Nishino H, et al. Homozygous Machado-Joseph disease presenting as REM sleep behaviour disorder and prominent psychiatric symptoms. Eur J Neurol 2002;9(1):97–100.

34. Friedman JH. Presumed rapid eye movement behavior disorder in Machado-Joseph disease (spinocerebellar ataxia type 3). Mov Disord 2002;17(6):1350–3.

35. Syed BH, Rye DB, Singh G. REM sleep behavior disorder and SCA-3 (Machado-Joseph disease). Neurology 2003;60(1):148.

36. Friedman JH, Fernandez HH, Sudarsky LR. REM behavior disorder and excessive daytime somnolence in Machado-Joseph disease (SCA-3). Mov Disord 2003;18(12):1520–2.

37. Kumru H, Santamaria J, Tolosa E, et al. Rapid eye movement sleep behavior disorder in parkinsonism with parkin mutations. Ann Neurol 2004;56(4):599–603.

38. Limousin N, Konofal E, Karroum E, et al. Restless legs syndrome, rapid eye movement sleep behavior disorder, and hypersomnia in patients with two parkin mutations. Mov Disord 2009;24(13):1970–6.

39. Arnulf I, Nielsen J, Lohmann E, et al. Rapid eye movement sleep disturbances in Huntington disease. Arch Neurol 2008;65(4):482–8.

40. Lo Coco D, Caruso G, Mattaliano A. REM sleep behavior disorder in patients with DJ-1 mutations and parkinsonism-dementia-ALS complex. Mov Disord 2009;24(10):1555–6.

41. Anderson K, Shneerson J, Smith I. Möbius syndrome in association with the REM sleep behaviour disorder. J Neurol Neurosurg Psychiatr 2007;78(6): 659–60.

42. Kohyama J, Shimohira M, Kondo S, et al. Motor disturbance during REM sleep in group A xeroderma pigmentosum. Acta Neurol Scand 1995;92:91–5.

43. Zambelis T, Paparrigopoulos T, Soldatos CR. REM sleep behaviour disorder associated with a neurinoma of the left pontocerebellar angle. J Neurol Neurosurg Psychiatr 2002;72(6):821–2.

44. Plazzi G, Montagna P. Remitting REM sleep behavior disorder as the initial sign of multiple sclerosis. Sleep Med 2002;3(5):437–9.

45. Tippmann-Peikert M, Boeve BF, Keegan BM. REM sleep behavior disorder initiated by acute brainstem multiple sclerosis. Neurology 2006;66(8):1277–9.

46. Kimura K, Tachibana N, Kohyama J, et al. A discrete pontine ischemic lesion could cause REM sleep behavior disorder. Neurology 2000;55(6):894–5.

47. Xi Z, Luning W. REM sleep behavior disorder in a patient with pontine stroke. Sleep Med 2009;10(1):143–6.

48. Iranzo A, Aparicio J. A lesson from anatomy: focal brain lesions causing REM sleep behavior disorder. Sleep Med 2009;10(1):9–12.

49. Iranzo A, Graus F, Clover L, et al. Rapid eye movement sleep behavior disorder and potassium channel antibody-associated limbic encephalitis. Ann Neurol 2006;59(1):178–81.

50. Lin FC, Liu CK, Hsu CY. Rapid-eye-movement sleep behavior disorder secondary to acute aseptic limbic encephalitis. J Neurol 2009;256(7):1174–6.
51. Manni R, Terzaghi M. REM behavior disorder associated with epileptic seizures. Neurology 2005;64(5):883–4.
52. Manni R, Terzaghi M, Zambrelli E, et al. Interictal, potentially misleading, epileptiform EEG abnormalities in REM sleep behavior disorder. Sleep 2006;29(7):934–7.
53. Manni R, Terzaghi M, Zambrelli E. REM sleep behavior disorder and epileptic phenomena: clinical aspects of the comorbidity. Epilepsia 2006;47(Suppl 5): 78–81.
54. Manni R, Terzaghi M, Zambrelli E. REM sleep behaviour disorder in elderly subjects with epilepsy: frequency and clinical aspects of the comorbidity. Epilepsy Res 2007;77(2-3):128–33.
55. Thirumalai SS, Shubin RA, Robinson R. Rapid eye movement sleep behavior disorder in children with autism. J Child Neurol 2002;17(3):173–8.
56. Trajanovic NN, Voloh I, Shapiro CM, et al. REM sleep behaviour disorder in a child with Tourette's syndrome. Can J Neurol Sci 2004;31(4):572–5.
57. Minz M, Autret A, Laffont F, et al. A study on sleep in amyotrophic lateral sclerosis. Biomedicine 1979;30:40–6.
58. Schenck CH, Mahowald MW. Motor dyscontrol in narcolepsy: rapid-eye-movement (REM) sleep without atonia and REM sleep behavior disorder. Ann Neurol 1992;32(1):3–10.
59. Nightingale S, Orgill JC, Ebrahim IO, et al. The association between narcolepsy and REM behavior disorder (RBD). Sleep Med 2005;6(3):253–8.
60. Dauvilliers Y, Rompré S, Gagnon JF, et al. REM sleep characteristics in narcolepsy and REM sleep behavior disorder. Sleep 2007;30(7):844–9.
61. Fantini ML, Michaud M, Gosselin N, et al. Periodic leg movements in REM sleep behavior disorder and related autonomic and EEG activation. Neurology 2002; 59(12):1889–94.
62. Manconi M, Ferri R, Zucconi M, et al. Time structure analysis of leg movements during sleep in REM sleep behavior disorder. Sleep 2007;30(12):1779–85.
63. Tachibana N, Yamanaka K, Kaji R, et al. Sleep bruxism as a manifestation of subclinical rapid eye movement sleep behavior disorder. Sleep 1994;17(6): 555–8.
64. Attarian HP, Schenck CH, Mahowald MW. Presumed REM sleep behavior disorder arising from cataplexy and wakeful dreaming. Sleep Med 2000;1: 131–3.
65. Gagnon JF, Postuma RB, Montplaisir J. Update on the pharmacology of REM sleep behavior disorder. Neurology 2006;67(5):742–7.
66. Schenck CH, Mahowald MW, Kim SW, et al. Prominent eye movements during NREM sleep and REM sleep behavior disorder associated with fluoxetine treatment of depression and obsessive-compulsive disorder. Sleep 1992;15:226–35.
67. Winkelman JW, James L. Serotonergic antidepressants are associated with REM sleep without atonia. Sleep 2004;27:317–21.
68. Schutte S, Doghramji K. REM behavior disorder seen with venlafaxine (Effexor). Sleep Res 1996;25:364.
69. Onofrj M, Luciano AL, Thomas A, et al. Mirtazapine induces REM sleep behavior disorder (RBD) in parkinsonism. Neurology 2003;60:113–5.
70. Iranzo A, Santamaria J. Bisoprolol-induced rapid eye movement sleep behavior disorder. Am J Med 1999;107(4):390–2.
71. Hishikawa Y, Sugita Y, Teshima Y, et al. Sleep disorders in alcoholic patients with delirium tremens and transient withdrawal hallucinations—reevaluation of the

REM rebound and intrusion theory. In: Karacan I, editor. Psychophysiological aspects of sleep. Park Ridge (NJ): Noyes Medical Publishers; 1981. p. 109–22.

72. Vorona RD, Ware JC. Exacerbation of REM sleep behavior disorder by chocolate ingestion: a case report. Sleep Med 2002;3(4):365–7.

73. Stolz SE, Aldrich MS. REM sleep behavior disorder associated with caffeine abuse. Sleep Res 1991;20:341.

74. Mahowald MW. Does "idiopathic" REM sleep behavior disorder exist? Sleep 2006;29(7):874–5.

75. Uchiyama M, Isse K, Tanaka K, et al. Neuropsychological assessment in idiopathic REM sleep behavior disorder (RBD): does the idiopathic form of RBD really exist? Neurology 2004;62(1):41–5.

76. Schenck CH, Mahowald MW. REM sleep behavior disorder: clinical, developmental, and neuroscience perspectives 16 years after its formal identification in SLEEP. Sleep 2002;25(2):120–38.

77. Britton TC, Chaudhuri KR. REM sleep behavior disorder and the risk of developing Parkinson disease or dementia. Neurology 2009;72(15):1294–5.

78. Postuma RB, Gagnon JF, Vendette M, et al. Quantifying the risk of neurodegenerative disease in idiopathic REM sleep behavior disorder. Neurology 2009; 72(15):1296–300.

79. Postuma RB, Gagnon JF, Vendette M, et al. Idiopathic REM sleep behavior disorder in the transition to degenerative disease. Mov Disord 2009;24(15): 2225–32.

80. Fantini ML, Ferini-Strambi L, Montplaisir J. Idiopathic REM sleep behavior disorder: toward a better nosologic definition. Neurology 2005;64(5):780–6.

81. Fantini ML, Postuma RB, Montplaisir J, et al. Olfactory deficit in idiopathic rapid eye movements sleep behavior disorder. Brain Res Bull 2006;70(4–6):386–90.

82. Miyamoto T, Miyamoto M, Iwanami M, et al. Odor identification test as an indicator of idiopathic REM sleep behavior disorder. Mov Disord 2009; 24(2):268–73.

83. Postuma RB, Lang AE, Massicotte-Marquez J, et al. Potential early markers of Parkinson disease in idiopathic REM sleep behaviour disorder. Neurology 2006;66(6):845–51.

84. Massicotte-Marquez J, Décary A, Gagnon JF, et al. Executive dysfunction and memory impairment in idiopathic REM sleep behaviour disorder. Neurology 2008;70(15):1250–7.

85. Postuma RB, Gagnon JF, Montplaisir J. Cognition in REM sleep behavior disorder—A window into preclinical dementia? Sleep Med 2008;9(4):341–2.

86. Terzaghi M, Sinforiani E, Zucchella C, et al. Cognitive performance in REM sleep behaviour disorder: a possible early marker of neurodegenerative disease? Sleep Med 2008;9(4):343–51.

87. Gagnon JF, Vendette M, Postuma RB, et al. Mild cognitive impairment in rapid eye movement sleep behavior disorder and Parkinson's disease. Ann Neurol 2009;66(1):39–47.

88. Ferini-Strambi L, Oldani A, Zucconi M, et al. Cardiac autonomic activity during wakefulness and sleep in REM sleep behaviour disorder. Sleep 1996;19(5):367–9.

89. Lanfranchi PA, Fradette L, Gagnon JF, et al. Cardiac autonomic regulation during sleep in idiopathic REM sleep behaviour disorder. Sleep 2007;30(8): 1019–25.

90. Miyamoto T, Miyamoto M, Inoue Y, et al. Reduced cardiac 123I-MIBG scintigraphy in idiopathic REM sleep behavior disorder. Neurology 2006;67(12): 2236–8.

91. Kashihara K, Imamura T. Reduced myocardial 123I-MIBG uptake in a patient with idiopathic rapid eye movement sleep behavior disorder. Mov Disord 2007;22(1):150–1.

92. Koyama S, Tachibana N, Masaoka Y, et al. Decreased myocardial (123)I-MIBG uptake and impaired facial expression recognition in a patient with REM sleep behavior disorder. Mov Disord 2007;22(5):746–7.

93. Miyamoto T, Miyamoto M, Suzuki K, et al. 123I-MIBG cardiac scintigraphy provides clues to the underlying neurodegenerative disorder in idiopathic REM sleep behavior disorder. Sleep 2008;31(5):717–23.

94. Oguri T, Tachibana N, Mitake S, et al. Decrease in myocardial 123I-MIBG radio-activity in REM sleep behavior disorder: two patients with different clinical progression. Sleep Med 2008;9(5):583–5.

95. Miyamoto T, Miyamoto M, Suzuki K, et al. Comparison of severity of obstructive sleep apnea and degree of accumulation of cardiac 123I-MIBG radioactivity as a diagnostic marker for idiopathic REM sleep behavior disorder. Sleep Med 2009;10(5):577–80.

96. Miyamoto T, Miyamoto M, Iwanami M, et al. Three-year follow-up on the accumulation of cardiac (123)I-MIBG scintigraphy in idiopathic REM sleep behavior disorder. Sleep Med 2009;10(9):1066–7.

97. Stefanova N, Bücke P, Duerr S, et al. Multiple system atrophy: an update. Lancet Neurol 2009;8(12):1172–8.

98. Iranzo A, Luca Ratti P, Casanova-Molla J, et al. Excessive muscle activity increases over time in idiopathic REM sleep behavior disorder. Sleep 2009; 32(9):1149–53.

99. Postuma RB, Gagnon JF, Rompré S, et al. Severity of REM atonia loss in idiopathic REM sleep behavior disorder predicts Parkinson disease. Neurology 2010;74(3):239–44.

100. Fantini ML, Gagnon JF, Petit D, et al. Slowing of electroencephalogram in rapid eye movement sleep behavior disorder. Ann Neurol 2003;53(6):774–80.

101. Massicotte-Marquez J, Carrier J, Décary A, et al. Slow-wave sleep and delta power in rapid eye movement sleep behavior disorder. Ann Neurol 2005; 57(2):277–82.

102. Unger MM, Möller JC, Ohletz T, et al. Transcranial midbrain sonography in narcoleptic subjects with and without concomitant REM sleep behaviour disorder. J Neurol 2009;256(6):874–7.

103. Stockner H, Iranzo A, Seppi K, et al. Midbrain hyperechogenicity in idiopathic REM sleep behavior disorder. Mov Disord 2009;24(13):1906–9.

104. Boeve BF, Silber MH, Ferman TJ, et al. Association of REM sleep behavior disorder and neurodegenerative disease may reflect an underlying synucleinopathy. Mov Disord 2001;16(4):622–30.

105. Gjerstad MD, Boeve B, Wentzel-Larsen T, et al. Occurrence and clinical correlates of REM sleep behaviour disorder in patients with Parkinson's disease over time. J Neurol Neurosurg Psychiatr 2008;79(4):387–91.

106. Postuma RB, Gagnon JF, Vendette M, et al. REM sleep behaviour disorder in Parkinson's disease is associated with specific motor features. J Neurol Neurosurg Psychiatr 2008;79(10):1117–21.

107. Kumru H, Santamaria J, Tolosa E, et al. Relation between subtype of Parkinson's disease and REM sleep behavior disorder. Sleep Med 2007;8(7-8):779–83.

108. Postuma RB, Gagnon JF, Vendette M, et al. Manifestations of Parkinson disease differ in association with REM sleep behaviour disorder. Mov Disord 2008; 23(12):1665–72.

109. Gagnon JF, Fantini ML, Bédard MA, et al. Association between waking EEG slowing and REM sleep behavior disorder in PD without dementia. Neurology 2004;62(3):401–6.
110. Vendette M, Gagnon JF, Décary A, et al. REM sleep behavior disorder predicts cognitive impairment in Parkinson disease without dementia. Neurology 2007; 69(19):1843–9.
111. Pacchetti C, Manni R, Zangaglia R, et al. Relationship between hallucinations, delusions, and rapid eye movement sleep behavior disorder in Parkinson's disease. Mov Disord 2005;20(11):1439–48.
112. Sinforiani E, Zangaglia R, Manni R, et al. REM sleep behavior disorder, hallucinations, and cognitive impairment in Parkinson's disease. Mov Disord 2006; 21(4):462–6.
113. Sinforiani E, Pacchetti C, Zangaglia R, et al. REM behavior disorder, hallucinations and cognitive impairment in Parkinson's disease: a two-year follow up. Mov Disord 2008;23(10):1441–5.
114. Tachibana N, Kimura K, Kitajima K, et al. REM sleep motor dysfunction in multiple system atrophy: with special emphasis on sleep talk as its early clinical manifestation. J Neurol Neurosurg Psychiatr 1997;63(5):678–81.
115. Schenck CH, Garcia-Rill E, Skinner RD, et al. A case of REM sleep behavior disorder with autopsy-confirmed Alzheimer's disease: postmortem brain stem histochemical analyses. Biol Psychiatry 1996;40(5):422–5.
116. Schenck CH, Mahowald MW, Anderson ML, et al. Lewy body variant of Alzheimer's disease (AD) identified by postmortem ubiquitin staining in a previously reported case of AD associated with REM sleep behavior disorder. Biol Psychiatry 1997;42(6):527–8.
117. Ferman TJ, Boeve BF, Smith GE, et al. REM sleep behavior disorder and dementia: cognitive differences when compared with AD. Neurology 1999; 52(5):951–7.
118. Nevsimalova S, Prihodova I, Kemlink D, et al. REM behavior disorder (RBD) can be one of the first symptoms of childhood narcolepsy. Sleep Med 2007;8(7-8): 784–6.
119. Bonakis A, Howard RS, Williams A. Narcolepsy presenting as REM sleep behaviour disorder. Clin Neurol Neurosurg 2008;110(5):518–20.
120. Stiasny-Kolster K, Clever SC, Möller JC, et al. Olfactory dysfunction in patients with narcolepsy with and without REM sleep behaviour disorder. Brain 2007; 130(Pt 2):442–9.
121. Xu Z, Anderson KN, Shneerson JM. Association of idiopathic rapid eye movement sleep behavior disorder in an adult with persistent, childhood onset rhythmic movement disorder. J Clin Sleep Med 2009;5(4):374–5.
122. Stores G. Rapid eye movement sleep behaviour disorder in children and adolescents. Dev Med Child Neurol 2008;50(10):728–32.
123. Schenck CH, Bundlie SR, Smith SA, et al. REM behavior disorder in a 10 year old girl and aperiodic REM and NREM sleep movements in an 8 year old brother. Sleep Res 1986;15:162.
124. Turner R, Allen WT. REM sleep behavior disorder associated with narcolepsy in an adolescent: a case report. Sleep Res 1990;19:302.
125. Rye DB, Johnston LH, Watts RL, et al. Juvenile Parkinson's disease with REM sleep behavior disorder, sleepiness, and daytime REM onset. Neurology 1999;53(8):1868–70.
126. Mathis J, Hess CW, Bassetti C. Isolated mediotegmental lesion causing narcolepsy and rapid eye movement sleep behaviour disorder: a case evidencing

a common pathway in narcolepsy and rapid eye movement sleep behaviour disorder. J Neurol Neurosurg Psychiatr 2007;78(4):427–9.

127. Boeve BF, Silber MH, Saper CB, et al. Pathophysiology of REM sleep behaviour disorder and relevance to neurodegenerative disease. Brain 2007;130(Pt 11): 2770–88.

128. Desseilles M, Dang-Vu T, Schabus M, et al. Neuroimaging insights into the pathophysiology of sleep disorders. Sleep 2008;31(6):777–94.

129. Culebras A, Moore JT. Magnetic resonance findings in REM sleep behavior disorder. Neurology 1989;39:1519–23.

130. Shirakawa S, Takeuchi N, Uchimura N, et al. Study of image findings in rapid eye movement sleep behavioural disorder. Psychiatry Clin Neurosci 2002;56:291–2.

131. Mazza S, Soucy JP, Gravel P, et al. Assessing whole brain perfusion changes in patients with REM sleep behavior disorder. Neurology 2006;67:1618–22.

132. Miyamoto M, Miyamoto T, Kubo J, et al. Brainstem function in rapid eye movement sleep behavior disorder: the evaluation of brainstem function by proton MR spectroscopy (1H-MRS). Psychiatry Clin Neurosci 2000;54:350–1.

133. Iranzo A, Santamaria J, Pujol J, et al. Brainstem proton magnetic resonance spectroscopy in idopathic REM sleep behavior disorder. Sleep 2002;25:867–70.

134. Eisensehr I, Linke R, Noachtar S, et al. Reduced striatal dopamine transporters in idiopathic rapid eye movement sleep behaviour disorder. Comparison with Parkinson's disease and controls. Brain 2000;123(Pt 6):1155–60.

135. Eisensehr I, Linke R, Tatsch K, et al. Increased muscle activity during rapid eye movement sleep correlates with decrease of striatal presynaptic dopamine transporters. IPT and IBZM SPECT imaging in subclinical and clinically manifest idiopathic REM sleep behavior disorder, Parkinson's disease, and controls. Sleep 2003;26:507–12.

136. Stiasny-Kolster K, Doerr Y, Moller JC, et al. Combination of 'idiopathic' REM sleep behaviour disorder and olfactory dysfunction as possible indicator for alpha-synucleinopathy demonstrated by dopamine transporter FP-CIT-SPECT. Brain 2005;128:126–37.

137. Schenck CH, Garcia-Rill E, Segall M, et al. HLA class II genes associated with REM sleep behavior disorder. Ann Neurol 1996;39(2):261–3.

138. Onofrj M, Luciano AL, Iacono D, et al. HLA typing does not predict REM sleep behaviour disorder and hallucinations in Parkinson's disease. Mov Disord 2003; 18(3):337–40.

139. Schenck CH, Ullevig CM, Mahowald MW, et al. A controlled study of serum antilocus ceruleus antibodies in REM sleep behavior disorder. Sleep 1997;20(5): 349–51.

140. Stiasny-Kolster K, Mayer G, Schäfer S, et al. The REM sleep behavior disorder screening questionnaire—a new diagnostic instrument. Mov Disord 2007; 22(16):2386–93.

141. American Academy of Sleep Medicine. AASM manual for the scoring of sleep and associated events: rules, terminology and technical specifications 2007. AASM. Westchester (IL): American Academy of Sleep Medicine; 2007.

142. Lapierre O, Montplaisir J. Polysomnographic features of REM sleep behavior disorder: development of a scoring method. Neurology 1992;42(7):1371–4.

143. Consens FB, Chervin RD, Koeppe RA, et al. Validation of a polysomnographic score for REM sleep behavior disorder. Sleep 2005;28(8):993–7.

144. Burns JW, Consens FB, Little RJ, et al. EMG variance during polysomnography as an assessment for REM sleep behaviour disorder. Sleep 2007;30(12): 1771–8.

145. Mayer G, Kesper K, Ploch T, et al. Quantification of tonic and phasic muscle activity in REM sleep behaviour disorder. J Clin Neurophysiol 2008;25(1):48–55.
146. Ferri R, Manconi M, Plazzi G, et al. A quantitative statistical analysis of the submentalis muscle EMG amplitude during sleep in normal controls and patients with REM sleep behavior disorder. J Sleep Res 2008;17(1):89–100.
147. Bliwise DL, Rye DB. Elevated PEM (phasic electromyographic metric) rates identify rapid eye movement behavior disorder patients on nights without behavioral abnormalities. Sleep 2008;31(6):853–7.
148. Frauscher B, Iranzo A, Högl B, et al. Quantification of electromyographic activity during REM sleep in multiple muscles in REM sleep behavior disorder. Sleep 2008;31(5):724–31.
149. Iranzo A, Santamaría J. Severe obstructive sleep apnea/hypopnea mimicking REM sleep behavior disorder. Sleep 2005;28(2):203–6.
150. Manni R, Terzaghi M, Repetto A. The FLEP scale in diagnosing nocturnal frontal lobe epilepsy, NREM and REM parasomnias: data from a tertiary sleep and epilepsy unit. Epilepsia 2008;49(9):1581–5.
151. Derry CP, Davey M, Johns M, et al. Distinguishing sleep disorders from seizures: diagnosing bumps in the night. Arch Neurol 2006;63(5):705–9 [Erratum in: Arch Neurol 2006;63(7):1037].
152. Schenck CH, Boyd JL, Mahowald MW. A parasomnia overlap disorder involving sleepwalking, sleep terrors, and REM sleep behavior disorder in 33 polysomnographically confirmed cases. Sleep 1997;20(11):972–81.
153. Limousin N, Dehais C, Gout O, et al. A brainstem inflammatory lesion causing REM sleep behavior disorder and sleepwalking (parasomnia overlap disorder). Sleep Med 2009;10(9):1059–62.
154. Schuld A, Kraus T, Haack M, et al. Obstructive sleep apnea syndrome induced by clonazepam in a narcoleptic patient with REM-sleep-behavior disorder. J Sleep Res 1999;8(4):321–2.
155. Anderson KN, Shneerson JM. Drug treatment of REM sleep behavior disorder: the use of drug therapies other than clonazepam. J Clin Sleep Med 2009;5(3): 235–9.
156. Kunz D, Bes F. Melatonin effects in a patient with severe REM sleep behavior disorder: case report and theoretical considerations. Neuropsychobiology 1997;36(4):211–4.
157. Kunz D, Bes F. Melatonin as a therapy in REM sleep behavior disorder patients: an open-labeled pilot study on the possible influence of melatonin on REM-sleep regulation. Mov Disord 1999;14(3):507–11.
158. Takeuchi N, Uchimura N, Hashizume Y, et al. Melatonin therapy for REM sleep behavior disorder. Psychiatry Clin Neurosci 2001;55(3):267–9.
159. Boeve BF, Silber MH, Ferman TJ. Melatonin for treatment of REM sleep behavior disorder in neurologic disorders: results in 14 patients. Sleep Med 2003;4(4): 281–4.
160. Anderson KN, Jamieson S, Graham AJ, et al. REM sleep behaviour disorder treated with melatonin in a patient with Alzheimer's disease. Clin Neurol Neurosurg 2008;110(5):492–5.
161. Tan A, Salgado M, Fahn S. Rapid eye movement sleep behavior disorder preceding Parkinson's disease with therapeutic response to levodopa. Mov Disord 1996;11(2):214–6.
162. Yamauchi K, Takehisa M, Tsuno M, et al. Levodopa improved rapid eye movement sleep behavior disorder with diffuse Lewy body disease. Gen Hosp Psychiatry 2003;25(2):140–2.

163. Fantini ML, Gagnon JF, Filipini D, et al. The effects of pramipexole in REM sleep behavior disorder. Neurology 2003;61(10):1418–20.

164. Schmidt MH, Koshal VB, Schmidt HS. Use of pramipexole in REM sleep behavior disorder: results from a case series. Sleep Med 2006;7(5):418–23.

165. Kumru H, Iranzo A, Carrasco E, et al. Lack of effects of pramipexole on REM sleep behavior disorder in Parkinson disease. Sleep 2008;31(10):1418–21.

166. Ringman JM, Simmons JH. Treatment of REM sleep behavior disorder with donepezil: a report of three cases. Neurology 2000;55(6):870–1.

167. Bamford CR. Carbamazepine in REM sleep behavior disorder. Sleep 1993; 16(1):33–4.

168. Shinno H, Kamei M, Nakamura Y, et al. Successful treatment with Yi-Gan San for rapid eye movement sleep behaviour disorder. Prog Neuropsychopharmacol Biol Psychiatry 2008;32(7):1749–51.

169. Shneerson JM. Successful treatment of REM sleep behavior disorder with sodium oxybate. Clin Neuropharmacol 2009;32(3):158–9.

170. Takahashi T, Mitsuya H, Murata T, et al. Opposite effects of SSRIs and tandospirone in the treatment of REM sleep behaviour disorder. Sleep Med 2008;9(3): 317–9.

171. Schenck CH, Lee SA, Bornemann MA, et al. Potentially lethal behaviors associated with rapid eye movement sleep behavior disorder: review of the literature and forensic implications. J Forensic Sci 2009;54(6):1475–84.

Attention-deficit/ Hyperactivity Disorder and Sleep Disorders in Children

Ming-Horng Tsai, MD[a,b,c], Yu-Shu Huang, MD[c,d,e],*

KEYWORDS

- Sleep • Attention-deficit hyperactivity disorder
- Children • Alertness

Attention-deficit/hyperactivity disorder (ADHD) is a neurocognitive and behavior abnormality commonly seen in childhood and adolescence. Symptoms and consequences of ADHD and sleep problems frequently overlap, and their relationship is complex and bidirectional. ADHD-associated disrupted behavior may influence nighttime sleep with symptoms of bedtime struggles, insomnia, poor sleep quality, or insufficient sleep duration. Conversely, primary sleep disorders, such as obstructive sleep apnea (OSA), restless legs syndrome (RLS), and periodic limb movement disorder (PLMD), cause daytime neurobehavioral symptoms that resemble those of ADHD, especially in children.

This article looks at the association between sleep problems and ADHD, focusing on recent studies in children. It provides critical insights about the clinical management of sleep disturbances in ADHD; emphasizes new developments; presents an updated overview of the most relevant studies on the prevalence, causes, pathophysiology, and treatment strategies of sleep problems in children with ADHD; and discusses future research in this field.

[a] Division of Pediatric Hematology/Oncology, Department of Pediatrics, Chang Gung Memorial Hospital, Yunlin, Taiwan
[b] Division of Pediatric Neonatology, Department of Pediatrics, Chang Gung Memorial Hospital, Yunlin, Taiwan
[c] College of Medicine, Chang Gung University, Taoyuan, Taiwan
[d] Department of Child Psychiatry and Sleep Center, Chang Gung Memorial Hospital, Linkou, Taiwan No. 5, Fu-Shing Street, Kwei-Shan, Taoyuan 333, Taiwan
[e] Sleep Center, Chang Gung Memorial Hospital, Taoyuan, Taiwan
* Corresponding author. Department of Child Psychiatry and Sleep Center, Chang Gung Memorial Hospital, Linkou, Taiwan No. 5, Fu-Shing Street, Kwei-Shan, Tapyuan 333.
E-mail address: hu1109s@yahoo.com.tw

Med Clin N Am 94 (2010) 615–632
doi:10.1016/j.mcna.2010.03.008
0025-7125/10/$ – see front matter © 2010 Elsevier Inc. All rights reserved.

medical.theclinics.com

CLINICAL FEATURES AND EPIDEMIOLOGY OF ADHD

ADHD is a common childhood-onset neuropsychiatric disorder, with reported prevalence rates of between 5% and 12% in school-aged children.[1–3] According to the *Diagnostic and Statistical Manual of Mental Disorders* (Fourth Edition) (*DSM-IV*), Text Revision,[4] ADHD is characterized by developmentally inappropriate symptoms of inattention, hyperactivity, and impulsivity that begin before the age of 7 years and causes impairment to age-appropriate academic performance, intellectual functioning, social skills, driving, and occupational functioning in 2 or more settings (eg, at school and at home). Although symptoms of ADHD may lessen with age, it is estimated that 15% to 65% of children with ADHD have symptoms that persist into adulthood.[5,6] The prevalence of ADHD[1] is estimated at approximately 3.8% to 9.4% in prepubertal children (*Diagnostic and Statistical Manual of Mental Disorders* [Third Edition Revised] [*DSM-III-R*]) in Canada (Montreal); 3.4% of prepubertal children (*DSM-III-R*) in Australia; 6.7% of young children and 2% to 3% of teenagers (*DSM-III-R*) in New Zealand; 4.2% of children (*International Classification of Diseases, Ninth Revision*) in Germany; 5% to 29% of children (*Diagnostic and Statistical Manual of Mental Disorders* [Third Edition]) in India; 7.5% of children in Taiwan[7]; 6% to 9% of children (*DSM-III-R*) in China; 1.3% of teenagers (*DSM-III-R*) in the Netherlands; 9.5% of children and teenagers (*DSM-III*) in Puerto Rico; 7.7% of children (*DSM-III-R* ratings) in Japan; 2% to 13% of children (*DSM-IV* ratings) in Colombia; and 5.8% of 12 to 14 year olds (*DSM-IV*) in Brazil. These different incidences may be due to the diagnostic criteria used, cultural differences, and methodological limitations. Moreover, the prevalence of ADHD is higher in boys, with a male-to-female ratio of between 4:1 and 9:1 throughout the world.[4,8,9]

SLEEP PROBLEMS IN CHILDREN WITH ADHD
General Considerations

In recent years, there has been growing interest in sleep problems associated with ADHD. Sleep problems are reported in an estimated 25% to 50% of children and adolescents with ADHD.[10] Some sleep disorders, such as periodic limb movements of sleep (PLMS) and sleep-disordered breathing (SDB), are associated with inattention[11] and hyperactivity,[11,12] which are often mistaken for the symptoms seen in ADHD.[11,12] Symptoms of ADHD and sleep disorders overlap, and ADHD and sleep problems cause neurocognitive and behavioral problems and impaired academic performance.[13,14]

Although many early studies reported that sleep alterations in children with ADHD are due mainly to the effects of ADHD drugs (in particular stimulants),[15,16] available evidence suggests that ADHD drugs are only 1 of the possible causes of sleep disturbances in children with ADHD. Although a recent meta-analysis study concluded that children with ADHD had significantly higher bedtime resistance, more sleep-onset difficulties, nighttime awakenings, difficulties with morning awakenings, SDB, and daytime sleepiness compared with the control patients,[17] another study demonstrated that adults with ADHD more often experienced daytime sleepiness and sleep disturbances not attributable to ADHD pharmacotherapy.[18] Thus, the sleep problems in ADHD patients are multifactorial.

Objective Measurement of Sleep Problems in Children with ADHD

Objective tools for measurement of sleep in children with ADHD include polysomnography (PSG), actigraphy, and multiple sleep latency testing (MSLT). Sleep studies, possibly performed with video-PSG, have been used as part of the diagnostic screening for ADHD.[19] The most common PSG findings in children with ADHD are increased rates of movement and respiratory disturbance during sleep, although most results reporting objective sleep parameters, such as sleep-onset latency, sleep duration, or most aspects of sleep architecture, are inconsistent.[20–22] Some studies have shown rapid eye movement (REM) sleep abnormalities in children with ADHD, but the conclusions are inconsistent, including reports of increased[23,24] and of decreased or delayed REM.[25,26]

Sleep Patterns, Nocturnal Activity, and Sleep Disturbances in Children with ADHD

Children with ADHD symptoms have unstable sleep patterns or inconsistency in their sleep and wake times.[27,28] Longer[16,29] or shorter[30,31] sleep durations, more frequent night wakenings,[30] delayed sleep onset,[32] and increased instability in sleep onset[33] have been found by parental reports when compared with healthy children. Although most of the objective studies did not find any difference in total sleep time and other sleep variables but revealed an increase in intraindividual day-to-day variability in children with ADHD,[27,28,34] recent studies have demonstrated that children with ADHD experienced shorter actual sleep time (defined as time in minutes from sleep onset to final morning awakening),[17,31] more total interrupted sleep time,[31] longer sleep latency,[32] lower sleep efficiency,[17] and more sleep disturbance[35] on PSG than normal control children, which suggest that children with ADHD have both reduced sleep quantity and quality.

Children[22] and adults[36] with ADHD were found to have significantly higher levels of nocturnal activity than controls. This higher number of sleep movements was also demonstrated in a recent review of the literature.[37] These movements may not actually result in sleep disruption, however, because no significant differences in PSG variables between children with ADHD and controls were observed.[22] Several studies demonstrated that the use of late afternoon methylphenidate (MPH) doses reduced nocturnal activity and improved sleep quality by consolidating sleep.[38,39]

Approximately one-third of children with ADHD are reported to experience chronic sleep-onset insomnia.[40–42] In addition, bedtime resistance, more sleep-onset difficulties, less refreshing sleep, and difficulties wakening in the morning have been documented in children with ADHD.[17,31]

Daytime Sleepiness and ADHD

Excessive sleepiness in adolescents and young adults often has a profound negative effect on school performance, cognitive function, and mood and has been associated with other serious consequences, such as automobile crashes.[43] Daytime sleepiness is associated with inattention and probably hyperactivity.[43,44] The problem of daytime sleepiness is assumed to be the consequence of a delayed sleep pattern,[45–47] and sleep disruption, related to an underlying SDB[48,49] or dyssomnia.[50] The presence of these is reported to be associated with an increased risk of problematic behaviors suggestive of ADHD.[12,48,49,51] Sleepy children may try to stay awake and alert by attention shifting and excessive motor activity, which resembles inattention and hyperactivity.[44,52]

A parent-reported ADHD symptomatology study demonstrated that children with ADHD presented with more daytime sleepiness, but neither hyperactive-impulsive nor inattentive ADHS symptomatology was uniquely related to parent-reported problems involving sleep resistance, parasomnias, or dyssomnias.[53] Using an objective measure: the MSLT, children with ADHD had shorter sleep-onset latency during daytime and excessive daytime sleepiness.[34,50] In conclusion, children and adolescents with ADHD tend to feel more sleepy than general children and have shorter sleep-onset latency during the daytime MSLT.[17,34,50]

SDB and ADHD

Although some sleep problems or disorders are well documented as associated with the diagnosis of ADHD[16,22] or ADHD-related symptoms,[11,51] others are not.[11,16,51] The most well studied sleep problems are SDB (OSA), PLMS, and RLS.

Table 1 summarizes recent investigations of SDB and ADHD. Although some studies support the association of SDB with ADHD-related symptoms,[12,44,49,51–53,57] such an association with the diagnosis of ADHD is controversial.[56,59] Children with OSA or habitual snoring due to adenotonsillar hypertrophy often present with inattentive and hyperactive symptoms, and approximately one-third of children who have frequent, loud snoring or SDB show significant inattention or hyperactivity.[60–63] After tonsillectomy and treatment of these respiratory sleep problems, symptoms of ADHD, including excessive daytime sleepiness and all neurobehavioral morbidities, generally improved.[64,65]

The reasons why the relationship of ADHD and SDB is inconclusive lies not only in the confounding factors of comorbid oppositional defiant disorder and the use of psychostimulants[16,66] but also in the overlapping symptoms of SDB and ADHD. Because children with sleep problems are often inattentive or hyperactive, it is possible that some may be misdiagnosed as having ADHD. Huang and colleagues[57] identified complicating factors, however, such as higher rates of SDB in children who had ADHD. In a study of 88 ADHD children and 27 school controls, ADHD children had a higher apnea-hypopnea index (AHI) (AHI >1, 56.8%, and AHI >5, 19.3%) than the control children (only 1 child's AHI was equal to 1.2/h). ADHD children with OSA had significantly increased symptoms of hyperactivity than those without OSA. Golan and colleagues[50] found that ADHD children had more signs of SDB than controls and 50% of children with ADHD exhibited a respiratory disturbance index exceeding 2 compared with only 22% of controls. A continuous investigation by Huang and colleagues[56] of treatment outcome in ADHD children, with treatment options including MPH, adenotonsillectomy for children with OSA, or no treatment, showed that improvement in inattentive and hyperactivity symptoms was significant in surgical and MPH groups and that the surgical group had significantly more improvement in inattention than the MPH group. Dillon and colleagues[64] also reported that children with ADHD and an AHI greater than 1 and fewer than 5 events per hour improved significantly more after adenotonsillectomy than after stimulant treatment.

Combining the results of the studies of Huang and colleagues[56,57] and Dillon and colleagues,[64] OSA may be a cause of ADHD symptoms rather than a consequence of inattention and hyperactivity in some children. This assumption is supported by the reduction in inattention, hyperactivity, and neurocognitive deficits after treating OSA by adenotonsillectomy.[56,65] OSA, however, could be an aggravating factor for ADHD, because persistent OSA still can be found in few patients even after adenotonsillectomy.[67]

PLMS and ADHD

Excessive PLMS in association with ADHD has been reported by several investigators (**Table 2**). Studies by Huang and colleagues[57] (10.2%) and Golan and colleagues[50] (15%) provided an objective support for the assumption that ADHD children are more restless during nighttime sleep, in agreement with parental reports. Although ADHD and PLMS may present with daytime symptoms of inattentiveness due to poor sleep, daytime sleepiness, and decreased school performance,[71] another study demonstrated that patients with ADHD without symptoms suggestive of a primary disorder or daytime sleepiness have normal sleep on PSG.[26]

The current studies[11,19,26,50,57,68,71–74] focused on the relationship of PLMS and ADHD and concluded that children with ADHD had a higher incidence of PLMS or that symptoms of ADHD were associated with more PLMS in children. Few studies, however, evaluated the treatment strategies for the coexistence of PLMS and ADHD. Because the presence of PLMS and ADHD is, in some surveys, associated with a low serum iron level in children,[72] and because low iron is a possible contributing cause of ADHD in children,[73,74] future trials of iron supplementation for abnormal sleep motor activity in children with ADHD can be suggested.

RLS in Children with ADHD

RLS is characterized by an irresistible urge to move the legs accompanied by uncomfortable sensations in the legs or other body parts with a clear circadian distribution of symptoms. In a recent literature review,[20] approximately 44% of patients with ADHD have been found to have RLS or RLS symptoms, and up to 26% of patients with RLS have been found to have ADHD or ADHD symptoms. RLS occurs in 5% to 10% of adults in the United States and Western Europe. The prevalence of RLS in children is unknown, but most reports found that the majority of adults with RLS had these symptoms since childhood.[75,76] A recent study found that some aspects of RLS, especially clinical sleep disturbance, can occur long before the full diagnostic criteria are present,[77] and Rajaram and colleagues[78] suggested that some children with growing pains may actually have RLS.

Recent studies discussing the relationship of RLS and ADHD are summarized in **Table 3**. Patients with RLS often complain of insomnia due to leg discomfort, and RLS leg discomfort or poor quality of sleep may lead to inattentiveness, moodiness, and paradoxic overactivity.[20,82] Diurnal manifestations of RLS, including restlessness and inattention, might mimic ADHD symptoms. In addition to ADHD, the comorbidities of RLS include parasomnias, ADHD, oppositional defiant disorder, anxiety, and depression.[77] ADHD patients with RLS were found to have more severe ADHD symptoms than those without RLS.[83]

Some dopamine-receptor agonists (such as pramipexole, ropinirole, cabergoline, piribedil, and α-dihydroergocryptine) and dopaminergic agents, amantadine and selegiline, may be effective in the treatment of RLS.[84] Because a common dopamine dysfunction is considered to be shared by these 2 conditions,[20] children with symptoms of RLS and ADHD may benefit from treatment with dopaminergic agents.[85,86] Dopaminergic agents, however, are not approved for use in children with RLS and are only prescribed off label. Another treatment strategy is the usage of iron supplementation (iron is a cofactor for 1 of the major enzymes in the dopamine synthesis pathway). Iron deficiency may be a possible common pathophysiologic mechanism for RLS and ADHD. A pilot, randomized, controlled trial of the effectiveness of iron therapy in the treatment of ADHD in children with RLS was recently published[74]; however, it would be worthwhile to conduct larger, randomized, placebo-controlled trials of iron supplementation for RLS and ADHD in children.

Sleep Disturbances and Psychiatric Comorbidities in ADHD

There are psychiatric comorbidities, including oppositional disorder, conduct disorder, mood disorders, anxiety disorders, learning disorders, developmental coordination disorder, tic, and Tourette syndrome, they are common in subjects with ADHD and that may contribute to sleep problems in children with ADHD.[15,87–89] Sleep problems are common in children with bipolar disorder, Tourette syndrome, anxiety, and depression,[15,90] and the presence of psychiatric comorbid conditions increases the risks for insomnia and nightmares.[91] Psychiatric comorbidities can partially explain

Table 1
Studies investigating the association between ADHD symptoms/ADHD diagnosis and SDB/OSA in children and adolescents

Study	Sample Size	Age	Study Design	Measures/Assessment of SDB and OSA	Major Findings
ADHD symptoms					
Gau, 2006[54]	2463	7–15	Cross sectional, community based	Parent reports	SDB was associated with inattention and hyperactivity/impulsivity.
O'Brien, 2003[12]	117	5–7	Cross sectional, community based	PSG	SDB was highly prevalent in children with mild ADHD symptoms but not in those with significant ADHD symptoms.
Gottlieb, 2003[49]	3019	5	Cross sectional, community based	Parent report	Children with SDB symptoms were more likely to have hyperactivity, inattention, and aggressiveness.
Chervin, 2002[51]	866	2–14	Cross sectional, community based	Parent report	Inattention and hyperactivity were associated with snoring and other symptoms of SDB.
Chervin, 2001[55]	59	2–18	Cross sectional, clinic based	PSG	Hyperactivity showed no significant associations with the rate of apneas and hypopneas.
ADHD diagnosis					
Huang, 2007[56]	86	6–12	Cross sectional, clinic based, ADHD children with mild OSA	PSG	Inattention and hyperactivity reduced after treating OSA by adenotonsillectomy or treating ADHD with stimulant.

Study	N	Age	Design	Method	Findings
Sangal, 2005[26]	40	6–14	Cross sectional, clinic based	PSG	Normal sleep on PSG was noted in patients with ADHD without symptoms of primary sleep disorder.
Kirov, 2004[24]	34	8–15	Cross sectional, clinic based	PSG	Apnea and hypopnea during sleep were not significantly different in ADHD compared with controls.
Golan, 2004[50]	66	12.4 ± 4.6	Cross sectional, clinic based	PSG	ADHD children had more signs of SDB compared with the control group.
Huang, 2004[57]	88	6–12	Cross sectional, clinic based	PSG	ADHD children had a higher AHI (56.8% AHI >1, 19.3% AHI >5) than control children.
Cooper, 2004[58]	38	4–16	Cross sectional, clinic based	PSG	ADHD group is normal in AHI and had no difference from controls.
O'Brien, 2003[25]	149	ADHD from clinical/community samples: 8.0 ± 1.6/6.6 ± 0.4, control: 6.7 ± 0.4	Cross sectional, community and clinical samples	PSG	AHI and apnea index did not differ in the 3 groups.

Data from Chiang HL, Huang YS, Gau SS. Association between symptoms/diagnosis of attention deficit/hyperactivity disorder and sleep problems/disorders—focus on Taiwan's studies. Taiwanese J Psychiatry 2009;23:90–103.

Table 2
Studies investigating the association between ADHD symptoms/ADHD diagnosis and PLMS/PLMD in children and adolescents

Study	Sample Size	Age	Study Design	Measures/Assessment of PLMS	Major Findings
ADHD symptoms					
Silvestri, 2009[19]	55	8.9 ± 2.7	Cross sectional, clinic based	Nocturnal video-PSG	Strong significant correlations emerged for PLMS indexes, hyperactivity, opposition scores, and ADHD subtypes.
Chervin, 2002[11]	866	2–14	Cross sectional, community based	Parent report	Inattention and hyperactivity in general pediatric patients are associated with symptoms of PLMS.
Chervin, 2001[55]	59	2–18	Cross sectional, clinic based	PSG	Hyperactivity was associated with the presence of 5 or more PLMS per hour.
ADHD diagnosis					
Goraya, 2009[68]	33	3–16	Retrospective, clinic based	PSG	PLMS was common (30%) in children with ADHD who have symptoms of disturbed sleep.
Sangal, 2005[26]	40	6–14	Cross sectional, clinic based	PSG	PLMS in not a common underlying disorder or etiologic factor in patients with ADHD; normal sleep on PSG was noted in patients with ADHD without symptoms of primary sleep disorder.
Kirov, 2004[24]	34	8–15	Cross sectional, clinic based	PSG	Total movement time during sleep was not significantly different in ADHD compared with controls.

	N	Age	Design	Method	Findings
Huang, 2004[57]	88	6–12	Cross sectional, clinic based	PSG	Nine (10.2%) of the ADHD group had 5 or more PLMS per hour, but none in the control group.
Golan, 2004[50]	66	12.4 ± 4.6	Cross sectional, clinic based	PSG	Five (15%) of the ADHD group had PLMS versus none in the control group.
Cooper, 2004[58]	38	4–16	Cross sectional, clinic based	PSG	PLMS in the ADHD group was not different from the control group.
O'Brien, 2003[25]	149	ADHD from clinical/communitiy samples: 8.0 ± 1.6/6.6 ± 0.4, control: 6.7 ± 0.4	Cross sectional, community and clinic samples	PSG	PLMS with associated arousals was higher in clinical referred ADHD than the other groups, but there were no differences between community ADHD samples and controls.
Crabtree, 2003[69]	142	5–7	Cross sectional, community and clinic samples, PLMD with/ without ADHD	PSG	Children with PLMD and ADHD had a significantly greater number of arousals associated with PLMS than children with PLMD only.
Konofal, 2001[22]	49	5–10	Cross sectional, clinic based	PSG	ADHD children have higher levels of nocturnal activity than controls.
Picchietti, 1999[70]	24	5–12	Cross sectional, clinic based	PSG	The prevalence of PLMS was higher in the children with ADHD than in controls.
Picchietti, 1998[71]	56	2–15	Cross sectional, clinic based	PSG	The prevalence of PLMS was higher in the children with ADHD than in controls.

Table 3
Studies investigating the association between ADHD symptoms/ADHD diagnosis and RLS in children and adolescents

Study	Sample Size	Age	Study Design	Measures/Assessment of RLS	Major Findings
ADHD symptoms					
Picchietti, 2008[77]	18	Age at definite RLS diagnosis: 8.1–24.3	Retrospective review of children with RLS	National Institutes of Health–specific pediatric criteria	Clinical sleep disturbance preceded full appearance of RLS, and ADHD is a common comorbidity of RLS.
Konofal, 2007[79]	32	5.3–12	Cross sectional, clinic based	National Institutes of Health–specific pediatric criteria	Children with ADHD and a positive family of RLS are at risk of severe ADHD symptoms.
Gamaldo, 2007[80]	262	<18	Case controlled	Validated diagnostic telephone interview	ADHD was not related to RLS. Restless sleep in childhood was the only consistent factor related to the occurrence of RLS.
Rajaram, 2004[78]	11	6–16	Clinic based, ADHD children with growing pain referred	Parent interview	Some ADHD children with growing pains may actually have RLS.
Chervin, 2002[11]	866	2–14	Cross sectional, community based	Validated pediatric sleep questionnaire	Inattention and hyperactivity in general pediatric patients are associated with symptoms of RLS.
Chervin, 1997[7,81]	143	2–18	Cross sectional, clinic based	Parent report	The complaint of restless legs and a composite score for daytime sleepiness showed some evidence of an association with inattention and hyperactivity.
ADHD diagnosis					
Picchietti, 1999[70]	24	5–12	Cross sectional, clinic based	Parent interview	The parents (32%) of the children with ADHD were more likely to have RLS.
Picchietti, 1998[71]	56	2–15	Cross sectional, clinic based	From parental history	RLS-associated sleep disruption and the motor restlessness of RLS while awake could contribute to inattention and hyperactivity in a subgroup of ADHD-diagnosed children.

the relationship between ADHD and sleep problems. Undoubtedly, these psychiatric comorbidities, as well as the medications used to help them, can be confounding factors in the studies of the relationships between ADHD and sleep problems, emphasizing the need to take them into account when looking at sleep disorders in ADHD patients.[15,23,32] These comorbidities associated with ADHD may have an impact on treatment compliance, treatment response, and patients insights. For example, children with ADHD and conduct disorder have higher rates of antisocial personality and coexisting anxiety, which seem to attenuate impulsivity in ADHD.[92] Therefore, it is necessary to assess sleep and comorbid psychiatric conditions in children with ADHD, even until their adolescent period far after initial diagnosis, as suggested by Gau and Chiang[91] in a recent study.

Medications of ADHD or Its Comorbid Conditions Affect Sleep

The first-line Food and Drug Administration–approved medications for ADHD, including MPH, amphetamine, dextroamphetamine, and pemoline, are known to cause sleep problems in short- or long-term clinical trials.[93–95] MPH prescribed at standard doses (0.3 to 0.7mg/kg/dose, rounded to the nearest 2.5 or 5 mg) in school-aged children with ADHD were reported to result in reduced total sleep time, increased sleep-onset latency,[94,95] and thus reduced sleep efficiency.[95] Another study of long-term MPH use on children with ADHD showed a 14.7% prevalence of insomnia.[96]

Extended-release mixed amphetamine salts using forced-dose titration in a 4-week placebo-controlled trial for adolescences with ADHD showed 12% of patients developed insomnia,[97] although another study demonstrated that pediatric patients with bipolar disorder and concurrent ADHD can be safely and effectively treated with mixed amphetamine salts after their manic symptoms are stabilized with divalproex sodium.[98] An earlier study also concluded with a higher rate of insomnia during amphetamine treatment than with MPH treatment in children with ADHD.[99] The side effects of sleep disruption in patients with ADHD may be dose related,[97,100] however, and drawbacks are not always present with the use of these stimulants. Use of these medications to treat the psychiatric comorbidities of ADHD may improve the associated sleep problem, and this improvement may come from the drug effects or be secondary to the improved behavior.

Another nonamphetaminic stimulant, atomoxetine (ATX) is a useful option in the treatment of ADHD in children and adolescents, especially for patients at risk of substance abuse as well as those who have comorbid anxiety or tics.[101] A low incidence of 5.1% sleep-onset insomnia and 8.5% somnolence was reported in a recent meta-analysis study of long-term treatment with ATX in young children with ADHD.[102] Another study also demonstrated a lower rate of insomnia when ATX was prescribed twice a day rather than MPH 3 times a day for treatment of ADHD children (6.3% vs 26.6%).[103]

Treatment of Sleep Problems in Children with ADHD

At the exception to studies reporting on treatment of specific sleep problems such as PLM and RLS, with dopaminergic agents or iron supplementation and simultaneously treating the sleep problem associated with ADHD per se, there are few studies focusing on the treatment of sleep disorders in ADHD children. Several recent trials suggested the effectiveness of low-dose melatonin in alleviating ADHD-related insomnia.[40,104] Significant improvements in sleep-onset latency and increased total sleep time have also been reported for children who have stimulant-treated ADHD after treatment with melatonin (at doses of 3 to 6 mg) at bedtime.[40]

Other medications reported effective for treatment of ADHD-associated insomnia include clonidine, diphenhydramine, cyproheptadine, trazodone, mirtazapine, guanfacine, and tricyclic antidepressants.[105] Mullane and Corkum[106] reported the effectiveness of structured behavioral interventions as primary treatment of insomnia in children with ADHD.

Effect of ADHD Subtype on Sleep Problems/Disorders

According to the *DSM-IV* diagnostic criteria,[4] there are 3 subtypes of ADHD: Children with ADHD-inattentive type (ADHD-IA), children with ADHD-hyperactive impulsive type (ADHD-HI) and children with ADHD-combined type (ADHD-C). Studies examining the association between ADHD core symptoms[12] and subtypes[11,16,107,108] and sleep problems showed inconsistent results.[12,16] Some studies showed that SDB is strongly linked to hyperactive symptoms,[12] and chronic nocturnal snoring was greater in children with ADHD-HI.[108] Other studies, however, did not demonstrate an association between abnormal breathing pattern and ADHD subtypes.[107] Chervin and colleagues[11] and Corkum and colleagues[16] concluded that there is a positive relationship between ADHD-C and sleep-related involuntary movements due to the close association between RLS and PLMS and inattention and hyperactivity symptoms, but this was not supported by other studies.[107]

SUMMARY

ADHD-related symptoms and the diagnosis of ADHD are frequently associated with sleep problems/disorders, such as PLMS, RLS, SDB, and insomnia, but not with parasomnia. To avoid inappropriate diagnosis and inadequate management, mental health professionals should assess sleep problems and disorders in children, adolescents, and adults with ADHD-related symptoms and in those with a diagnosis of ADHD, regardless of *DSM-IV* subtypes and severity of current ADHD symptoms.[109] Screening for other psychiatric comorbidities and the side effects of medications, such as psychostimulants, is necessary when considering sleep complaints, because both of them have adverse effects on sleep. A prospective cohort study demonstrating a causal relationship between sleep problems and ADHD-related symptoms, while taking potential confounders into consideration, is needed to fill the gap of understanding of the underlying mechanisms present between these 2 common problems in children and adolescents.

REFERENCES

1. Faraone SV, Sergeant J, Gillberg C, et al. The worldwide prevalence of ADHD: is it an American condition? World Psychiatry 2003;2(2):104–13.
2. Biederman J. Attention-deficit/hyperactivity disorder: a selective overview. Biol Psychiatry 2005;57(3):1215–20.
3. Froehlich TE, Lanphear BP, Epstein JN, et al. Prevalence, recognition, and treatment of attention-deficit/hyperactivity disorder in a national sample of US children. Arch Pediatr Adolesc Med 2007;161(9):857–64.
4. American Psychiatric Association. Diagnostic and statistical manual of mental disorders. 4th edition. Washington, DC: American Psychiatric Association; 2000. Text revision: DSM-IVTR.
5. Faraone SV, Biederman J, Mick E. The age-dependent decline of attention deficit hyperactivity disorder: a meta-analysis of follow-up studies. Psychol Med 2006;36(2):159–65.
6. Lara C, Fayyad J, de Graaf R, et al. Childhood predictors of adult attention-deficit/hyperactivity disorder: results from the world health organization world mental health survey initiative. Biol Psychiatry 2009;65(1):46–54.

7. Gau SS, Chong MY, Chen TH, et al. A 3 year panel study of mental disorders among adolescents in Taiwan. Am J Psychiatry 2005;162:1344–50.
8. Leung PW, Hung SF, Ho TP, et al. Prevalence of DSM-IV disorders in Chinese adolescents and the effects of an impairment criterion: a pilot community study in Hong Kong. Eur Child Adolesc Psychiatry 2008;17(7):452–61.
9. Döpfner M, Breuer D, Wille N, et al. How often do children meet ICD-10/DSM-IV criteria of attention deficit-/hyperactivity disorder and hyperkinetic disorder? Parent-based prevalence rates in a national sample—results of the BELLA study. Eur Child Adolesc Psychiatry 2008;17(Suppl 1):59–70.
10. Owens J. The ADHD and sleep conundrum: a review. J Dev Behav Pediatr 2005; 26(4):312–22.
11. Chervin RD, Archbold KH, Dillon JE, et al. Associations between symptoms of inattention, hyperactivity, restless legs, and periodic leg movements. Sleep 2002;25(2):213–8.
12. O'Brien LM, Holbrook CR, Mervis CB, et al. Sleep and neurobehavioral characteristics of 5- to 7-year-old children with parentally reported symptoms of attention-deficit/hyperactivity disorder. Pediatrics 2003;111(3):554–63.
13. Chervin RD, Dillon JE, Archbold KH, et al. Conduct problems and symptoms of sleep disorders in children. J Am Acad Child Adolesc Psychiatry 2003;42(2): 201–8.
14. Gozal D, Pope DW Jr. Snoring during early childhood and academic performance at ages thirteen to fourteen years. Pediatrics 2001;107(6):1394–9.
15. Mick E, Biederman J, Jetton J, et al. Sleep disturbances associated with attention deficit hyperactivity disorder: the impact of psychiatric comorbidity and pharmacotherapy. J Child Adolesc Psychopharmacol 2000;10(3):223–31.
16. Corkum P, Moldofsky H, Hogg-Johnson S, et al. Sleep problems in children with attention-deficit/hyperactivity disorder: impact of subtype, comorbidity, and stimulant medication. J Am Acad Child Adolesc Psychiatry 1999;38(10):1285–93.
17. Cortese S, Faraone S, Konofal E, et al. Sleep in children with Attention-Deficit/Hyperactivity Disorder: meta-analysis of subjective and objective studies. J Am Acad Child Adolesc Psychiatry 2009;48(9):894–908.
18. Surman CB, Adamson JJ, Petty C, et al. Association between attention-deficit/hyperactivity disorder and sleep impairment in adulthood: evidence from a large controlled study. J Clin Psychiatry 2009;70(11):1523–9.
19. Silvestri R, Gagliano A, Aricò I, et al. Sleep disorders in children with Attention-Deficit/Hyperactivity Disorder (ADHD) recorded overnight by video-polysomnography. Sleep Med 2009;10(10):1132–8.
20. Cortese S, Konofal E, Lecendreux M, et al. Restless legs syndrome and attention-deficit/hyperactivity disorder: a review of the literature. Sleep 2005;28(8): 1007–13.
21. Gruber R. Sleep characteristics of children and adolescents with attention deficit-hyperactivity disorder. Child Adolesc Psychiatr Clin N Am 2009;18(4):863–76.
22. Konofal E, Lecendreux M, Bouvard MP, et al. High levels of nocturnal activity in children with attention-deficit hyperactivity disorder: a video analysis. Psychiatry Clin Neurosci 2001;55(2):97–103.
23. Kirov R, Kinkelbur J, Banaschewski T, et al. Sleep patterns in children with attention-deficit/hyperactivity disorder, tic disorder, and comorbidity. J Child Psychol Psychiatry 2007;48(6):561–70.
24. Kirov R, Kinkelbur J, Heipke S, et al. Is there a specific polysomnographic sleep pattern in children with attention deficit/hyperactivity disorder? J Sleep Res 2004;13(1):87–93.

25. O'Brien LM, Ivanenko A, Crabtree VM, et al. Sleep disturbances in children with attention deficit hyperactivity disorder. Pediatr Res 2003;54(2):237–43.

26. Sangal RB, Owens JA, Sangal J. Patients with attention-deficit/hyperactivity disorder without observed apneic episodes in sleep or daytime sleepiness have normal sleep on polysomnography. Sleep 2005;28(9):1143–8.

27. Gruber R, Sadeh A, Raviv A. Instability of sleep patterns in children with ADHD. J Am Acad Child Adolesc Psychiatry 2000;39(4):495–501.

28. Gruber R, Sadeh A. Sleep and neurobehavioral functioning in children with attention-deficit/hyperactivity disorder and no reported breathing problems. Sleep 2004;27(2):267–73.

29. Corkum P, Tannock R, Moldofsky H, et al. Actigraphy and parental ratings of sleep in children with attention-deficit/hyperactivity disorder (ADHD). Sleep 2001;24(3):303–12.

30. Owens JA, Maxim R, Nobile C, et al. Parental and self-report of sleep in children with attention-deficit/hyperactivity disorder. Arch Pediatr Adolesc Med 2000; 154(6):549–55.

31. Owens J, Sangal RB, Sutton VK, et al. Subjective and objective measures of sleep in children with attention-deficit/hyperactivity disorder. Sleep Med 2009; 10(4):446–56.

32. Hvolby A, Jørgensen J, Bilenberg N. Actigraphic and parental reports of sleep difficulties in children with attention-deficit/hyperactivity disorder. Arch Pediatr Adolesc Med 2008;162(4):323–9.

33. Hvolby A, Jørgensen J, Bilenberg N. Parental rating of sleep in children with attention-deficit/hyperactivity disorder. Eur Child Adolesc Psychiatry 2009; 18(7):429–38.

34. Lecendreux M, Konofal E, Bouvard M, et al. Sleep and alertness in children with ADHD. J Child Psychol Psychiatry 2000;41(6):803–12.

35. Gruber R, Xi T, Frenette S, et al. Sleep disturbances in prepubertal children with attention deficit hyperactivity disorder: a home polysomnography study. Sleep 2009;32(3):343–50.

36. Philipsen A, Feige B, Hesslinger B, et al. Sleep in adults with attention-deficit/hyperactivity disorder: a controlled polysomnographic study including spectral analysis of the sleep EEG. Sleep 2005;28(7):877–84.

37. Cortese S, Konofal E, Yateman N, et al. Sleep and alertness in children with attention-deficit/hyperactivity disorder: a systematic review of the literature. Sleep 2006;29(4):504–11.

38. Konofal E, Lecendreux M, Bouvard M, et al. Effects of vesperal methylphenidate (MPH) administration on diurnal and nocturnal activity in ADHD children: an actigraphic study [abstract supplement, 363.G]. Sleep 2001.

39. Kooij JJ, Middelkoop HA, van GK, et al. The effect of stimulants on nocturnal motor activity and sleep quality in adults with ADHD: an open-label case-control study. J Clin Psychiatry 2001;62(12):952–6.

40. Van der Heijden KB, Smits MG, Van Someren EJ, et al. Effect of melatonin on sleep, behavior, and cognition in ADHD and chronic sleep-onset insomnia. J Am Acad Child Adolesc Psychiatry 2007;46(2):233–41.

41. Bendz LM, Scates AC. Melatonin treatment for insomnia in pediatric patients with attention-deficit/hyperactivity disorder. Ann Pharmacother 2010;44(1): 185–91.

42. Van der Heijden KB, Smits MG, Van Someren EJ, et al. Idiopathic chronic sleep onset insomnia in attention-deficit/hyperactivity disorder: a circadian rhythm sleep disorder. Chronobiol Int 2005;22(3):559–70.

43. Millman RP. Excessive sleepiness in adolescents and young adults: causes, consequences, and treatment strategies. Pediatrics 2005;115(6):1774–86.
44. Fallone G, Acebo C, Arnedt JT, et al. Effects of acute sleep restriction on behavior, sustained attention, and response inhibition in children. Percept Mot Skills 2001;93(1):213–29.
45. Gau SF, Soong WT. The transition of sleep-wake patterns in early adolescence. Sleep 2003;26(4):449–54.
46. Yang CK, Kim JK, Patel SR, et al. Age-related changes in sleep/wake patterns among Korean teenagers. Pediatrics 2005;115(Suppl 1):250–6.
47. Gibson ES, Powles AC, Thabane L, et al. "Sleepiness" is serious in adolescence: two surveys of 3235 Canadian students. BMC Public Health 2006;2(6):116.
48. Johnson EO, Roth T. An epidemiologic study of sleep-disordered breathing symptoms among adolescents. Sleep 2006;29(9):1135–42.
49. Gottlieb DJ, Vezina RM, Chase C, et al. Symptoms of sleep-disordered breathing in 5-year-old children are associated with sleepiness and problem behaviors. Pediatrics 2003;112(4):870–7.
50. Golan N, Shahar E, Ravid S, et al. Sleep disorders and daytime sleepiness in children with attention-deficit/hyperactivity disorder. Sleep 2004;27(2):261–6.
51. Chervin RD, Archbold KH, Dillon JE, et al. Inattention, hyperactivity, and symptoms of sleep-disordered breathing. Pediatrics 2002;109(3):449–56.
52. Weinberg WA, Brumback RA. Primary disorder of vigilance: a novel explanation of inattentiveness, daydreaming, boredom, restlessness, and sleepiness. J Pediatr 1990;116(5):720–5.
53. Willoughby MT, Angold A, Egger HL. Parent-reported attention-deficit hyperactivity disorder symptomatology and sleep problems in a preschool-age pediatric clinic sample. J Am Acad Child Adolesc Psychiatry 2008;47(9):1086–94.
54. Gau SS. Prevalence of sleep problems and their association with inattention/hyperactivity among children aged 6-15 in Taiwan. J Sleep Res 2006;15(4):403–14.
55. Chervin RD, Archbold KH. Hyperactivity and polysomnographic findings in children evaluated for sleep-disordered breathing. Sleep 2001;24(3):313–20.
56. Huang YS, Guilleminault C, Li HY, et al. Attention-deficit/hyperactivity disorder with obstructive sleep apnea: a treatment outcome study. Sleep Med 2007; 8(1):18–30.
57. Huang YS, Chen NH, Li HY, et al. Sleep disorders in Taiwanese children with attention deficit/hyperactivity disorder. J Sleep Res 2004;13(3):269–77.
58. Cooper J, Tyler L, Wallace I, et al. No evidence of sleep apnea in children with attention deficit hyperactivity disorder. Clin Pediatr (Phila) 2004;43(7):609–14.
59. Sadeh A, Pergamin L, Bar-Haim Y. Sleep in children with attention-deficit hyperactivity disorder: a meta-analysis of polysomnographic studies. Sleep Med Rev 2006;10(6):381–98.
60. Archbold K, Giordani B, Ruzicka D, et al. Cognitive executive dysfunction in children with mild sleep-disordered breathing. Biol Res Nurs 2004;5(3):168–76.
61. O'Brien L, Mervis C, Holbrook C, et al. Neurobehavioral implications of habitual snoring in children. Pediatrics 2004;114(1):44–9.
62. O'Brien L, Mervis C, Holbrook C, et al. Neurobehavioral correlates of sleep-disordered breathing in children. J Sleep Res 2004;13(2):165–72.
63. Bass J, Corwin M, Gozal D, et al. The effect of chronic or intermittent hypoxia on cognition in children: a review of the evidence. Pediatrics 2004;114(3):805–16.
64. Dillon JE, Elunden S, Ruzicka DL, et al. DSM-IV diagnoses and obstructive sleep apnea in children before and 1 year after adenotonsillectomy. J Am Acad Child Adolesc Psychiatry 2007;46(11):1425–36.

65. Chervin RD, Ruzicka DL, Giordani BJ, et al. Sleep-disordered breathing, behavior, and cognition in children before and after adenotonsillectomy. Pediatrics 2006;117(4):e769–78.

66. O'Brien LM, Ivanenko A, Crabtree VM, et al. The effect of stimulants on sleep characteristics in children with attention deficit/hyperactivity disorder. Sleep Med 2003;4(4):309–16.

67. Mitchell RB. Adenotonsillectomy for obstructive sleep apnea in children: outcome evaluated by pre- and postoperative polysomnography. Laryngoscope 2007;117(10):1844–54.

68. Goraya JS, Cruz M, Valencia I, et al. Sleep study abnormalities in children with attention deficit hyperactivity disorder. Pediatr Neurol 2009;40(1):42–6.

69. Crabtree VM, Ivanenko A, O'Brien LM, et al. Periodic limb movement disorder of sleep in children. J Sleep Res 2003;12(1):73–81.

70. Picchietti DL, Underwood DJ, Farris WA, et al. Further studies on periodic limb movement disorder and restless legs syndrome in children with attention-deficit hyperactivity disorder. Mov Disord 1999;14(6):1000–7.

71. Picchietti DL, England SJ, Walters AS, et al. Periodic limb movement disorder and restless legs syndrome in children with attention-deficit hyperactivity disorder. J Child Neurol 1998;13(5):588–94.

72. Simakajornboon N, Gozal D, Vlasic V, et al. Periodic limb movements in sleep and iron status in children. Sleep 2003;26(6):735–8.

73. Cortese S, Konofal E, Bernardina BD, et al. Sleep disturbances and serum ferritin levels in children with attention-deficit hyperactivity disorder. Eur Child Adolesc Psychiatry 2009;18(7):393–9.

74. Konofal E, Lecendreux M, Deron J, et al. Effects of iron supplementation on attention-deficit hyperactivity disorder in children. Pediatr Neurol 2008;38(1):20–6.

75. Picchietti D, Allen RP, Walters AS, et al. Restless legs syndrome: prevalence and impact in children and adolescents. The peds REST study. Pediatrics 2007;120(2):253–66.

76. Picchietti MA, Picchietti DL. Restless legs syndrome and periodic limb movement disorder in children and adolescents. Semin Pediatr Neurol 2008;15(2):91–9.

77. Picchietti DL, Stevens HE. Early manifestations of restless legs syndrome in childhood and adolescence. Sleep Med 2008;9(7):770–81.

78. Rajaram SS, Walters AS, England SJ, et al. Some children with growing pains may actually have restless legs syndrome. Sleep 2004;27(4):767–73.

79. Konofal E, Cortese S, Marchand M, et al. Impact of restless legs syndrome and iron deficiency on attention-deficit/hyperactivity disorder in children. Sleep Med 2007;8(7–8):711–5.

80. Gamaldo E, Benbrook BE, Allen RP, et al. Childhood and adult factors associated with restless legs syndrome (RLS) diagnosis. Sleep Med 2007;8(7-8):716–22.

81. Chervin RD, Dillon JE, Bassetti C, et al. Symptoms of sleep disorders, inattention, and hyperactivity in children. Sleep 1997;20(12):1185–92.

82. Wagner ML, Walters AS, Fisher BC. Symptoms of attention-deficit hyperactivity disorder in adults with restless legs syndrome. Sleep 2004;27(8):1499–504.

83. Zak R, Fisher B, Couvadelli BV, et al. Preliminary study of the prevalence of restless legs syndrome in adults with attention deficit hyperactivity disorder. Percept Mot Skills 2009;108(3):759–63.

84. Littner MR, Kushida C, Anderson WM, et al. Practice parameters for the dopaminergic treatment of restless legs syndrome and periodic limb movement disorder. Sleep 2004;27(3):557–9.

85. Walters AS, Mandelbaum DE, Lewin DS, et al. Dopaminergic therapy in children with restless legs/periodic limb movements in sleep and ADHD. Dopaminergic Therapy Study Group. Pediatr Neurol 2000;22(3):182–6.

86. Konofal E, Arnulf I, Lecendreux M, et al. Ropinirole in a child with attention-deficit/hyperactivity disorder and restless legs syndrome. Pediatr Neurol 2005; 32(5):350–1.

87. Pliszka S. Practice parameter for the assessment and treatment of children and adolescents with attention-deficit/hyperactivity disorder. J Am Acad Child Adolesc Psychiatry 2007;46(7):894–921.

88. Wilens TE, Biederman J, Brown S, et al. Psychiatric comorbidity and functioning in clinically referred preschool children and school-age youths with ADHD. J Am Acad Child Adolesc Psychiatry 2002;41(3):262–8.

89. Spencer TJ. ADHD and comorbidity in childhood. J Clin Psychiatry 2006; 67(Suppl 8):27–31.

90. Mehl RC, O'Brien LM, Jones JH, et al. Correlates of sleep and pediatric bipolar disorder. Sleep 2006;29(2):193–7.

91. Gau SS, Chiang HL. Sleep problems and disorders among adolescents with persistent and subthreshold attention-deficit/hyperactivity disorders. Sleep 2009;32(5):671–9.

92. Pliszka SR. Comorbidity of attention-deficit/hyperactivity disorder with psychiatric disorder: an overview. J Clin Psychiatry 1998;59(Suppl 7):50–8.

93. Charach A, Lckowicz A, Schachar R. Stimulant treatment over five years: adherence, effectiveness, and adverse effects. J Am Acad Child Adolesc Psychiatry 2004;43(5):559–67.

94. Schwartz G, Amor LB, Grizenko N, et al. Actigraphic monitoring during sleep of children with ADHD on methylphenidate and placebo. J Am Acad Child Adolesc Psychiatry 2004;43(10):1276–82.

95. Galland BC, Tripp EG, Taylor BJ. The sled off methylphenidate:ep of children with attention deficit hyperactivity disorder on an a matched case-control study. J Sleep Res 2009. [Epub ahead of print].

96. Wilens T, Pelham W, Stein M, et al. ADHD treatment with once-daily OROS methylphenidate: interim 12-month results from a long-term open-label study. J Am Acad Child Adolesc Psychiatry 2003;42(4):424–33.

97. Spencer TJ, Wilens TE, Biederman J, et al. Efficacy and safety of mixed amphetamine salts extended release (Adderall XR) in the management of attention-deficit/hyperactivity disorder in adolescent patients: a 4-week, randomized, double-blind, placebo-controlled, parallel-group study. Clin Ther 2006;28(2): 266–79.

98. Scheffer RE, Kowatch RA, Carmody T, et al. Randomized, placebo-controlled trial of mixed amphetamine salts for symptoms of comorbid ADHD in pediatric bipolar disorder after mood stabilization with divalproex sodium. Am J Psychiatry 2005;162(1):58–64.

99. Efron D, Jarman F, Barker M. Side effects of methylphenidate and dexamphetamine in children with attention deficit hyperactivity disorder: a double-blind, crossover trial. Pediatrics 1997;100(4):662–6.

100. Stein MA, Sarampote CS, Waldman ID, et al. A dose-response study of OROS methylphenidate in children with attention-deficit/hyperactivity disorder. Pediatrics 2003;112(5):e404.

101. Garnock-Jones KP, Keating GM. Atomoxetine: a review of its use in attention-deficit hyperactivity disorder in children and adolescents. Paediatr Drugs 2009;11(3):203–26.

102. Kratochvil CJ, Wilens TE, Greenhill LL, et al. Effects of long-term atomoxetine treatment for young children with attention-deficit/hyperactivity disorder. J Am Acad Child Adolesc Psychiatry. 2006;45(8):919–27.
103. Sangal RB, Owens J, Allen AJ, et al. Effects of atomoxetine and methylphenidate on sleep in children with ADHD. Sleep 2006;29(12):1573–85.
104. Tjon Pian Gi CV, Broeren JPA, Starreveld JS, et al. Melatonin for treatment of sleeping disorders in children with attention-deficit/hyperactivity disorder: a preliminary open label study. Eur J Pediatr 2003;162(7–8):554–5.
105. Kratochvil CJ, Lake M, Pliszka SR, et al. Pharmacological management of treatment-induced insomnia in ADHD. J Am Acad Child Adolesc Psychiatry 2005; 44(5):499–501.
106. Mullane J, Corkum P. Case series: evaluation of a behavioral sleep intervention for three children with attention-deficit/hyperactivity disorder and dyssomnia. J Atten Disord 2006;10(2):217–27.
107. Wiggs L, Montgomery P, Stores G. Actigraphic and parent reports of sleep patterns and sleep disorders in children with subtypes of attention-deficit hyperactivity disorder. Sleep 2005;28(11):1437–45.
108. LeBourgeois MK, Avis K, Mixon M, et al. Snoring, sleep quality, and sleepiness across attention-deficit/hyperactivity disorder subtypes. Sleep 2004;27:520–5.
109. Chiang HL, Huang YS, Gau SS. Association between symptoms/diagnosis of attention deficit/hyperactivity disorder and sleep problems/disorders-focus on Taiwan's studies. Taiwanese J Psychiatry 2009;23:90–103.

Index

Note: Page numbers of article titles are in **boldface** type.

Med Clin N Am 94 (2010) 633–643
doi:10.1016/S0025-7125(10)00065-9
0025-7125/10/$ – see front matter © 2010 Elsevier Inc. All rights reserved.

medical.theclinics.com

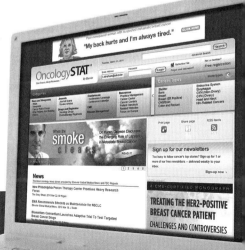

Moving?

Make sure your subscription moves with you!

To notify us of your new address, find your **Clinics Account Number** (located on your mailing label above your name), and contact customer service at:

Email: journalscustomerservice-usa@elsevier.com

800-654-2452 (subscribers in the U.S. & Canada)
314-447-8871 (subscribers outside of the U.S. & Canada)

Fax number: 314-447-8029

Elsevier Health Sciences Division
Subscription Customer Service
3251 Riverport Lane
Maryland Heights, MO 63043

*To ensure uninterrupted delivery of your subscription, please notify us at least 4 weeks in advance of move.

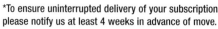

ELSEVIER